THE ROAD TO NURSING

Second edition

Being an effective and well-rounded nurse in Australia is not just about technical skills – it is also about thinking like a nurse. *The Road to Nursing* helps students develop clinical reasoning and critical reflection skills, understand the philosophical and ethical considerations necessary to care for clients and reflect on how to provide care that meets the unique needs of each client.

The three parts – beginning, becoming and being – guide students through their transition to university, formation of a professional identity and progression to professional practice. The revised structure improves the transition between topics and a new chapter explores the ever-changing Australian health landscape, including recent technological innovations. There is expanded coverage of topics including culture and diversity; nursing roles and career pathways; communication and interpersonal skills; and standards, regulation and the law.

Each chapter includes definitions of key terms, reflection questions, perspectives from nurses, end-of-chapter review questions, a research topic and resources that connect students with the real-world practice of nursing.

Written by healthcare experts, *The Road to Nursing* is a fundamental resource for students making the transition into the nursing profession.

Nick Arnott is a registered nurse and teaching fellow in health and community services at the University of Tasmania.

Penny Paliadelis is a registered nurse and professor with an academic career spanning more than 20 years.

Mary Cruickshank is a professor of nursing at Federation University.

Cambridge University Press acknowledges the Australian Aboriginal and Torres Strait Islander peoples of this nation. We acknowledge the traditional custodians of the lands on which our company is located and where we conduct our business. We pay our respects to ancestors and Elders, past and present. Cambridge University Press is committed to honouring Australian Aboriginal and Torres Strait Islander peoples' unique cultural and spiritual relationships to the land, waters and seas, and their rich contribution to society.

THE ROAD TO NURSING

EDITED BY

NICK ARNOTT
PENNY PALIADELIS
MARY CRUICKSHANK

SECOND EDITION

CAMBRIDGE
UNIVERSITY PRESS

CAMBRIDGE
UNIVERSITY PRESS

University Printing House, Cambridge CB2 8BS, United Kingdom

One Liberty Plaza, 20th Floor, New York, NY 10006, USA

477 Williamstown Road, Port Melbourne, VIC 3207, Australia

314–321, 3rd Floor, Plot 3, Splendor Forum, Jasola District Centre, New Delhi – 110025, India

103 Penang Road, #05–06/07, Visioncrest Commercial, Singapore 238467

Cambridge University Press is part of the University of Cambridge.

It furthers the University's mission by disseminating knowledge in the pursuit of
education, learning and research at the highest international levels of excellence.

www.cambridge.org
Information on this title: www.cambridge.org/9781009003476

First published 2019
Second edition 2022

Cover designed by Cate Furey
Typeset by Integra Software Services Pvt. Ltd
Printed in Singapore by Markono Print Media Pte Ltd, September 2021

A catalogue record for this publication is available from the British Library

A catalogue record for this book is available from the National Library of Australia

ISBN 978-1-009-00347-6 Paperback

Additional resources for this publication at www.cambridge.org/highereducation/isbn/9781009003476/resources

Contents

17 Preparing for the transition to registered nursing practice — 333
Jackie Lea

18 Conclusion: What now? Where to from here? — 353
Penny Paliadelis

Figures and tables

Figures

Tables

Contributors

Nick Arnott is a registered nurse and teaching fellow in health and community services at the University of Tasmania. In a career spanning more than 30 years, he has held clinical, policy and executive roles in acute care, community and primary health care, disability support and international health and development. Since moving into academia in 2009, Nick has maintained a research interest in nursing education, gratitude and the health of vulnerable and marginalised population groups but his main passion is teaching, mentoring and empowering the next generation of nurses and community support professionals.

Penny Paliadelis is a registered nurse who has had an academic career spanning more than 20 years, including senior leadership roles such as Acting Deputy Vice-Chancellor (Academic), Professor of Nursing and Executive Dean, Faculty of Health at Federation University Australia, and Acting Head of School of Health, University of New England. She is Managing Director of Paldyne Consulting Pty Ltd, a higher education and leadership consultancy, and she holds the position of Adjunct Professor at Federation University and DeakinCo. Penny is listed on the national register of Tertiary Education Quality Standards Agency (TEQSA) experts for healthcare curriculum design and is a graduate of the Australian Institute of Company Directors. Penny's research focus is on building leadership roles in health, and she has conducted a number of funded projects to develop collaborative interprofessional health education using digital storytelling approaches, always with a focus on workforce capacity-building.

Mary Cruickshank is employed as a professor of nursing at Federation University on a part-time basis, supervising PhD candidates, and is a director of a higher education board in Melbourne, Victoria. Mary is also Adjunct Professor at the ASEAN Institute for Health Development at Mahidol University in Bangkok, Thailand, where she supervises postgraduate students in the health disciplines. She was previously head of the School of Nursing, Midwifery and Healthcare at Federation University Australia. Mary has published widely, both internationally and nationally, and has conducted numerous research projects on rural health topics, health education, evidence-based practice and organisational and workplace culture.

Suzanne Bliss was a lecturer in philosophy and healthcare ethics at the University of Tasmania. She has a background as a registered nurse and a Bachelor of Arts majoring in philosophy and anthropology. She completed a PhD in philosophy in 2008. Her research interests include moral pedagogy – particularly with respect to students of nursing and other health professions. She has taught legal and ethical issues in health care to nursing and paramedicine students, and ethics, metaphysics and epistemology to philosophy students.

Patricia Bromley is a lecturer in nursing at the University of Tasmania. She teaches in the Bachelor of Nursing and is unit coordinator of the Postgraduate Certificate in Neonatal Intensive Care (PG Cert NIC). She has a doctorate in education, which explored the concept of capability in postgraduate nursing students in Australian neonatal intensive care.

Nicole Coombs is a lecturer at Federation University Australia and has ten years of clinical experience in emergency nursing. She is particularly interested in primary health and health promotion, as well as the teaching and learning of future nurses. Combining these areas of nursing, Nicole's research interests include patient education in the emergency department, health promotion and nursing education.

Rhian Cramer is program coordinator of the Graduate Diploma of Midwifery at Federation University Australia. Rhian is an experienced clinician, having practised in a variety of metropolitan, regional and remote settings. Her areas of special interest and research focus are women's health, lactation, and community and tertiary education.

Melanie Eslick is a registered nurse specialising in cancer. She works as a content author at eviQ, the Australian government's online resource for cancer treatment protocols, which was developed by multidisciplinary teams of cancer specialists, for use by cancer clinicians and nurses, and where she specialises in cancer genetics and cancer patient/carer education. Melanie is also a tutor in the University of Tasmania's School of Nursing and is Education Officer for the Cancer Nurses of Australia NSW branch. She spent much of 2020 conducting contact tracing during the COVID-19 pandemic. Prior to that she was clinical editor at the Leukaemia Foundation, and she practised as an oncology and haematology nurse, and clinical trials coordinator at the Royal Hobart Hospital. Melanie is undertaking postgraduate studies in public health. Her key interests are cancer control and education, compassionate care models and promotion of the role and importance of research to nurses and student nurses.

Swapnali Gazula is a nursing lecturer and international Nursing Student Coordinator in the School of Health at Federation University Australia. With over 15 years in academia and industry, she has numerous academic and service accolades, the most recent being Vice Chancellor's Award for outstanding contribution to student learning.

Diana Guzys is a lecturer in nursing in the School of Nursing, College of Health and Medicine at the University of Tasmania. After relocating to a rural environment and taking up a community health nursing role, Diana embraced a change in her professional practice and career direction. Health education and health promotion were the mainstay of her practice for over two decades, first as a generalist community health nurse and later as a secondary school nurse. Her research has demonstrated a return by communities to improving and optimising the health of rural communities, and supporting nurses working in community nursing roles.

Joyce Hendricks is an associate professor in the School of Nursing, Midwifery and Social Sciences at Central Queensland University. She has worked in the academic sector for 20 years. She has held high-level positions in industry, mostly related to the education of nurses, midwives, doctors, allied health, corporate and other supporting staff. This hands-on industry experience has provided her with a realistic appreciation of real-world issues related to research, competence assessment and maintaining up-to-date knowledge and skills of a multidisciplinary workforce providing frontline care.

Kylie Hoffman is a teaching-intensive academic in the School of Health Sciences at the University of Tasmania, where she has been involved in bioscience education for undergraduate nursing and paramedic students for more than 14 years.

Kerry Howells is a thought-leader, author, award-winning educator and experienced researcher who has spent over 25 years researching, teaching and practising gratitude. School leaders and teachers at all levels of education, as well as whole-school communities, have reported flourishing relationships and improved resilience through their gratitude practices. Some of these case studies can be read in her book, *Gratitude in Education: A Radical View*, which has been used globally to guide educational programs, pedagogy and many professional book clubs. Kerry has a particular interest in cross-cultural lenses of gratitude and their implications for communication, and has studied this in Australian Indigenous and African cultures. Her research incorporates the role of gratitude in palliative care settings.

Elisabeth Jacob is an experienced clinical nurse, educationalist and researcher. Her clinical links provide essential networks for her research in areas of evidence-based practice, nursing education and the nursing workforce. In her position as Head of School, Nursing, Midwifery and Paramedicine (Victoria) at the Australian Catholic University, Elisabeth is responsible for the leadership of nursing, midwifery and paramedicine programs across multiple campuses. Her research has made a significant contribution to the body of literature on nursing education, transition to practice and various nursing workforce roles and responsibilities. Her research includes investigating the evidence for the collection of blood samples through peripheral intravenous cannulas, simulation in health education and the development of critical thinking skills in nursing students.

Jeong-ah Kim is an academic at Federation University Australia with expertise in the fields of nursing, public and occupational health, and patient safety, acquired over the past 20 years. She has broad experience in teaching nursing and other health discipline programs and has achieved significant results in promoting nursing and occupational health and safety at national and international conferences. She is particularly interested in how different systems, methods, environments and social issues influence society, our wellbeing and patient safety.

Carolyn King is the course coordinator for the Associate Degree in Applied Health and Community Support at the University of Tasmania, where she has been teaching for the past 13 years. She has a PhD in neuroscience and her research interests include open and online education, engaging non-traditional learners and educational neuroscience.

Jackie Lea is an associate professor and Associate Head of Teaching, Learning and Student Success in the School of Nursing and Midwifery at the University of Southern Queensland, based in Toowoomba. As a registered nurse and active researcher, Jackie's research interests include the transition from student to beginning-level clinician, clinical education and workplace learning in health, quality and safety in health care.

Judith Lyons is an associate professor and Associate Dean Accreditation in the School of Health at Federation University Australia. Her experience and expertise are in academic development in higher education, nursing and midwifery practice and education, curriculum design, flexible learning and evaluation. Judith is an award-winning teacher, having received an Australian National Citation Award for Outstanding Contribution to Student Learning. The focus of her research is the scholarship of learning and teaching, including curriculum design and development, learning and teaching pedagogical innovations in nursing and midwifery education within the higher education context.

Margaret McAllister is Emeritus Professor of Nursing at Central Queensland University. Her research interests are in nursing education, nursing history and mental health nursing. She has published seven books and 150 refereed journal articles.

Alicia J. Perkins has over 30 years' nursing experience as a clinician, manager and educator, specialising in cardiothoracic intensive care and cardiovascular catheterisation since 1990. From 2000 until 2008 she worked as a nurse unit manager at Cardiovascular Catheter Laboratories. In addition to being a registered nurse, she holds a Bachelor of Psychological Science and postgraduate qualifications in trauma and critical care. She is focused on empowering nurses through the acquisition of knowledge and strives to motivate all nursing students to share this passion.

Maryanne Podham is a lecturer in nursing at Charles Sturt University, with over 20 years' experience in clinical nursing in rural practice. She is passionate about student-centred education and improving clinical practice across the lifespan.

Joanne Porter is an associate professor and Director of the Collaborative Evaluation Unit in the School of Health at Federation University Australia. She has worked in both metropolitan and regional health facilities, predominantly in emergency departments and intensive care units. Her research interests include deteriorating patient outcomes, simulation and emergency care research.

Gina Richards is a lecturer in the School of Nursing and Midwifery at Edith Cowan University. She began as an enrolled nurse then undertook further studies to become a registered nurse. Her research interests include nursing professionalism, curriculum design, online and blended-learning strategies and student support measures. Gina is an Australian and Nursing Midwifery Council national accreditor, a reviewer for *Nurse Education Today* and a committee member of the global professional nursing organisation Sigma Theta Tau.

David Stanley trained as a registered nurse and midwife in South Australia. In 1993 he completed the Bachelor of Nursing at Flinders University. He then worked as a volunteer midwife in Zimbabwe before moving to the United Kingdom and working as a coordinator of children's services and a nurse practitioner. He has a Master of Health Science and a doctorate in nursing, and has been a director of nursing for remote health services in Alice Springs. David has taught nursing since 1987. In 2011 he was awarded the Pearson Nurse Educator of the Year and he is an adjunct professor at Charles Sturt University. His research interests include interprofessional socialisation, men in nursing, rural nursing and clinical leadership.

Karen Stanley nursed in the United Kingdom for 20 years, then emigrated to Australia in 2009. Her teaching interests include assessment in clinical education, communication and counselling skills, and research and evidence-based practice. Her research interests include interprofessional socialisation practices within higher education, men in nursing, rural nursing and clinical leadership. Karen has a PhD from Curtin University and is committed to nursing, as well as promoting interprofessional collaboration for students and health educators, in clinical practice and higher education. Karen is now a freelance nurse educator.

Kathleen Tori is an endorsed nurse practitioner and completed her PhD studies in the research area of advanced practice nursing. Kathy's research interests include all facets of the Australian Nurse Practitioner models of care: transitional processes of the role, barriers and enablers that challenge successful implementation, economic impact and sustainability of emerging nurse-led health care, particularly in rural areas. Kathy has been employed by the University of Tasmania as an associate professor in the School of Nursing since 2018. She has a several professional affiliations and has served on several professional and nursing accreditation boards. She is also a founding director of a nurse practitioner-led model of healthcare service that provides equitable, accessible, efficient and effective health care to meet the needs of small rural communities.

Lolita Wikander is a lecturer at Charles Darwin University. She is an experienced educator with a background and interests in remote health, the assessment of simulated clinical skills and the retention and engagement of first-year undergraduate nursing students, especially in the online environment.

Acknowledgements

The editors and Cambridge University Press would like to thank the following for permission to reproduce material in this book.

Figure 5.1: © 2016 Gravity Consulting Services Pty Ltd. Reproduced with permission. **Figure 8.1:** © Getty Images/traveler1116. **Figure 8.3:** © Getty Images/George Marks. **Figure 9.6:** reproduced with permission from material © McGraw Hill. **Figure 12.1:** © Nursing and Midwifery Board of Australia. Reproduced with permission. For up-to-date information, standards, codes and guidelines for nurses and midwives, see the NMBA website: www.nursingmidwiferyboard.gov.au. **Figure 14.1:** reproduced from Levett-Jones, T., Reid-Searl, K. & Bourgeois, S. (2018). *The clinical placement: An essential guide for nursing students*, 4th edn. Sydney: Elsevier. © Elsevier 2018. Reproduced under STM guidelines. **Figure 17.2:** © Judy Duchscher. Reproduced with permission.

Chapter 18 Nursing perspective: this extract from Rogers, M. (2017). Political refugee dedicates nursing career to giving back. *Griffith News*, 12 September is © Griffith University. Reproduced with permission.

Every effort has been made to trace and acknowledge copyright. The publisher apologises for any accidental infringement and welcomes information that would redress this situation.

Using your VitalSource enhanced eBook

Once you have redeemed your VitalSource access code (see the inside front cover for instructions), the enhanced eBook will be available through your VitalSource account, accessible through the VitalSource Bookshelf website or the VitalSource Bookshelf app, available on all major platforms. The navigation instructions below provide a general overview of the main features available in the enhanced eBook. Note that all solution pop-ups can be moved about the page.

VitalSource features

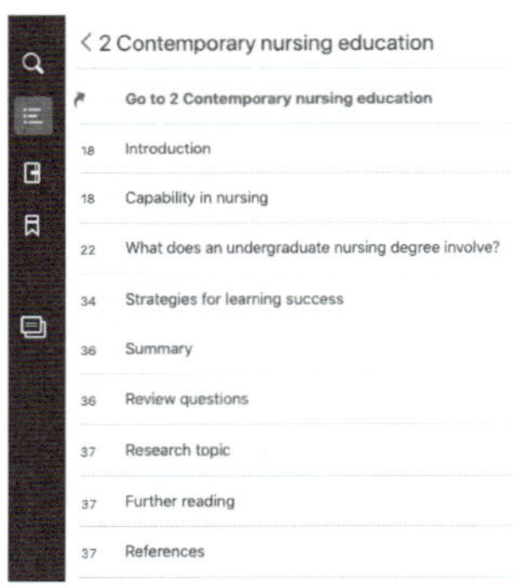

Navigation and search

Move between pages and sections in multiple ways, including via the linked table of contents and the search tool.

Highlight

Highlight text with one click in your choice of colours. Add notes to the highlighted passages.

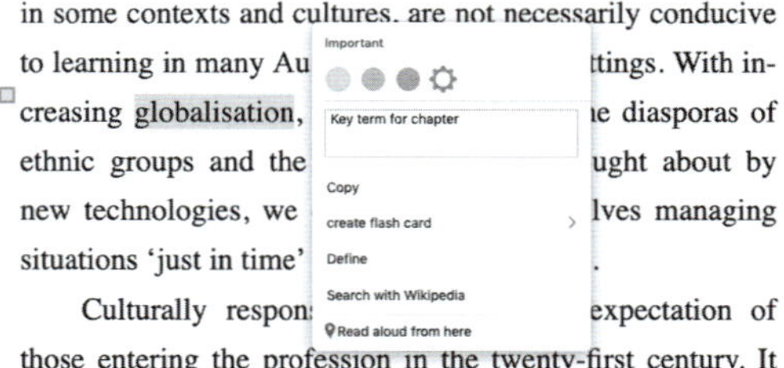

Read aloud

VitalSource Bookshelf includes a read-aloud feature. Controls can be used to increase or decrease the reading speed, or to alter the voice. The feature will remember where you left off and will not be disrupted by navigation to other sections of the book.

Book features

Icon

This icon is used throughout the book to indicate the presence of an interactive component in the eBook. The accompanying descriptor indicates the type of content available.

Margin definitions

Click on terms set in **bold** to display pop-up definitions of key terms.

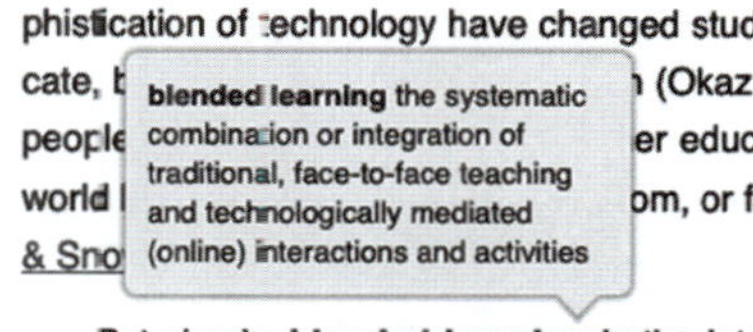

Multiple-choice questions

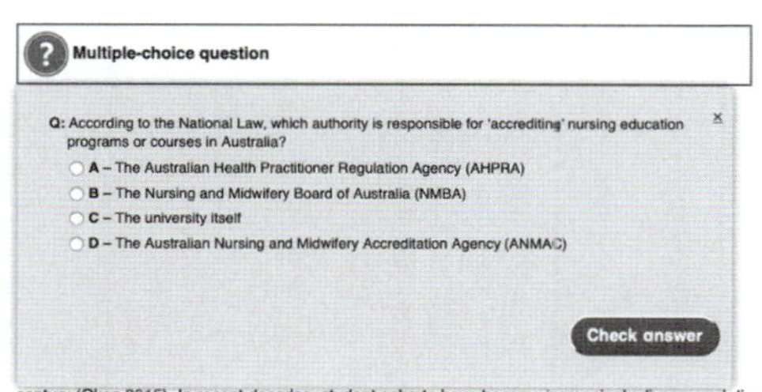

Open the pop-up box for multiple-choice questions, select the correct answers and click 'Check answer' to assess your results. Note that this box can be moved about the page so you can read the text while choosing your responses.

Short-answer questions

Read the question and key your answer into the box. Submit your answers to view the guided solutions and assess your results.

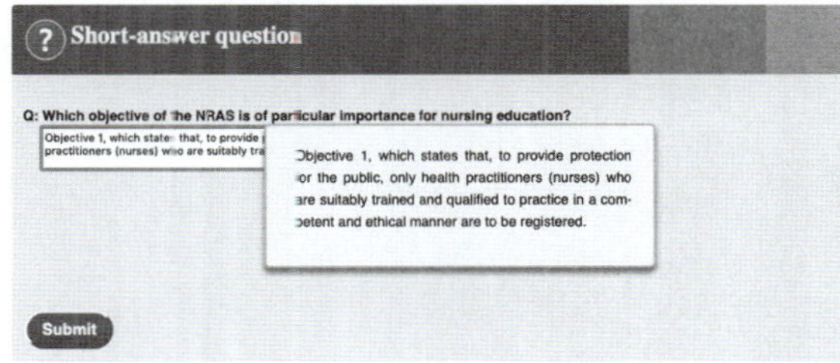

Connecting with practice

Visit industry-related websites to see and understand real-world examples of the theories and concepts covered in the text. Each resource is accompanied by a question to prompt your learning.

Videos and podcasts

To extend your knowledge on the topics presented in the book, click the icon to access relevant video or podcast content. Each resource is accompanied by a question to prompt your learning.

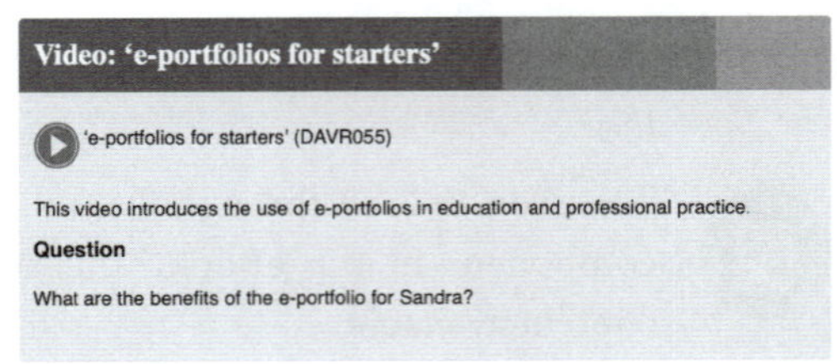

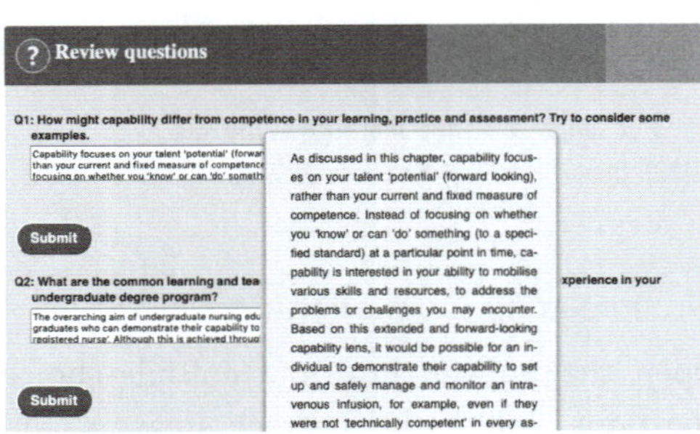

Review questions

Respond to the review questions at the end of each chapter and use the guided solutions to assess your responses.

PART 1

Beginning

1 The journey begins

Nick Arnott, Penny Paliadelis
and Mary Cruickshank

LEARNING OBJECTIVES

At the completion of this chapter, you should be able to:

1 Reflect on your personal motivation and passion for nursing, and formulate a 'beginning' definition of nursing, recognising that this is a continuing process of discovery and refinement.
2 Describe the purpose, structure and features of this book.
3 Discuss the key concepts and ideas that underpin your undergraduate nursing journey.

Introduction

Congratulations on choosing nursing as a profession. Whatever your interests and motivations, nursing is certain to be a career that rewards, challenges and inspires you throughout life. Nursing requires the seamless blending of theoretical and technical knowledge with a way of being and behaving (moral comportment), leading to clinical wisdom, or deep understanding, that supports the highest possible quality of care for individuals, families and communities (Benner, Hooper-Kyriakidis & Stannard 2011; Benner et al. 2010).

The Classical Greek philosopher Socrates is said to have described education as 'the kindling of a flame, not the filling of a vessel'. All the contributors to this book – along with the other authors, teachers, clinical facilitators and mentors you will encounter along the way – are absolutely committed to preparing the very best future custodians and leaders of this profession we love. However, we recognise that not all knowledge can be derived from teachers or external authorities – or indeed a textbook. Knowledge is constructed, not given, and students learn by critically thinking about, sharing, discussing, appraising, questioning, debating, reflecting and practising the concepts, ideas, skills and behaviours that are relevant to contemporary nursing practice (Gottlieb & Gottlieb 2012). Rather than offering a theoretical and technical resource focused on what we want or expect you to *know* or *be able to do,* this book is intended to be a 'journey of discovery', or *to kindle your learning flame.* We present a range of nursing knowledge and perspectives that we believe are important for professional nursing practice in contemporary Australian health care. We encourage you to engage in your own theorising and reflections about what it really means to *be* and *act* as a nurse, with the aim of discovering and nurturing your own passion for nursing (Benner et al. 2010; Gottlieb & Gottlieb 2012, p. 4).

This opening chapter aims to set the scene for your undergraduate nursing journey. We welcome you to the wonderful, dynamic and diverse profession of nursing and encourage some initial thinking about what nursing is, why you have chosen this career and the sort of nurse you hope to be. We also outline the purpose, structure and features of this book, and introduce you to the key concepts and ideas underpinning your learning journey, many of which are emphasised and explored further in subsequent chapters.

Welcome to nursing

It would be difficult to find someone whose life has not been touched in some way by a nurse. We all interact with different professions as we navigate our way through various life events or stages, but by virtue of the diversity in nursing roles and the settings in which they work, nursing is one of the few professions that appears and reappears (sometimes in the foreground and sometimes in the background) across the entire lifespan. At the risk of sounding clichéd, nurses may be present at birth and at death, and at almost every major transition and circumstance in between – through wellness, illness, recovery and dying. Nurses have privileged access to people's lives, bearing witness to the best and the worst of times. They share in some of our most precious, intimate and transformative moments; times of great happiness and triumph but also of great pain, suffering and loss. This privilege comes with enormous rewards and carries great responsibility to uphold the trust and confidence that the community has in our profession.

You have most likely come to this program of study with an existing conception of nursing, informed by various influences and experiences. Perhaps you have friends or family members who are nurses, or you have worked alongside nurses in a related role. Perhaps you have been a direct recipient of nursing care yourself, or have witnessed a nurse's patience, humility and compassion in their care of a loved one. Maybe your views have been shaped by stereotypes, or the ways in which nurses are depicted in film, television, literature or the media. Your initial conception probably enables you to describe what you think nursing is and to explain why you are here and where you would like to take your career. In reality, though, quality learning (and practice) requires a willingness to critically examine the status quo (what you think right now) as a means of informing, guiding and refining what you believe and how you act as you progress through your studies and into practice. This is not to say that your existing conception is flawed; rather, it is just a reminder that a critical mindset through which you analyse, question and evaluate the things you learn, observe and experience is not only important for your success as a student but also key to being a safe, effective and professionally accountable registered nurse.

REFLECTION 1.1

- Why nursing? What were the influences that motivated your decision to become a nurse?
- What are you expecting or hoping for from your career in nursing?

Defining nursing

Nurses (and the public) know, and research evidence confirms, that skilled nursing makes a difference. However, recognising and putting into words exactly what this difference is, and to whom or how it is done, remains elusive (Royal College of Nursing (RCN) 2014). A meaningful definition of nursing can inform the way nursing is perceived, practised and regulated in our rapidly changing healthcare environment, and how the profession differentiates and 'positions' itself as a key stakeholder and leader in continuing healthcare reform. As an undergraduate student, a definition can provide a useful frame of reference to guide and contextualise your learning and reflection. While the need or rationale for a definition may be clear, coming up with a universally accepted definition of nursing is a complex and difficult undertaking. Simply providing a recognised definition would be contrary to the 'critical engagement' we called for earlier, so below we discuss some established definitions, to stimulate the critical thinking needed to inform your own beginning definition of nursing for the learning journey ahead.

The International Council of Nurses (ICN), a coalition of peak nursing associations from more than 100 countries, promotes a short-form definition that captures the complex nature of nursing:

> Nursing encompasses autonomous and collaborative care of individuals of all ages, families, groups and communities, sick or well and in all settings. Nursing includes the promotion of health, prevention of illness, and the care of ill, disabled and dying people. Advocacy, promotion of a safe environment, research, participation in shaping health policy and in patient and health systems management, and education are also key nursing roles (ICN n.d.).

In 2003, following extensive research and consultation, the Royal College of Nursing (RCN) in the United Kingdom published the following definition, which was subsequently reviewed and reconfirmed in 2014:

> Nursing is the use of clinical judgement in the provision of care to enable people to improve, maintain, or recover health, to cope with health problems, and to achieve the best possible quality of life, whatever their disease or disability, until death (RCN 2014, p. 3).

Although concise, the RCN definition is supported by six defining characteristics, which emphasise the purpose, values and interventions of nursing, the importance of relationships and a commitment to partnerships. While other health professions share some of these characteristics, the uniqueness of nursing lies in their combination (RCN 2014). The full document, *Defining Nursing,* is well worth reading: it provides an explanation of how and why this definition was developed and a detailed overview of the defining characteristics.

The above definitions aim to capture both the essence and functions of nursing. They reflect nursing's complexity and diversity, emphasising a focus across the lifespan, in all settings, on health, not only sickness; on the care of individuals, families, groups and communities; and on responses to actual and potential health problems, combining direct care, advocacy, health promotion, health policy and systems improvement.

Although implied, these definitions do not clearly account for the 'roles within roles' that many individual nurses need to assume as they attempt to enact nursing's core focus in different clinical contexts and settings. Along with serving as primary caregivers, nurses often fulfil a number of different roles as clinicians, technicians, advocates, translators, mediators, counsellors, teachers, researchers and leaders – to name just a few. We may develop the ability to move seamlessly between such roles, but it can distort our personal concept of what nursing really is, what it is for and how we do it. This may not only affect our sense of professional identity and purpose, but also our capacity to uphold the profession's social mandate to make clear to the public (and other health professions) the nature of the service we offer, what differentiates us from other health professions and what they can expect from a registered nurse (RCN 2014).

Videos: Campaigns to promote nursing

These definitions also fall short when it comes to addressing the eternal debates about whether nursing is more about theory or practice, the head or the heart. Although the literature is replete with sound arguments on both sides, our view is that nursing involves the seamless blending of **science** and **art**, evidence and intuition, thinking and doing. Nursing certainly requires scientific knowledge and technical know-how, but also the ability to 'artfully' apply this through caring, compassionate and strengths-based practice, which emphasises person-focused care, empowerment, health promotion and collaborative partnerships that support clients, families and communities to heal, cope, develop, grow, thrive and transform (Gottlieb 2017; Stein-Parbury 2018).

Nursing is a wonderful career choice, and we welcome you with open arms. We hope that this is the start of a lifelong journey that constantly surprises, enthrals, humbles and rewards you, as it has us. You will undoubtedly experience challenges and frustrations along the way, and there may even be moments when you want to walk away and never return, but through it all nursing keeps you in touch with your humanity through experiences of tragedy and extreme joy, and offers a limitless and fulfilling career that is everchanging (Wilson & Wilson 2011).

NURSING PERSPECTIVE

There is a lot of useful and sometimes lighthearted information to assist new (and more experienced) nurses to reflect on their role, identity and value.

Here is one example of some simple thoughts that go a long way towards capturing the enduring values of nurses:

Welcome to nursing
Be proud, but check your ego at the door.
Be brave, but seek strength in others.
Be open, but share with caution.
Be humble, but know your worth.
Be kind, but assertive.
Be firm, but malleable.
Be professional, but human.
Be informed, but teachable.
Be selfless, but honour self.
Be you, not who you think you should be.

Above all, do not allow the behaviour of others to cause you to lose sight of why you became a nurse. Deflect any unwelcomed or negative energy. Find your tribe of people and hold them tight. Cry when you need to. Speak up when it is necessary. And last but not least, buy a pair of sensible shoes!

Source: Boggan (2016).

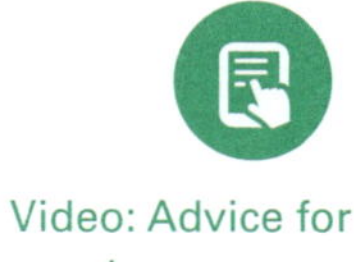

Video: Advice for graduate nurses

About this book

This book focuses on the entire undergraduate 'journey', rather than just individual or discrete units or topics of study. Our vision was to create a companion guide for your learning journey – not dissimilar to a travel guide – that integrates core information with useful tips and resources, and the opinions and stories (lived experience) of actual travellers (in this case, other students, practising nurses and educators). It is likely that some material in this book will be more relevant to particular parts of the course or journey than others; however, we want you to engage deeply in all aspects of your learning and hope to stimulate and encourage thinking, reflection and debate that will guide and inform your transition from beginning student to registered nurse.

Many learning and teaching models emphasise development of the knowledge, skills and attitudes necessary for learning and practising a particular discipline. Billett (2015) extends and reframes this by describing three dimensions of knowledge required to support readiness for healthcare practice: (1) **conceptual knowledge**; (2) **procedural knowledge**; and (3) **dispositional knowledge**. While conceptual and procedural knowledge are obviously important for many aspects of nursing practice, Billett (2015) claims an individual's ability to draw upon and use that knowledge effectively is underpinned by their dispositional readiness. This type of readiness is premised on personal factors such as the value an individual places on particular activities, how interested they are in engaging in such activities or interactions, and the conscious effort and energy they direct towards that engagement. Thus, dispositional knowledge is central to what you do and learn, and, perhaps more critically, to how effective or successful you are in these goal-directed activities. For example, you may *know* about the actions required for person-centred and interprofessional practice, but if you do not value working in such ways, you are unlikely to exercise the effort required for these interactions to be effective, or to benefit from the learning that may come from these endeavours.

In your program of study, much of your conceptual and procedural knowledge will be developed through topical or specialist texts and units of study in areas such as bioscience, health assessment and nursing or clinical skills. This book will sit alongside these other resources, introducing and exploring some of the foundational or universal concepts, skills and theories that are relevant to contemporary nursing practice, but with a particular focus on cultivating your dispositional knowledge or readiness for practice, which is essential for effectively translating the *knowing* of nursing to the *doing* and *being* of nursing. Your attitudes and dispositions are, of course, your own. This book suggests, prompts and models certain ways of thinking and acting; however, the emphasis should be on the meaning *you* make of things: what things really mean to you in different situations and contexts; how this meaning is established; why particular knowledge is necessary or important; and how all this informs your learning, practice and formation of your professional identity (developing your own conception of what it really means to be and act as a nurse).

The book is divided into three sections, reflective of the undergraduate 'journey':

- *beginning* – transitioning to university studies (thinking and acting like a university student)
- *becoming* – forming a professional identity (thinking and acting like a student of nursing)
- *being* – transitioning to professional practice (thinking and acting like a registered nurse).

Although the book adopts a traditional format in which content is presented in a linear or sequential manner, this is not necessarily the way you will engage with this text.

---

conceptual knowledge includes concepts, facts and propositions. This may be superficial knowledge – for example, the names of anatomical structures or certain health conditions – or deep understanding of the links and associations required to comprehend and explain these things, make decisions, select actions or interventions, and evaluate outcomes (e.g. clinical reasoning) (Billett 2015).

procedural knowledge the knowledge required to achieve goals (specific tasks and procedures) through thinking and action; may include physical actions (e.g. psychomotor skills) as well as other cognitive or strategic processes such as planning, selecting and monitoring these acts (Billett 2015)

dispositional knowledge the attitudes, values, interests and intentions that direct and guide an individual's conscious thinking and acting, and therefore their learning (Billett 2015)

Sticking with the 'travel guide' analogy for a moment, you may sometimes backtrack or take unexpected detours on your travels, and may revisit your 'favourite' places over and over again. Each time, you are likely to see different things, encounter different situations and meet different people – not to mention bringing different perspectives, intentions and expectations of your own. All of this conspires to influence and vary your actual experience – or, in the context of this book, your learning. The 'beginning' section of this book is perhaps akin to the preparatory reading you might do *before* your journey, so you may choose to work through it sequentially. For the rest, however, we fully expect (and hope) that you will move in and out, and backwards and forwards, throughout your undergraduate journey and into practice. For example, Chapter 7 presents some of the philosophical perspectives and ideas that underpin nursing practice. At first view, these concepts may seem quite difficult to grasp, but they are likely to take on more meaning and significance as you contextualise, link and apply them to new learning or experiences as your studies progress.

Core concepts underpinning this journey (and the book)

Professional nursing identity

professional identity the acquiring and embodying of the knowledge, values, norms and ways of behaving of a professional group

Learning and acculturation in nursing informs the development of your **professional identity**. It is not our intention to propose a distinct or defined nursing 'identity'; rather, this book introduces some of the knowledge and ideas that, through critical thinking, observation, reflection and practice, will see your professional identity emerge and develop. Some of the knowledge and ideas represent shared or collective wisdom that has developed within the discipline of nursing itself, but this will inevitably be influenced and nuanced by public images and stereotypes (see Chapter 8), your emotional capacities and awareness of self and others (see Chapter 10), and your developing capability as a nurse (see Chapter 2).

'Identity' was once considered a sole, distinct and fixed concept, but it is now seen as a more dynamic conception of multiple identities that are assembled and disassembled throughout one's life in response to our interpersonal relationships and interactions with others, the different roles we adopt and our unique interpretations of lived experiences (Cardoso, Batista & Graca 2014; Johnson et al. 2012). More specifically, identity can be described as 'a set of self-relevant meanings held as standards for the identity in question' (Burke 2006, p. 81), and thus professional identity can be defined as the negotiation of, and commitment to, the knowledge, values, beliefs and practices that are shared with others in a particular professional group (Moola 2017; Willetts & Clarke 2014).

In undergraduate nursing programs, professional identity is often conceptualised in relation to the development of 'professionalism', or the knowledge, skills and attitudes necessary to assume the professional nursing role. While most courses focus on facilitating the development, and even mastery, of such knowledge and skills, the formation of professional identity is as much about *how we come to know* and the *meaning we make* of things, as what we *actually know* or *can do* – especially when viewed and understood from an ontological perspective involving one's conception of what it really means to be and act as a nurse (Johnson et al. 2012; Maginnis 2018; Willetts & Clarke 2014).

The formation of a professional identity has been conceptualised, researched and debated from a range of theoretical perspectives, many deriving from social psychology, which considers identity-formation to be mainly social and relational in nature (Maginnis 2018; Moola 2017; Willetts & Clarke 2014). In this context, acculturation or socialisation into nursing is a process of developing a sense of occupational or professional identity, including 'the development of perceptual abilities, the ability to draw on disciplinary-knowledge and skilled know-how, and a way of being and acting in practice and in the world' (Benner et al. 2010, p. 166).

A nursing identity cannot be taught or imposed. Professional socialisation is a complex process involving the internalisation and reconciliation of the knowledge, values, attitudes and norms of the professional group with the public's perception and expectations of nurses (ten Hoeve, Jansen & Roodbol 2014) and one's own beliefs, behaviours and self-conception (Maginnis 2018; Moola 2017). While this involves a process of construction and deconstruction throughout one's nursing life, the undergraduate journey from beginning student to graduate and registered nurse is of particular significance. This is a formative period in which your existing conception of nurses and nursing is likely to be both affirmed and challenged by the things you learn, observe, experience and do as a student.

Critical thinking

Critical thinking in nursing is a central component of professional accountability and quality nursing care (Wong & Kowitlawakul 2020). For nursing students, it is an essential cognitive skill that enables you to achieve better academic and clinical performance, and improved outcomes for your clients (Chan 2019). It is in our very nature to think but often our decisions and actions are based on intuition, emotions, habits or assumptions. This does not necessarily represent faulty thinking – and we can, of course, be well served by such thought processes in certain situations. However, without the 'critical lens' highlighted earlier in this chapter, our thoughts or responses can sometimes be biased, distorted, uninformed, prejudiced or even dangerous (Paul & Elder 2019).

Critical thinking demands that we question the status quo, or what we may usually take for granted. It is a mode of thinking and reasoning about any subject, content or problem in which a person improves the quality of their thinking (and therefore their actions and/or the outcomes achieved) by applying the cognitive skills of analysis, interpretation, inference, explanation, evaluation and self-regulation, in order to reach an informed judgement about what to believe or do in a given situation or context (Ennis 2015; Paul & Elder 2019).

Chapter 9 explores the 'what, why and how' of critical thinking in greater depth. Various questions, case studies, reflections and activities are also included throughout the text to encourage your critical thinking.

critical thinking self-directed, self-disciplined and self-regulatory thinking and reasoning that informs and guides what to believe and how to act in a given situation or context

REFLECTION 1.2

- As you begin this journey, what do you think about your own thinking?
- How might you begin to develop your critical thinking skills?

Reflective practice

Reflective practice in nursing involves a continuous (and intentional) cycle of examining your experiences, feelings, assumptions and actions, with the aim of developing, expanding and improving the knowledge, skills and behaviours needed for quality learning and practice (Caldwell & Grobbel 2013; Sadlon 2018). Reflection is closely linked to critical thinking. While they are not identical, it is essential that reflection has a 'critical intent' – in other words, it is imperative that your reflections draw upon the critical thinking skills of questioning, analysing and evaluating your actions and assumptions. Without this critical intent, reflection can be reduced to simply 'describing' certain situations or experiences, or to expressing a personal opinion – neither of which necessarily leads to change or improvement in perspective or action. Examining these things against the views of others and what the literature and evidence have to say provides the critical perspectives needed to ensure that your decisions, actions and behaviours are better informed and contribute to transformative change.

Chapter 9 provides further details and strategies for developing your skills as a reflective learner and practitioner, including some models and frameworks that can be used to guide your reflective practice and reflective writing. Reflection questions are also included throughout the book to prompt and encourage this critical approach to your learning and development.

Self-care

The learning and practice of nursing involve complex and demanding work in constantly changing and emotionally charged situations and environments. Although rewarding, it can also be inherently stressful. As such, *caring for the caregiver* (**self-care**) is emphasised and encouraged throughout this book. Specific strategies such as reflection and journalling (Chapter 9), self-compassion (Chapter 7), self-awareness, self-management and mindfulness (Chapter 10), clinical supervision (Chapter 14) and gratitude (Chapter 7) are explored; however self-care is essentially a personal matter and everyone's approach is likely to be different.

Self-care is often described as an essential survival skill for health professionals. It refers to activities, practices and strategies with which we can engage on a regular basis to reduce stress and to maintain and enhance our health and wellbeing (Blum 2014). Self-care is necessary and valuable in many ways but in the context of nursing practice (and education) it is about fulfilling the need to balance personal wellness with one's professional life. By engaging in self-care we assert our right to be well, ensure our own needs are clearly considered in our professional work and model health-promoting behaviours to others, including helping clients and colleagues to deal with their own stress (Crane & Ward 2016). Self-care has become even more vital for health professionals in recent times as the world has witnessed a significant disruption to people's lives as a result of the COVID-19 pandemic (Wallace et al. 2020). The COVID-19 pandemic has presented the world with many challenges, including emotional, behavioural and psychological conditions, so preventative and supportive measures are needed for many vulnerable groups (Pedrosa et al. 2020; Horesh & Brown 2020).

Stress is a natural human response to any stimulus that evokes a change. It can be the catalyst for a positive response that stimulates us to perform well under pressure, but it can often have negative repercussions, affecting our ability to think clearly or act decisively, and sometimes leading to pain, anxiety, exhaustion or burnout (Gomathi, Jasmindebora & Baba 2017).

Emotional labour is one such stressor that is common in service or helping roles like nursing. Emotional labour is the process of regulating or managing emotional expressions and feelings within our work role, often in accordance with organisationally defined rules and guidelines. Given that people experience a wide range of emotions during any given work day, emotions that are felt and those that are required or expected to be expressed may not always be congruent. The mismatch between felt emotion and what an employee is required to display (e.g. feeling angry, but having to maintain a cheerful and caring attitude) can be draining and can often lead to stress, burnout or emotional dissonance (a discrepancy between expressed and felt emotions), which can be detrimental to one's wellbeing, both personally and professionally (Kinman & Leggetter 2016; Lartey, Amponsah-Tawiah & Osafo 2019).

Compassion fatigue is another stressor that nurses may experience in response to constant demands to feel and express empathy in our support of clients, who are suffering in some way (Jakimowicz, Perry & Lewis 2018; Zhang, et al. 2018). Therapeutic relationships are characterised as 'helping relationships' focused on the needs of the client rather than the professional, so compassion fatigue may reflect a failure to acknowledge one's own emotions and needs, or a deeper inability to 'say no' on the part of the caregiver (Kelly, Runge & Spencer 2015; Mills et al. 2015). Without effective self-care, compassion fatigue may contribute to the negative manifestations of stress and may eventually lead to burnout, and even the ending of one's career (Alharbi, Jackson & Usher 2020).

'Burnout' is a term used to describe what happens when a practitioner becomes increasingly 'inoperative' in the work environment (Smullens 2012). It is usually characterised by a state of heightened stress and complete physical and emotional exhaustion, which often renders the person unable to perform their professional role to the standards expected or required (Crane & Ward 2016; Mudallal, Othman & Al Hassan 2017). Common symptoms of burnout include absenteeism, poor morale and physical illness, along with many adverse psychological consequences, including resignation, irritability, anger, depression, anxiety and paranoia. If left unrecognised or unresolved, burnout can cause people to leave or to be forced out of a promising career they have worked hard to attain (Gomathi et al. 2017). Again, self-care strategies that help to manage professional and personal stress are essential for preventing or reversing the effects of burnout.

As already noted, everyone's approach to self-care may be different. Your personal strategies might involve things you do at work or outside of work. From a broad perspective, self-care endeavours may fall into a number of core categories, including (Gomathi et al. 2017; Crane & Ward 2016; University of Buffalo 2016):

- *physical strategies* – activities that help you to stay fit, healthy and energised so you can effectively meet your work and personal commitments
- *emotional and psychological strategies* – activities that promote self-awareness and allow you to feel clear-headed and able to intellectually engage with professional

and personal challenges, and to safely experience and express a full range of emotions

- *social and relational strategies* – activities that enable you to establish, maintain and nurture healthy, supportive and diverse relationships, both within and outside the workplace
- *spiritual strategies* – activities that involve having a sense of perspective or belief that extends beyond day-to-day life
- *workplace and professional strategies* – activities that help you to consistently work to the professional standards expected, and to create a supportive work environment.

Video: Stress management

A word on language and style

This book is a collection of different perspectives and voices. While all contributors share a common intention to stimulate, guide and shape your learning, some perspectives may represent contentious or conflicting views. Our editorial decision regarding such content has been to leave it largely unchanged, recognising that different or conflicting beliefs, ideas and approaches are in fact accurate and realistic reflections of the world in which we live and work. We believe that critical thinking and debate about these different views contribute to deeper learning and improved readiness for your future practice.

Similar perspectives regarding language or terminology also exist. For example, some practitioners use the term 'patient', while others prefer 'person', 'client' or 'consumer' (some may use different terms interchangeably, and others might use an individual term as being 'inclusive' of clients, families and significant others). Throughout this book we have chosen to use the term 'client' to describe people who are consumers of healthcare services. Gender and gendered language also receive much attention in nursing. In this book, some contributors have used the pronouns she/he, her/his, they/them; others have tried to avoid pronouns or gender stereotypes altogether; and yet others have opted to use a single term (e.g. 'her' or 'his') as a 'universal' reference.

Again, these will likely reflect what you commonly hear and see in health care, and we hope that the varied use in this text will stimulate some reflection about the terminology you would like to use in your own practice.

Having different contributors also means there are some subtle differences in style; however, each chapter follows a standard format and supports learning through pedagogical features including case studies, nursing perspectives, reflections, key terms, review questions and research topics.

REFLECTION 1.3

- What's in a name?
- How would you like to refer to or describe the people you care for as a nurse?

SUMMARY

- This chapter welcomes you to the wonderful and diverse profession of nursing. Whatever your interests and motivations, nursing is certain to be a career that rewards, challenges and inspires you throughout life. Establishing a universal definition of nursing is a complex and difficult undertaking. This chapter explores some contemporary definitions that aim to capture both the essence and functions of nursing. They reflect nursing's complexity and diversity, emphasising a focus across the lifespan; in all settings; on health, not only sickness; on the care of individuals, families, groups and communities; and on responses to actual and potential health problems, combining direct care, advocacy, health promotion, health policy and systems improvement. We ask you to reflect upon the features of these definitions that most resonate for you and your existing conception of nursing, and to use this emerging knowledge to formulate your own beginning definition of nursing to help guide and contextualise the learning journey that lies ahead of you.
- This book is designed as a companion guide for your undergraduate learning journey. It focuses on the entire undergraduate 'journey', rather than just individual or discrete units or topics of study. This book will sit alongside other learning resources, introducing and exploring some of the foundational or universal concepts, skills and theories that are relevant to contemporary nursing practice. The book is divided into three sections:
  - *beginning*, which sets the scene for your learning journey through a focus on 'thinking and acting' like a university student
  - *becoming*, which emphasises your emerging identity and capability as a nurse, or 'thinking and acting' like a student of nursing, and
  - *being*, which focuses on 'thinking and acting' like a registered nurse and the concepts and ideas that will support your successful transition to professional practice.
- We want you to engage deeply in all aspects of your learning, and hope this book will stimulate and encourage thinking, reflection and debate that guides and informs your transition from beginning student to registered nurse.
- This book covers a range of content areas; however, we believe that there are some key concepts and ideas that underpin or empower your learning journey: professional identity-formation, critical thinking, reflective practice and self-care. These concepts are introduced in this chapter and are emphasised throughout the book, sometimes directly and other times implicitly.

REVIEW QUESTIONS

1 What are the core defining features or characteristics of nursing?
2 How is professional identity formed or developed?
3 What is a key difference between critical thinking and everyday thinking?
4 What does it mean to be a reflective practitioner?
5 Why is self-care important for health professionals?

Suggested responses

FURTHER READING

Alharbi, J., Jackson, D. & Usher, K. (2020). Personal characteristics, coping strategies and resilience impact on compassion fatigue in critical care nurses: A cross-sectional study. *Nursing and Health Sciences*, 22(1), 20–7.

Blum, C. (2014). Practising self-care for nurses: A nursing program initiative. *Online Journal of Issues in Nursing*, 19(3), Manuscript 3. Available from https://www.ncbi.nlm.nih.gov/pubmed/26824151.

Devine, C.A. & Chin, E.D. (2018). Integrity in nursing students: A concept analysis. *Nursing Forum*, 60, 133–8.

Fasbinder, A., Shidler, K. & Carboral-Stevens, M. (2020). A concept analysis: Emotional regulation of nurses. *Nursing Forum*, 55(2), 118–27.

Jackson, D., Bradbury-Jones, C., Baptiste, D., Gelling, L., Morin, K., Neville, S. & Smith, G.D. (2020). Life in the pandemic: Some reflections on nursing in the context of COVID-19. *Journal of Clinical Nursing*, 29(13–14), 2041–3.

Paul, R. & Elder, L. (2019). *The miniature guide to critical thinking concepts and tools*, 8th edn. Tomales, CA: Foundation for Critical Thinking.

Schmidt, B.J. & McArthur, E.C. (2018). Professional nursing values: A concept analysis. *Nursing Forum*, 53(1), 69–75.

REFERENCES

Alharbi, J., Jackson, D. & Usher, K. (2020). The potential for COVID-19 to contribute to compassion fatigue in critical care nurses. *Journal of Clinical Nursing*, 29(15–16), 2762–4.

Benner, P., Hooper-Kyriakidis, P. & Stannard, D. (2011). *Clinical wisdom and interventions in acute and critical care: A thinking-in-action approach*. New York: Springer.

Benner, P., Sutphen, M., Leonard, V. & Day, L. (2010). *Educating nurses: A call for radical transformation*. San Francisco: Jossey-Bass.

Billett, S. (2015). Readiness and learning in health care education. *The Clinical Teacher*, 12, 367–72.

Blum, C. (2014). Practising self-care for nurses: A nursing program initiative. *Online Journal of Issues in Nursing*, 19(3), Manuscript 3. Retrieved from https://www.ncbi.nlm.nih.gov/pubmed/26824151.

Boggan, L. (2016). Welcome to nursing. *Mighty Nurse Blog*. Retrieved from http://www.mightynurse.com/welcome-to-nursing-stories.

Burke, P.J. (2006). Identity change. *Social Psychology Quarterly*, 69(1), 81–96.

Caldwell, L. & Grobbel, C.C. (2013). The importance of reflective practice in nursing. *International Journal of Caring Sciences*, 6(3), 319–26.

Cardoso, I., Batista, P. & Graca, A. (2014). Professional identity in analysis: A systematic review of the literature. *The Open Sports Sciences Journal*, 7, 83–97.

Chan, Z.C.Y. (2019). Nursing students' view of critical thinking as 'own thinking, searching for truth, and cultural influences'. *Nurse Education Today*, 78, 14–18.

Crane, P.J. & Ward, S.F. (2016). Self-healing and self-care for nurses. *AORN Journal*, 104(5), 386–400.

Ennis, R.H. (2015). Critical thinking: A streamlined conception. In M. Davies & R. Barnett (eds), *The Palgrave handbook of critical thinking in higher education*. New York: Palgrave Macmillan.

Gomathi, S., Jasmindebora, S.V. & Baba, V. (2017). Impact of stress on nursing students. *International Journal of Innovative Research and Advanced Studies*, 4(4),107–10.

Gottlieb, L.N. (2017). Strengths-based nursing: A process for implementing a philosophy into practice. *Journal of Family Nursing*, 23(3), 319–40.

Gottlieb, L.N. & Gottlieb, B. (2012). *Strengths-based teaching and learning: An instructor's manual*. New York: Springer.

Horesh, D. & Brown, A.D. (2020). Traumatic stress in the age of COVID-19: A call to close critical gaps and adapt to new realities. *Psychological Trauma: Theory, Research, Practice, and Policy*, 12(4), 331–5.

International Council of Nurses (ICN) (n.d.). Definition of nursing. Retrieved from http://www.icn.ch/who-we-are/icn-definition-of-nursing.

Jakimowicz, S., Perry, L. & Lewis, J. (2018). Compassion satisfaction and fatigue: A cross-sectional survey of Australian intensive care nurses. *Australian Critical Care*, 3(6), 395–405.

Johnson, M., Cowin, L.S., Wilson, I. & Young, H. (2012). Professional identity in nursing: Contemporary theoretical developments and future research challenges. *International Nursing Review*, 59, 562–9.

Kelly, L., Runge, J. & Spencer, C. (2015). Predictors of compassion fatigue and compassion satisfaction in acute care nurses. *Journal of Nursing Scholarship*, 47(6), 522–8.

Kinman, G. & Leggetter, S. (2016). Emotional labour and wellbeing: What protects nurses? *Healthcare*, 4(4), 89.

Lartey, J.K.S., Amponsah-Tawiah. K. & Osafo, J. (2019). The moderating effect of perceived organizational support in the relationship between emotional labour and job attitudes: A study among health professionals *Nursing Open*, doi: 10.1002/nop2.295.

Maginnis, C. (2018). A discussion of professional identity development in nursing students. *Journal of Perspectives in Applied Academic Practice*, 6(1), 91–7.

Mills, J., Wand, T. & Fraser, J.A. (2015). On self-compassion and self-care in nursing: Selfish or essential for compassionate care? *International Journal of Nursing Studies*, 52(4), 791–3.

Moola, S. (2017). Crafting, constructing and developing a nurse's professional identity scale (NPIS). *Global Journal of Health Sciences*, 9(8), 21–31.

Mudallal, R.H., Othman, W.M. & Al Hassan, N.F. (2017). Nurses' burnout: The influence of leader empowering behaviors, work conditions, and demographic traits. *The Journal of Health Care Organization, Provision, and Financing*, 54, 1–10.

Paul, R. & Elder, L. (2019). *The miniature guide to critical thinking concepts and tools*, 8th edn. Tomales, CA: Foundation for Critical Thinking.

Pedrosa, A.L., Bitencourt, L., Froes, A.C.F., Cazumba, M.L., Campos, R.G.B., Soares de Brito, S.B.C. & Simoes e Silva, A.C. (2020). Emotional, behavioral, and psychological impact of the COVID-19 pandemic. *Frontiers in Psychology*, 11, 1–18.

Royal College of Nursing (RCN) (2014). *Defining nursing*. London: RCN. Retrieved from https://www.rcn.org.uk/professional-development/publications/pub-004768.

Sadlon, P.P. (2018). The process of reflection: A principle-based concept analysis. *Nursing Forum*, 53(3), 364–8.

Smullens, S. (2012) What I wish I had known: Burnout and self-care in our social work profession. *New Social Worker*, 19(4), 6–9.

Stein-Parbury, J. (2018). *Patient and person: Interpersonal skills in nursing*, 6th edn. Sydney: Elsevier.

ten Hoeve, Y.T., Jansen, G. & Roodbol, P. (2014). The nursing profession: Public image, self-concept and professional identity – a discussion paper. *Journal of Advanced Nursing*, 70(2), 295–309.

University of Buffalo (2016). *Self-care starter kit*. Retrieved from https://socialwork .buffalo.edu/resources/self-care-starter-kit.html.

Wallace, C.L., Wladkowski, S.P., Gibson, A. & White, P. (2020). Grief during the COVID-19 pandemic: Considerations for palliative care providers. *Journal of Pain and Symptom Management*, 60(1), 70–6.

Willetts, G. & Clarke, D. (2014). Constructing nurses' professional identity through social identity theory. *International Journal of Nursing Practice*, 20(2), 164–9.

Wilson, A. & Wilson, M. (2011). What I wish I knew about nursing. Retrieved from http://www.whatiwishiknew.com.

Wong, S. & Kowitlawakul, Y. (2020). Exploring perceptions and barriers in developing critical thinking and clinical reasoning of nursing students: A qualitative study. *Nurse Education Today*, 95, 104600.

Zhang, Y., Zhang, C., Han, X., Li, W. & Wang, Y. (2018). Determinants of compassion satisfaction, compassion fatigue and burnout in nursing. *Medicine*, 97(26), 1–7.

Contemporary nursing education

Nick Arnott, Carolyn King,
Patricia Bromley and Kylie Hoffman

LEARNING OBJECTIVES

At the completion of this chapter, you should be able to:

1 Explain the notion of 'capability' in nursing education and practice.
2 Describe the common features and components of a contemporary undergraduate nursing degree.
3 Apply various resources and strategies to optimise your learning success.

Introduction

Florence Nightingale's legacy to the nursing profession is discussed in detail in Chapter 8, but one such legacy was her advocacy for, and establishment of, a formal system of training for nurses. At the request of the then-colonial government, a delegation of Nightingale nurses arrived in Australia in the late 1800s, with a brief to improve the standard of nursing and introduce a nurse training program at the Sydney Infirmary (Willetts 2015). This vocational, or apprenticeship, model of training rapidly spread, with hospital-based training schools being set up across the country. This approach continued largely unchanged until the 1980s and early 1990s (the timing varied in different jurisdictions) when, in response to the growing body of nurse-specific knowledge and nurses assuming greater autonomy and increased responsibility for aspects of health care, nursing education moved into the higher education sector as a discrete academic discipline. This chapter is not about the historical approach, nor the political or professional factors that brought about the change to nursing education models; however, the snapshot above gives some context to the profession you are now entering. You are likely to encounter nurses from both of these educational backgrounds and being cognisant of the *what, why* and *how* of your own education will help you to navigate your way through the rigorous and often passionate debates on the merits (or otherwise) of these two systems.

This chapter introduces the core elements and considerations in 'contemporary' nursing education. We link this to the notion of 'capability in nursing' and provide an overview of what you can expect as you undertake your degree, with links to other chapters where these concepts and ideas are explored in depth. We conclude the chapter with a brief look at some of the resources and strategies that can be used to optimise your learning success.

Capability in nursing

In order to practise in Australia, nurses and midwives must be registered with the Australian Health Practitioner Regulation Agency (AHPRA) and meet the professional standards specified by the Nursing and Midwifery Board of Australia (NMBA 2016). Chapter 12 provides more details about the regulatory context and environment for nursing in Australia. These standards outline the expected practice and conduct of nurses and midwives in Australia, and are therefore reflected in the learning activities, assessment tasks and outcomes of accredited undergraduate (and many postgraduate) nursing degrees. In 2016, the Registered Nurse Standards for Practice (NMBA 2016) superseded a set of 'competency standards'. These revised standards adopted a **capability** mindset, which emphasises an individual's ability to address new or unexpected challenges and achieve desired outcomes, rather than focusing on the testing or measurement of knowledge, skills or performance against a specifically and often narrowly defined benchmark. While all the standards for practice are interlinked, Standard 3 explicitly requires nurses to 'maintain their capability for practice' (NMBA 2016).

capability a forward-looking concept that focuses on a person's talent and potential, rather than only their cognitive or technical competence; it emphasises the individual's ability to address new or unexpected challenges or problems in order to achieve optimal outcomes

What is meant by 'capability'?

Bromley (2017) undertook a review of capability in the context of nursing education, as summarised below. Building on earlier work on capability and quality in higher education from the 1990s, Stephenson and Yorke (2012) declared capability to be a much broader concept than that of competence:

> Capability embraces competence but is also forward looking, concerned with the realization of potential … Capability is an integration of knowledge, skills, personal qualities and understanding used appropriately and effectively – not just in familiar and highly focused specialist contexts but in response to new and changing circumstances … to take actions in uncertainty, and to see initial failure as a basis of learning how to do better (2012, pp. 2–3).

Contemporary definitions of capability have evolved from these original ideas. Scott, Chang and Grebennikov (2010, pp. 27–8) found that capability 'involves a mixture of emotional and cognitive intelligence including the ability to determine when and when not to deploy these competencies'. Brewer and colleagues (2014, p. 30) suggested that capability extends well beyond disciplinary knowledge and understanding: '[It includes] communication, reflective skills, team function, conflict resolution and client-centred care … [requiring] a sophisticated, integrated set of capabilities that encompass more than discipline specific knowledge, skills and understandings'. O'Connell, Gardner and Coyer (2014) considered what this would involve or look like in individuals, asserting that capable people are 'creative, have a high degree of self-efficiency, know how to learn, can take appropriate and effective action to formulate and solve problems, can apply competencies in unfamiliar and familiar situations, and work well with others' (p. 2731).

Short-answer question

Preparing capable graduates

Capable graduates are required to be 'work-ready', with easily transferable skills and capabilities (Foundation for Young Australians 2016). Higher education requires the development of graduates who are employable in a rapidly changing occupational world (Coetzee 2014). In fact, the Foundation for Young Australians (2016) stated that these 'transferable skills … enable young people to engage with a complex working world and … [are] a powerful predictor of long-term job success' (p. 8).

Coetzee (2014) identified eight core skills and attributes that constitute *graduateness* (capable graduates) within the three domains of scholarship (problem-solving and decision-making skills, analytical thinking skills, enterprising skills); global and moral citizenship (ethical and responsible behaviour, presenting and applying information skills, interactive skills); and lifelong learning (goal-directed behaviour and continuous learning orientation). Similarly, Scott, Chang and Grebennikov (2010) identified capabilities of the successful graduate as personal and interpersonal capabilities, cognitive abilities, and generic skills and knowledge. In her research on capability in neonatal nurses, Bromley (2018) identified similar characteristics. She conceptualised capability as a combination of professionalism, interpersonal relationships, and knowledge and skills, which are closely interlinked and interdependent – like the gears on a wheel, where the movement of one gear initiates the movement of another (Figure 2.1).

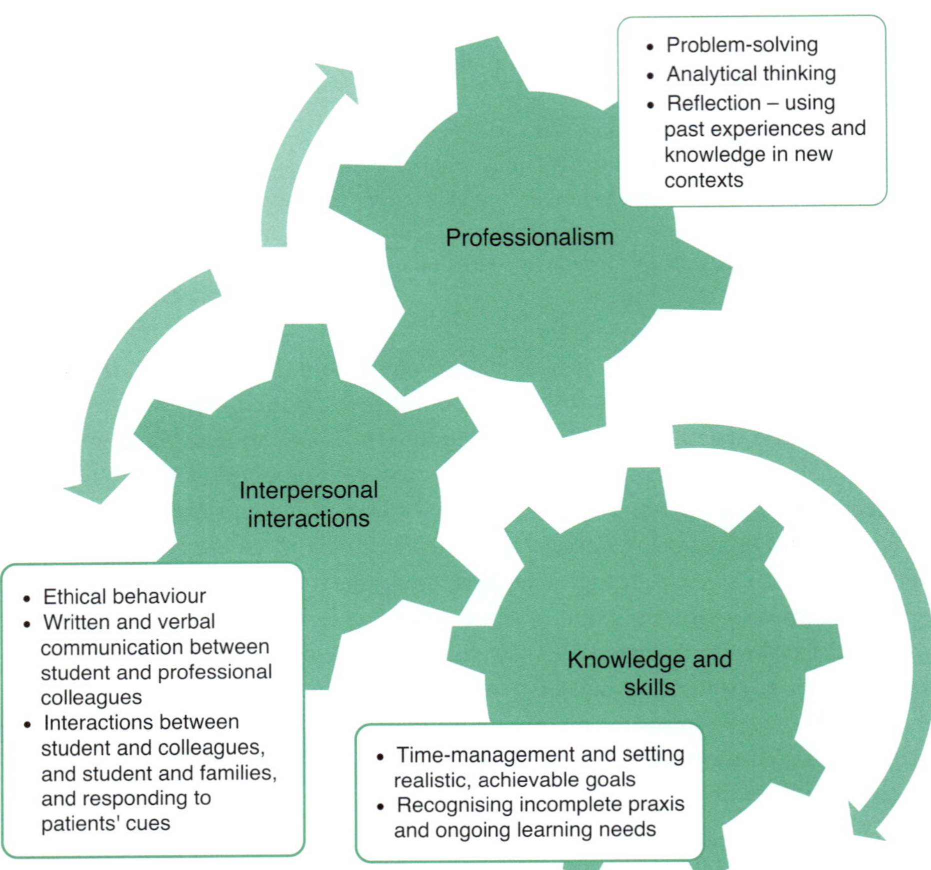

Figure 2.1   The gears of capability for student nurses

Source: Adapted from Bromley (2018).

Capable graduates possess both a high level of technical competence and personal, interpersonal and cognitive capabilities that support their readiness for practice and promote continuous learning, improvement and the development of greater mastery over time (Scott et al. 2010; Bromley 2018). From this perspective, mentors (clinical educators, preceptors or facilitators) appraise the student's application of knowledge and their skill in navigating the complexities of the work context, as demonstrated through their verbal and non-verbal actions and behaviours in the practice environment (Bromley 2018).

These mentors interpret student behaviours in a clinical context to evaluate their skills in managing different (often unfamiliar or uncertain) situations, which in turn informs their view of the student's overall capability for managing future situations (Bromley 2018).

In other words, appraising capability allows the mentors to make decisions or judgements about the student's potential.

Bromley (2018) represents this conceptualisation of capability in a capability wheel (Figure 2.2). The gears of capability (Figure 2.1) sit at the centre of the wheel, propelling capability forward. Continuing this analogy, a wheel has spokes that revolve around the geared hub. According to Bromley, the spokes, which incorporate essential capability requisites, 'play an important role in maintaining strength and stability in the wheel' (Bromley 2018, p. 97). In Bromley's research, the spokes represent 20 neonatal intensive care (NIC) capability requisites. They connect to the gears and are essential for functional capability in the specific work context or environment. The specific capability requisites are powered through the gears of capability – or, in other words,

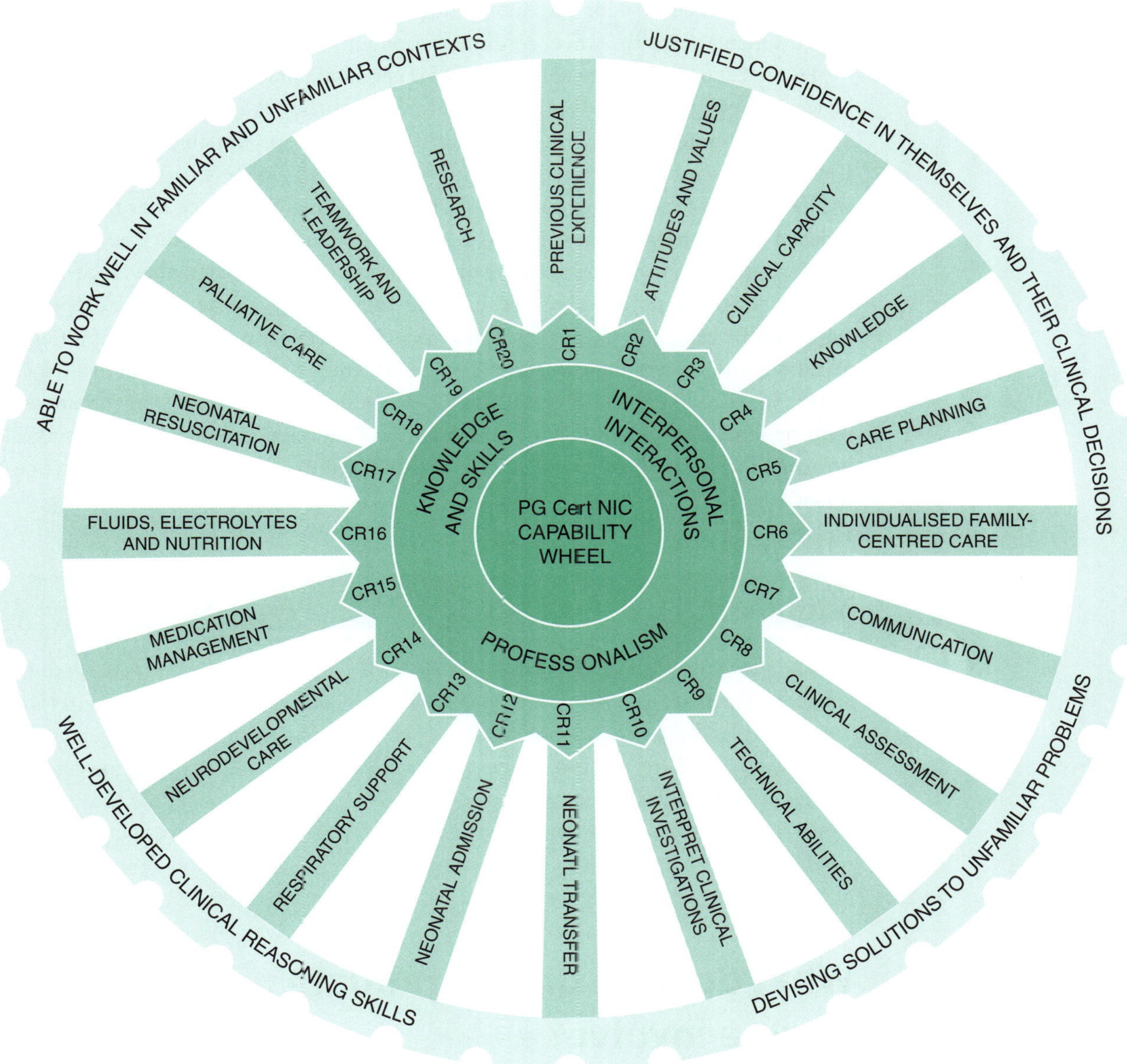

Figure 2.2   The Postgraduate Certificate in NIC capability wheel: The embodiment of a capable neonatal nurse
Source: Bromley (2018).

the interaction between 'professionalism, interpersonal interactions, knowledge and skills' (Bromley 2018, p. 97). The spokes also connect to the tyre, which is 'the interface with the road' (Bromley 2018, p. 97). The tyre represents the interface with practice – how capability is seen, or demonstrated, in practice. In Bromley's (2018) research, the capability wheel describes the embodiment of a capable neonatal nurse – one who utilises knowledge, interpersonal interactions and professionalism at all times; can be relied on to work just as well in familiar as in unfamiliar environments or contexts; has a justified confidence in their clinical decision-making; and possesses well-developed clinical reasoning skills as the means to devise novel solutions to unfamiliar problems.

Each part of the capability wheel is dependent on the other parts to be functional: straight spokes, well-greased gears and good rubber on the tyre. The capability wheel moves the nurse forward along the path of capability (continuous learning and improvement), so as the wheel continues, capability continues to develop.

Figure 2.2 presents a capability wheel for neonatal nurses (Bromley 2018). You may be wondering how or why this is relevant to your journey as an undergraduate nursing student. As noted earlier, the regulatory framework for nursing in Australia (see Chapter 12) requires all nurses – including students – to develop and demonstrate their capability for nursing practice, whatever that area of practice may be. Although focused on neonatal nurses, Figure 2.2 helps to illustrate capability as a forward-moving concept involving a number of interdependent parts that focus on an individual's 'talent potential', rather than only their cognitive or technical competence. Importantly, capability requisites 1–10 and 19–20 reflect 'universal capabilities' for all nurses and closely align with the Registered Nurse Standards for Practice (NMBA 2016). So, too, do capability requisites 11–18, which broadly represent the universal requirements of problem-solving ability and well-developed clinical reasoning skills; however, these have been nuanced or contextualised to a particular area of practice in this wheel.

REFLECTION 2.1

Have a go at applying the capability wheel in Figure 2.2 to different units of study and the practice placements you undertake as an undergraduate student. Insert the particular 'capability requisites' that you think are pertinent to this area of practice (replacing 11–18, or however many you think are necessary). Regularly revisit this wheel to reflect upon your developing capability, how you demonstrate this in your learning and practice, and ways in which you might extend and improve your capability in the future.

What does an undergraduate nursing degree involve?

In the recent independent review of nursing education in Australia, Schwartz (2019) stated that:

> There is much that is excellent about Australian nursing education, and the fundamentals of high-quality nursing education are already in place. Australia has a system of national standards for course accreditation. It also has a diverse set of educational institutions that have developed innovative curricula to meet those standards (p. 3).

In 2009, the *Health Practitioner Regulation National Law Act 2009* (the National Law) was created to establish a national registration and accreditation scheme (NRAS) for health practitioners (AHPRA 2009). The scheme has six objectives, with the first being of primary importance for nursing education:

> to provide for the protection of the public by ensuring that only health practitioners who are suitably trained and qualified to practice in a competent and ethical manner are registered (AHPRA 2009, p. 25).

In accordance with the National Law, to apply to become a registered nurse in Australia, individuals must first complete a program of study that is accredited and monitored by the Australian Nursing and Midwifery Accreditation Council (ANMAC) and approved by the NMBA. These programs of study (sometimes referred to as 'entry-to-practice' programs) are delivered by accredited universities or higher education providers, and lead to the award of a bachelor's or master's degree in nursing (ANMAC 2012; Schwartz 2019).

Short-answer question

ANMAC is the independent accrediting authority for nursing and midwifery education under the NRAS outlined above (also see Chapter 12). ANMAC 'helps to protect the health and safety of the Australian community by establishing high-quality standards of nursing and midwifery education, training and assessment' (ANMAC 2017, p. 2).

The overarching aim of undergraduate (or entry-to-practice) nursing education is to prepare graduates who can demonstrate their capability to 'think and act like a registered nurse'. While these accreditation standards ensure the quality and consistency of nursing education programs, every program is unique, with each university or provider having the scope to tailor aspects of its curriculum and approach (Schwartz 2019). A typical nursing course (program of study) 'may cover an extensive range of topics: anatomy, physiology, microbiology, psychology, cultural diversity, informatics, public health, mental health, pharmacology, ethics, clinical reasoning, Aboriginal health care, and child development as well as clinical practice skills and knowledge' (Schwartz 2019, p. 12). The COVID-19 pandemic has seen an expanded focus on the fundamentals of infection prevention and control (Morin 2020), and some programs are also devoting increased teaching time to topics such as chronic conditions, disability, ageing, end-of-life care and substance abuse. However, in an already busy curriculum, many of these remain the focus of postgraduate study, where students build on the strong generalist base of their registered nursing education.

Given these differences, it is not our intention in this chapter to discuss every possible topic of study (refer to the recommended textbooks and readings in your own program of study). However, despite the differences, every program is likely to share some common features or components (Figure 2.3), which we explore in this chapter.

Multiple-choice question

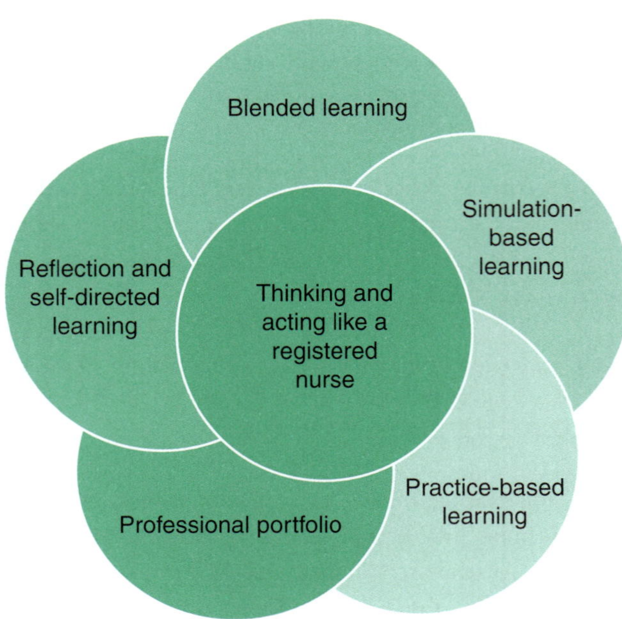

Figure 2.3   Common learning and teaching framework for an undergraduate nursing degree

Blended learning

Face-to-face lectures and classroom instruction have been the mainstay of university teaching for over a century (Okaz 2015). In recent decades, student cohorts have become increasingly diverse and dispersed, making these traditional models of learning and teaching less conducive to their needs and preferences, and posing challenges for education providers in meeting the growing expectations and demands for flexible, high-quality learning experiences and outcomes (Alammary, Sheard & Carbone 2014; Bower et al. 2014). At the same time, the increasing presence and sophistication of technology have changed students' behaviours and attitudes, and have altered the ways in which they engage, learn and communicate, both in and outside of the classroom (Okaz 2015, p. 601). Information and communication technologies (ICT) are transforming the ways in which people live, work and learn, and higher education institutions are rising to the challenge of helping students to thrive in this technologically based world by 'blending' traditional classroom, or face-to-face, learning with online and mobile learning approaches (Bower et al. 2014; El-Mowafy, Kuhn & Snow 2013; Hrastinski 2019).

blended learning the systematic combination or integration of traditional, face-to-face teaching and technologically mediated (online) interactions and activities

Put simply, **blended learning** is the integration of traditional learning (face-to-face teaching) with online activities or approaches (Hrastinski 2019). Bliuc, Goodyear and Ellis (2007) preferred a more rigorous definition:

> Blended learning describes learning activities that involve a systematic combination of copresent (face-to-face) interactions and technologically mediated interactions between students, teachers and learning resources (p. 234).

Alammary and colleagues (2014) proposed that blended learning courses or approaches (1) thoughtfully integrate different instructional methods such as lectures, discussion groups and self-paced activities; and (2) comprise both face-to-face and computer-mediated components. The emphasis in these definitions on *systematic combining* and *thoughtful integration* suggests that the design of blended learning requires a great deal of planning and forethought (Alammary et al. 2014; Branch & Dousay 2015).

Difficulties 'connecting' with teachers in computer-mediated learning settings; barriers to accessing online resources (e.g. having limited or no access to internet or wi-fi, or insufficient broadband width to access learning materials such as videos, voice-over slide presentations and high-fidelity simulations); limited IT-acuity of students or teachers; difficulties fostering cooperative learning; and the loss of a sense of connection, belonging and 'classroom community' have all been suggested as challenges or barriers to blended learning (Halasa et al. 2020; Leidl, Ritchie & Moslemi 2020; Morin 2020; Okaz 2015). However, in their meta-analysis of more than 1000 published studies, Means and colleagues (2009) concluded that blended learning is more effective than either online learning or face-to-face instruction alone, with similar claims or outcomes being reported in recent studies on blended learning in nursing education specifically (Halasa et al. 2020; Leidl et al. 2020).

Due to the threat of COVID-19, many institutions decided to cancel all face-to-face classes during the pandemic, including laboratory sessions, clinical placements and other learning experiences, to help keep their students, staff and the community safe during this public health emergency (Hodges et al. 2020). While a small number of nursing education programs were already operating fully online, these decisions were largely taken as a temporary 'emergency remote teaching' response (Hodges et al. 2020). While the design and use of particular technologies may vary from course to course, and even from unit to unit, blended learning is almost certain to be the type of course delivery you experience as an undergraduate nursing student.

Multiple-choice question

Flipped teaching and learning

The concept of 'flipped' teaching, or flipped classrooms, is a common blended-learning approach used in nursing education (Halasa et al. 2020). As the name suggests, **flipped learning** is when the traditional model of didactic teaching through lectures and tutorials, followed by homework or follow-up activities to extend and consolidate learning, is reversed, or flipped (El-Mowafy et al. 2013). Instead, students are provided with learning materials such as readings, recorded lectures, other audiovisual resources, e-assessments, quizzes and discussion forums in advance, with the expectation that they will prepare themselves as appropriate for the subsequent classroom (in-person or virtual) and/or practical activities. This enables classroom learning to shift from 'passive' teaching and provision of information to a focus on the specific questions and dilemmas raised by these *informed* students, and the promotion, reinforcement and application of the core concepts and outcomes of the subject matter under consideration (El-Mowafy et al. 2013). Flipped teaching is not simply about the ways in which learning materials and activities are ordered or sequenced: it must be pedagogically sound (concerned with the theory and practice of teaching, or what a teacher does to influence learning in others), as highlighted by Talbert (2017):

> Flipped Learning is a pedagogical approach in which first contact with new concepts moves from the group learning space [classroom] to the individual learning space in the

flipped learning a type of blended learning whereby online learning resources and activities are provided before (rather than after or during) classes, with the expectation that students will prepare themselves appropriately for the subsequent classroom activities, which can then focus on promoting, reinforcing and applying core concepts as opposed to 'teaching' them

form of structured activity [e.g. subject notes and readings; recorded lectures], and the resulting group space is transformed into a dynamic, interactive learning environment where the educator guides students as they apply concepts and engage creatively in the subject matter.

Although in theory flipped learning appears logical and straightforward, it does require a concerted effort from the student to actively engage and participate in this style of learning. Inevitably, there will be times when a student falls a bit behind or is unable to complete the necessary self-directed work in advance; however, if they are repeatedly unprepared or come with the attitude that 'I can catch up in class' or 'I pay you to teach me this stuff', this will not only undermine their own learning outcomes, but may also diminish the learning opportunities and experiences of their well-prepared peers.

Group-based learning

There are two important priorities for learning and assessment in a nursing (in fact, any) degree. First, the program needs to develop and evaluate theoretical and practical knowledge (subject-specific content knowledge and skills), which should also inform and enable course-level learning outcomes and graduate attributes. Second, and just as importantly for this degree, it needs to facilitate achievement of the professional standards established by the NMBA, which students must demonstrate in order to qualify for the degree and subsequently register to practise nursing in Australia (NMBA 2016).

A key requirement for both priorities is for students to demonstrate collaboration and their ability to work effectively in teams. The importance of effective teamwork in nursing and health care cannot be overemphasised (Barton, Bruce & Schreiber 2018). It has been shown to enhance client safety and the continuous quality improvement of care and services; improve efficiency and productivity; and promote care coordination, integration and innovation (Barton et al. 2018; Jackson et al. 2014).

The literature is replete with evidence and examples of the benefits that flow from students working collaboratively in groups. Working together has been shown to facilitate 'deep, active and collaborative learning' (Jackson et al. 2014, p. 117) and to have a positive influence on learning outcomes (Wong 2018). Group work promotes the development of learning communities and encourages peer interaction, dialogue and negotiation (Jackson et al. 2014). This provides opportunities for students to share their different experiences and perspectives, and to develop, refine and articulate their knowledge and understanding in various content domains (Barton et al. 2018), particularly authentic and contextualised knowledge and 'real-life' understanding (Biggs & Tang 2011). Collaborative work can also increase students' motivation for learning, and their sense of responsibility and accountability for themselves and others, and provides experiences of self-regulation and the evaluation of their own and others' work (Wong 2018).

Group work is likely to be a common feature throughout your degree program, sometimes as a means of facilitating critical thinking and debate about important content or topics, and at other times to prepare group projects or presentations for the purpose of assessment. While it may seem as though this should involve face-to-face contact and activities, group work is increasingly being facilitated through technology-mediated interactions, as part of a 'blended learning' approach. Online learning management systems (LMS) now incorporate a range of features to support collaborative learning, including discussion forums, web conferencing, media portals and virtual meeting spaces and classrooms. The rapid transition to remote, online learning during the COVID-19 pandemic also led to exponential growth in the use of publicly available platforms such as Zoom and Microsoft Teams (Morin 2020). Digitally literate students are able to readily and successfully extend their lessons and conversations beyond the traditional classroom (Kasraie & Alahmed 2014; Morin 2020). Of course, many students are also particularly adept when it comes to social media and other mobile technologies, so various social media platforms are commonly used (both formally and informally) to expedite collaborative learning, communication and a sense of connectedness and belonging in your nursing studies (see Chapter 14 for more information about the responsible use of social media as a health professional).

Simulation-based learning

In practice-based healthcare professions such as nursing, teaching and learning need to be focused on enabling students to assimilate clinical knowledge and skills, or to apply their classroom learning in clinical contexts (Bogossian et al. 2018; Schwartz 2019). You will engage in **simulation-based learning** throughout your studies as a strategy for achieving such outcomes. Simulation replaces 'real-life' experiences with guided and immersive experiences that replicate aspects of the real world in an authentic, safe and secure environment (Bogossian et al. 2018). In nursing education, simulation involves a variety of approaches and aids that help to replicate clinical situations, scenarios and skills (e.g. taking blood, priming an intravenous (IV) line or dressing a wound), thereby supporting the translation of theory into practice. Simulation supports the development of requisite capabilities in critical thinking and clinical reasoning (Levett-Jones 2018), and enables learners to participate in dynamic scenarios that support the integration of conceptual knowledge, technical or procedural skills, communication and interprofessional teamwork (Fernando et al. 2017; Schwartz 2019; Wilcox et al. 2017).

You are likely to experience low, medium and high levels of fidelity in simulation across your studies. The level of fidelity is the extent to which the simulation resembles the real-life scenario. Simulated activities include case studies and role-plays, immersive technologies and equipment (e.g. mannequins, virtual cases and models), task trainers (e.g. IV access simulators, airway-management trainers and simulated wounds) and human-client simulation using high-fidelity mannequins, virtual clients and/or human actors (Bogossian et al. 2016; Kononowicz et al. 2016).

Practice-based learning: Professional experience placements

Learning in the clinical environment is an essential component of nursing education. It complements the theoretical foundations and simulation-based learning provided at university (Birks et al. 2017). **Clinical placements** will form a significant part of your education program, with placements occurring in 'block' (full-time placements for a defined period) or distributed (one or two days per week over a semester or year)

simulation-based learning guided and immersive experiences that replicate aspects of the real world (clinical situations and scenarios) in an authentic, safe and secure learning environment

Multiple-choice question

Short-answer question

clinical placements planned opportunities to put theory into practice with real people, in real-world settings; they are designed to build students' knowledge, confidence and professional identity, and to develop and consolidate the capabilities required for registration

modes. Placements provide an opportunity for students to put newly acquired skills, behaviours and knowledge into practice, to immerse themselves in the professional culture of nursing and to gain a deep understanding of the diverse roles and 'identity' of the registered nurse within the Australian healthcare system. Each institution uses different models and has different expectations of professional experience placements, and therefore it is essential that you familiarise yourself and actively engage with all the preparatory requirements early in your degree.

This entire book aims to support your readiness for practice, but refer to Chapter 14 for some specific tips and resources regarding the aspects of your degree program that involve professional experience placement.

CASE STUDY

Practice-based learning

As a student nurse, one of my clinical placements was in a COVID-19 testing clinic at a major hospital, including a week at the drive-through testing clinic located in the carpark of a small suburban club. When I was told this would be my placement, I was excited to be a part of it but nervous about my own health and safety. I was also worried about the clients and what to expect. My parents were really concerned about me, and for a short time I considered asking to be reassigned.

My role in the clinic involved collecting data from clients, explaining the testing process, taking the swabs (under supervision) and entering notes and client data. The role was similar at the drive-through clinic but there we swabbed people in their cars. I learned so much about the importance of personal protective equipment (PPE) and hand hygiene, and also how to talk politely – but fast! The shifts were often hectic. After a few shifts I became tired and sometimes felt quite stressed trying to get through the volume of clients, particularly in the hospital clinic. It was hard to get much time or guidance from my preceptors but the university provided good support and checked in with me twice a week. I found it difficult having to wear a mask around the clock, and the learning opportunities were a bit limited as the work was busy but repetitive. Even so, working closely with members of the public, often with people who were also stressed or scared, was a great opportunity to further develop my client engagement, communication and education skills. It was also great to feel part of the team and to watch how well everyone adapted to changing rules and workloads.

QUESTIONS

1 What are you most and least looking forward to in regard to practice-based learning?

2 What can you start doing now to prepare yourself for the practice-based learning component of your nursing studies?

Professional portfolio

Chapter 9 provides some ideas about what a professional portfolio might look like, particularly in the context of reflective writing and practice. A professional portfolio is a tool to assist you in reflecting, storing, organising and sharing items from your learning and practice as a nurse. Although conceptually similar to a traditional journal or 'scrapbook', a contemporary professional portfolio is usually developed as an electronic record, enabling you to create, add and edit documents, graphics, audio files, videos, presentations, certificates, academic transcripts and the like in a single, readily accessible repository.

Most universities require you to create and maintain your own professional portfolio for your nursing degree. Even if it is not mandated by your institution, we strongly encourage you to establish a portfolio anyway, as it will be a valuable resource for your studies and provide a record of your learning and professional development throughout your working life, which is a mandated requirement in the yearly registration process for nurses. There are numerous e-portfolio platforms available, but many people have successfully established their portfolios using commonly available software applications, such as Microsoft's OneNote. We are reluctant to specify or recommend specific platforms because you really need to consider the features and access requirements that will best meet your needs. Some universities may have e-portfolios embedded in their online LMS, but these may not offer the 'portability' needed to continue or extend your portfolio beyond the term of your studies or enrolment.

While a student, your professional portfolio acts as a personal repository for information, activities, reflections, artefacts, skills, awards and qualifications that you prepare or acquire as part of your degree. This provides an evidence base or record of your academic achievements as well other information and evidence that may be required by future employers. Since it is a personal resource, your portfolio will not be accessed or viewed by teaching staff (or employers) without your expressed permission. However, from time to time you may be asked to draw upon certain experiences, events or records for the purposes of assessment, or to demonstrate your capability or competence in specified areas or domains, and having an e-portfolio will be helpful in doing so.

Although there may be a few more 'rules' or expectations of you while you undertake your studies, essentially it is up to you to decide what you want to include in your portfolio, how you want to organise it, and when and with whom you choose to share things. If you share items with your peers, teachers or potential employers, you will still retain the authority to determine the type and extent of access you permit. This may include the sharing of items that you have downloaded from ('taken out of') your portfolio; read-only access to specified resources within your portfolio; or perhaps permission for others to edit, add or respond to items, depending on the type of engagement and feedback you desire.

Reflection and self-directed learning

As highlighted in Chapter 1, reflection is emphasised, encouraged, observed and assessed throughout your degree, and is explored further in Chapter 9. **Reflective practice** in nursing involves a continuous cycle of examining your experiences,

Video: 'e-portfolios for starters'

reflective practice an intentional process of examining your experiences, feelings, assumptions and actions, with the aim of improving the knowledge, skills and behaviours needed for quality learning and practice

feelings, assumptions and actions, with the aim of developing your self-awareness and expanding your knowledge, skills and behaviours (Caldwell & Grobbel 2013; Nicol & Dosser 2016). Reflection is an important capability for students to develop, as it contributes to the depth of learning and understanding, acts as a professional motivator to 'do better' within practice, builds your sense of identity and confidence as a nurse, and enhances your ability to provide optimal client care (Nicol & Dosser 2016). In order for reflection to be effective, 'open-mindedness, courage, and a willingness to accept, and act on, criticism must be present' (Caldwell & Grobbel 2013, p. 319).

Taking responsibility for your own learning is a key to success in university education. Although you may have limited face-to-face contact in some subjects or units, a university's LMS is essentially designed as an extension of the classroom. A range of information and resources is usually provided through the LMS (and via other technologies) to guide and support your learning. The concept of flipped learning was discussed earlier, and you may be expected to engage with these resources and/or complete certain activities before (or in preparation for) your classes. You may also be encouraged to revisit these resources after class, and to complete follow-up activities to help consolidate and extend your learning. Additional learning or research will also be necessary in preparation for many of your assessment tasks. All this represents or requires a significant amount of **self-directed learning**. Although the requirements may vary for different units, it is suggested that for every hour of formal study (lectures, tutorials, practicals), you should undertake at least three hours of self-directed study to prepare, practise, reinforce, revise, consolidate and extend your knowledge and skills.

Other common features

Informatics

According to the Healthcare Information and Management Systems Society (HIMSS 2014), 'health informatics' is the term used to describe the design, development, adoption and application of information technology-based innovations in healthcare service delivery, management and planning. More specifically, nursing informatics is:

> a specialty that integrates nursing science with multiple information and analytical sciences to identify, define, manage, and communicate data, information, knowledge, and wisdom in nursing practice. Nursing informatics supports nurses, consumers, patients, the interprofessional healthcare team, and other stakeholders in their decision making in all roles and settings to achieve desired outcomes. This support is accomplished through the use of information structures, information processes, and information technology (ACN/HISA/NIA 2017, p. 1).

Informatics will be embedded in most of your units of study, and you will be required to learn about, understand and apply various information structures, processes and technologies in a range of contexts and settings. This may involve engagement with social media, electronic health records, e-health platforms, information repositories, data-management systems, research and evidence-based practice resources, computer and smartphone applications, and more.

Multiple-choice question

Connecting with practice:
Nurse Informatics
Position Statement

self-directed learning proactive engagement with learning resources and activities outside the classroom or structured class time; sometimes this engagement will be before or in preparation for class, and at other times after class to help extend and consolidate learning

Interprofessional learning

Interprofessional learning occurs when two or more professionals learn with, from and about each other to improve collaboration and the quality of care provided (ANMAC 2015; Barr et al. 2017). Throughout your degree, you will be encouraged to consider the teams of health professionals with which you will be working, and the ways in which these different roles interact, collaborate and communicate with one another to achieve safe, high-quality care. This may include shared-care arrangements (when various practitioners take responsibility for different aspects of a person's care), client-centred service coordination and the streamlining of referrals and transitions between different parts of the healthcare system.

More direct or formal interprofessional learning opportunities may also be offered during your degree. This might involve combined classes, simulation-based activities or on-the-job (practice-based) interactions and workshops (Fernando et al. 2017).

Assessment

Biggs and Tang (2011) described two kinds of knowledge that form the basis of learning and assessment in higher education: *declarative knowledge,* which engages students in key theories, models and frameworks, and *functioning knowledge,* which requires students to apply or enact knowledge, or to exercise active control over problems and decisions in relevant (and preferably authentic and contextualised) content domains. Declarative knowledge is obviously important in many nursing units or subjects; however, the ability to apply such knowledge to real-world problems is a priority for a practice-based discipline such as nursing.

You are likely to encounter a range of different assessment types or approaches in your degree program, some similar to your previous learning experiences and others new or less familiar. Written assignments such as essays, reports and case studies will be common, usually with an emphasis on higher-order thinking skills rather than simply recall of declarative knowledge. Some students are frustrated by such tasks, arguing that they will 'never need to write an essay in their practice'. While this is probably true, the ability to present clear, accurate and logical information in written form is essential in all areas of practice, and correlates with many of the Registered Nurse Standards for Practice (NMBA 2016). Thus, the development, refinement and assessment of such skills are both critical and important. Reflective writing and journalling are also increasingly common assessments used in nursing education, along with assessments such as presentations, posters and projects, individually or in groups, and in-person or online (e.g. video-based).

Examinations are common in many units of study. These are usually formal assessments involving a combination of multiple-choice, short-answer, extended-response and even reflective questions. Like the other written assessments already mentioned, exams are often designed to assess your critical thinking skills and ability to apply your knowledge to authentic and contextualised situations, and as such case-study or inquiry-based questions are commonly used. e-Assessments are also used in many units, especially online quizzes, which are used to assess your developing knowledge of core concepts and ideas. Online quizzes are increasingly used to 'incentivise' the flipped learning approach discussed earlier in this chapter, with weighted quizzes being set before a class to assess your preparedness for subsequent learning.

The assessment of clinical skills also features prominently in health professional education. This often occurs through the use of an objective structured clinical examination (OSCE), in which you will be required to demonstrate specific psychomotor skills and behaviours in a simulated professional scenario (Brighton et al. 2017). Some OSCEs focus only on technical or procedural competence, but most also assess the declarative and schematic knowledge associated with this, and core behaviours such as communication, teamwork and documentation.

REFLECTION 2.2

- What types of assessments are you familiar with from your previous studies? Do you prefer one type of assessment over others?
- How might you prepare for some of the less-familiar or less-appealing assessments that you may encounter in this degree program?

Learning bioscience

So far, this chapter has focused on the typical models and approaches in nursing education, rather than on specific topics or subject matter (content) you may encounter in your degree program, as these may vary between courses and universities. We have decided, however, to make a small exception and briefly explore bioscience education, because this content is common to all undergraduate nursing programs, and bioscience units are considered by many students to be the most challenging (McVicar, Andrew & Kemble 2015). The content covered is also regarded as among the most fascinating. While much of what you learn in undertaking a nursing degree is about understanding 'what' things are or 'how' to do something, the purpose of bioscience is to provide you with the understanding of 'why' you are doing it, so you can determine and articulate a clear rationale for your decision-making in practice (Taylor et al. 2015). Sometimes, this content is presented in separate, dedicated units, while other courses combine or integrate bioscience content with, for example, nursing skills.

REFLECTION 2.3

- How confident do you feel about the bioscience component of your degree program?
- What resources or strategies could you use to work through challenges you might encounter?

The bioscience component of an undergraduate nursing degree covers a diverse range of topics, including anatomy, physiology, cell biology, histology, microbiology, pathology, pathophysiology, pharmacology and genetics. You may encounter your first bioscience units in the first semester of your degree, or the start of bioscience teaching may be delayed to enable students to develop general skills for university-level learning and foundational nursing concepts or skills, prior to its introduction.

In your first year, you are likely to be introduced to basic anatomy and physiology, otherwise known as structure and function, or functional anatomy. The relationship between structure and function forms the core of understanding about human physiology. You will discover that every part of the body, from a blood cell to a bone, has a particular structure or shape that reflects its specific function. Keeping this relationship in mind will help you when considering injuries, illnesses and diseases that alter structure, and therefore change, function. You may also encounter cell biology (cellular structure and function), histology (groups of cells with common functions known as tissues), microbiology (micro-organisms such as bacteria and viruses) and aspects of genetics (genes and inheritance) in your first year.

In the second and third years of your degree program, you will progress to more advanced physiology (studying the functions of bodily systems in greater depth), pathology and pathophysiology (abnormal changes to structure and function associated with disease or injury), and pharmacology (uses, effects and modes of action of medicines).

Throughout your degree program, you will also learn what is essentially an entirely new vocabulary or language. The reason you need to know so many new terms is to ensure that you and your nursing colleagues, and everyone else with whom you interact as a member of the interprofessional healthcare team, share a common understanding. In general, the bioscientific terms you encounter will be descriptive (such as 'lateral' or 'pulmonary'); eponymous (named after a person – for example, 'Circle of Willis', 'Bowman's capsule'); derived from an ancient language such as Greek or Latin (for example, *card* = 'heart'); or may be presented as abbreviations (for example, GIT = gastrointestinal tract) or acronyms (for example, AIDS = Acquired Immune Deficiency Syndrome).

Connecting with practice: Language of bioscience

When learning a new term, it is best to break down the word into its component parts. Often, there is a 'root word' (the base of the term) that is derived from Latin or Greek, a prefix (letters appearing before the root word) and a suffix (letters appearing after the root word). For example, the word 'pericarditis' consists of the prefix *peri* = 'around', the root term *card* = 'heart' and the suffix *itis* = 'inflammation'. Therefore, 'pericarditis' means inflammation around the heart.

Connecting with practice: Link and story methods

Occasionally, in your study of bioscience, you will be introduced to concepts that seem quite abstract or difficult to relate to. For instance, some students find biological chemistry and cell biology difficult because they involve the study of structures that are too small to see with the human eye. One way to improve the relatability of structures that are very small is to 'upsize' them to something that is more tangible or familiar. For example, the immune system is the system of blood cells that protects the body from invading organisms. One person's approach to learning this system was to make every cell type a character from *The Simpsons* with a job related to that character's personality. For example, the 'macrophage' is a core part of the immune system and its name literally means 'big eater'. In the character analogy this was, of course, Homer Simpson. Creating stories is an excellent way to remember terms and concepts.

Connecting with practice: Interpreting data

Other students may be challenged by the interpretation of data, or understanding reference ranges and/or reading graphs and charts. These are skills that you will develop as part of your study of bioscience. Reference ranges refer to the values for a particular measurement, such as urine composition, blood pressure or bone density in a healthy person. These values are different in children and adults, and may change as part of normal ageing or due to other factors such as illness. By knowing these ranges and understanding the variation that may be considered normal between individuals, you will be able to determine when a client's measurements are outside of the normal range, to make sense of what this might mean and to assist in making decisions about appropriate interventions. It is also important to know that reference ranges may differ in the way they are expressed between countries. For example, blood glucose is measured in mmol/L (millimoles per litre) in Australia, while in the United States it is measured in mg/dL (milligrams per decilitre).

Strategies for learning success

To succeed in your studies, it is important for you to be organised, work consistently, develop effective study skills, manage your time effectively for a healthy study–life balance, make time for exercise and sleep, find a study group of like-minded people and be an active learner. **Active learning** is the process of actively engaging with content via reading, writing, talking, listening, practising, reflecting and problem-solving. The opposite of active learning is passive learning, where you might expect knowledge to sink into your brain automatically, just by listening to a lecture or turning up to a class. As you might imagine, passive learning is not an effective method of study. There is a strong correlation between active engagement with content and higher grade achievement (Freeman et al. 2014).

active learning the process of actively and critically engaging with learning resources or content via reading, writing, talking, listening, practising, reflecting and problem-solving

NURSING PERSPECTIVE

Critical thinking, research and reflection are all hallmarks of an active learner, but sometimes active learning is as simple as speaking up and asking questions. You will be surrounded by people with a diversity of experiences, perspectives and expertise, both in the classroom and the practice environment. Try to take advantage of this valuable learning resource.

My first charge nurse said to me, 'I would rather you ask me six stupid questions – and they may well be stupid because of how new you are – than make one stupid mistake.' I've never had a problem asking since (Alderton, cited in Wilson & Wilson 2011).

Another important concept to understand is that all brains are 'wired' a little differently, and not everyone has the same 'learning style' or preferred methods for learning. Theories about learning styles have been somewhat controversial. These theories essentially categorise or sort students into those who learn best visually, aurally, by reading or through hands-on experiences (Khazan 2018). While we may have preferences, the risk of categorisation is that our learning performance (successes and failures) can be viewed simply as the degree of alignment between the teaching style and the student's learning style. Instead, we need to focus on the ways in which we can adapt and tailor our own learning strategies and habits towards these preferences and, even more importantly, how we can build our capacity for the other learning styles, which we are almost certain to experience (Husmann & O'Loughlin 2019; Khazan 2018).

Play to your strengths as a learner by finding your best methods of learning and using them for maximum enjoyment and effectiveness. Some people concentrate better in the morning, while others prefer night times. Some people require absolute quiet, while others focus better with music in the background. There are dozens of different methods you can use to engage with content. For example, you may listen to recordings, take notes, read text out loud, study diagrams, draw or colour pictures, create flash cards, discuss material with others, make flow charts, complete quizzes, paste key words and definitions around the house, watch video clips, practise skills with a partner, read journal articles, engage in social media about relevant topics, and so on. Most importantly, you need to realise that every action you take in your learning journey is creating new connections in your brain and making you more capable as a learner. Basically, the more effort you put in, the 'bigger' and more efficient your brain will be.

A growth mindset

One of the approaches that can enhance your success in learning is your ability to understand and maintain a 'growth mindset'. A growth mindset is the belief that we are not limited by fixed talents, such as how intelligent, creative or artistic we are. Instead, those with a growth mindset believe that effort, failure and learning are the keys to increasing our skills and talents (Dweck 2006).

Your mindset has a profound effect on how you approach learning and work. The health sector is constantly evolving through new challenges, discoveries and changes. A growth mindset encourages us to put in the effort to grow with these changes, instead of simply sticking with what we know. If you believe your level of talent is fixed, you are always seeking to prove and protect your abilities. On the other hand, if you believe your skills improve through effort and (occasional) failure, you will seek out opportunities to grow them (Dweck 2006).

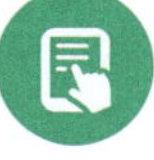

Video: 'Developing a growth mindset'

The opposite to a growth mindset is a 'fixed mindset'. Those with a fixed mindset believe traits such as intelligence, talent and abilities are innate and permanent. They say things like: 'You either have it or you don't'. This statement implies that it is not worth even trying for something if you are not immediately good at it. People with a fixed mindset avoid situations that may lead to failure or that threaten their skills and abilities. Because of this, they miss out on learning and growing to their full potential. How did you learn to ride a bike? How did you learn to walk? Did you fall and make mistakes? Of course you did! Failing and making mistakes is how we learn. With a growth mindset, we learn through effort and experience, and by making mistakes and asking for help and feedback along the way (Dweck 2006).

A growth mindset also reflects our contemporary view of the brain. Your brain is always changing, based on your experiences. This means your brain is not fixed; it evolves through experience and effort. It is exciting because, with a commitment to developing and practising a growth mindset, you have the power to grow and change your skills and potential.

Short-answer question

There will be times in your studies when you may feel the 'walls coming up' or the stress mounting. You might be plagued by doubts concerning your ability and worries about how much there is to learn, or you might feel yourself shutting down when topics arise that you have previously found difficult or that you do not 'relate to'. The most important thing you can do at these times is to recognise this state of mind, understand that it is a natural defensive reaction, allow it to pass and continue to remain open to the learning journey. By engaging with the unfamiliar in a state of curiosity rather than fear or defensiveness and maintaining a willingness to be changed by the knowledge you are developing every day, you are creating the optimal conditions for success.

Chapter 3 expands on these ideas further, providing a range of other tips and resources for optimising your learning success.

Connecting with practice: '25 ways to develop a growth mindset'

SUMMARY

- The regulatory framework for nursing in Australia requires all nurses (including students) to develop and demonstrate their 'capability' for nursing practice. Capability is a forward-looking concept that focuses on an individual's talent potential, rather than only their cognitive or technical competence. A *capability wheel* has been provided to help you understand and develop capability in your own learning and practice.
- The overarching aim of undergraduate nursing education is to prepare graduates who can demonstrate their capability to 'think and act like a registered nurse'. While every education program may look a little different, we have presented some of the common features and components that you are likely to experience, including blended learning, simulation-based learning, practice-based learning, reflection, self-directed learning and the creation and maintenance of a professional portfolio. We have also provided a 'primer' for your learning of bioscience, which will be a core focus of the curriculum, regardless of the university or program in which you are enrolled.
- Being an 'active' learner, developing a 'growth mindset', playing to your strengths, and finding and applying your best methods for learning have been highlighted as the keys to being a successful student. These tips and resources are expanded in Chapter 3.

REVIEW QUESTIONS

Suggested responses

1 How might capability differ from competence in your learning, practice and assessment? Try to consider some examples.
2 What are the common learning and teaching components or features that you are likely to experience in your undergraduate degree program?
3 What are some of the benefits of collaboration and group-based learning?
4 What are the two types of knowledge that are commonly assessed in university studies?
5 What does it mean to be an active learner?

RESEARCH TOPIC

Undertake some further research on 'capability in nursing' and the move from competence to capability that is now clearly recognised in the Registered Nurse Standards for Practice (NMBA 2016). Use the capability wheel presented in Figures 2.1 and 2.2 and discussed in this chapter to prepare (perhaps with some of your peers) a version of the wheel that represents the learning outcomes of your entire undergraduate degree. If you have an idea about future areas of specialisation, have a go at preparing a wheel for that too, which you can use as a guide as you work towards your goal.

FURTHER READING

Bromley, P. (2017). From competence to capability. *Australian Nursing and Midwifery Journal*, 25(2), 34.

Jackson, D., Hickman, L.D., Power, T., Disler, R., Potgieter, I., Deek, H. & Davidson, P.M. (2014). Small group learning: Graduate health students' views of challenges and benefits. *Contemporary Nurse*, 48(1), 117–28.

McVicar, A., Andrew, S. & Kemble, R. (2015). The 'bioscience problem' for nursing students: An integrative review of published evaluations of Year 1 bioscience, and proposed directions for curriculum development. *Nurse Education Today*, 35(3), 500–9.

REFERENCES

Alammary, A., Sheard, J. & Carbone, A. (2014). Blended learning in higher education: Three different design approaches. *Australasian Journal of Educational Technology*, 30(4), 440–54.

Australian College of Nursing, Health Informatics Society of Australia, and Nurse Informatics Australia (ACN/HISA/NIA) (2017). *Nursing Informatics Position Statement*. Retrieved from https://www.hisa.org.au/wp-content/uploads/2017/08/Nursing-Informatics-Position-Statement_06082017.pdf.

Australian Health Practitioner Regulation Agency (AHPRA) (2009). *Health Practitioner Regulation National Law Act 2009*. Retrieved from http://www.ahpra.gov.au/Legislationand-Publications/Legislation.aspx.

Australian Nursing and Midwifery Accreditation Council (ANMAC) (2012). *Registered Nurse Accreditation Standards 2012*. Retrieved from https://www.anmac.org.au/document/accreditation-standards-entry-program-registered-nurses-2012.

—— (2015). *Nurse Practitioner Accreditation Standards 2015*. Retrieved from https://www.anmac.org.au/sites/default/files/documents/Nurse_Practitioner_Accreditation_Standard_2015_FINAL_0.pdf.

—— (2017). *National Accreditation Guidelines: Nursing and midwifery education programs*. Retrieved from https://www.anmac.org.au/document/national-accreditation-guidelines.

Barr, H., Ford, J., Gray, R., Helme, M., Hutchings, M., Low, H., Machin, A. & Reeves, S. (2017). *Interprofessional education guidelines 2017*. Fareham, UK: Centre for the Advancement of Interprofessional Education (CAIPE). Retrieved from https://www.caipe.org/resources/publications/caipe-publications/caipe-2017-interprofessional-education-guidelines-barr-h-ford-j-gray-r-helme-m-hutchings-m-low-h-machin-reeves-s.

Barton, G., Bruce, A. & Schreiber, R. (2018). Teaching nurses teamwork: Integrative review of competency-based team training in nursing education. *Nurse Education in Practice*, 32, 129–37.

Biggs, J. & Tang, C. (2011). *Teaching for quality learning at university*, 4th edn. Maidenhead: Open University Press.

Birks, M., Bagley, T., Park, T., Burkot, C. & Mills, J. (2017). The impact of clinical placement model on learning in nursing: A descriptive exploratory study. *Australian Journal of Advanced Nursing*, 34(3), 16–23.

Bliuc, A., Goodyear, P. & Ellis, R. (2007). Research focus and methodological choices in studies into students' experiences of blended learning in higher education. *The Internet and Higher Education*, 10, 231–44.

Bogossian, F., Cooper, S., Kelly, M., Levett-Jones, T., McKenna, L., Slark, J. & Seaton, P. (2018). Best practice in clinical simulation education – are we there yet? A cross-sectional survey of simulation in Australian and New Zealand pre-registration nursing education. *Collegian*, 25(3), 327–34.

Bower, M., Kenney, J., Dalgarno, B., Lee, M.J.W. & Kennedy, G.E. (2014). Patterns and principles for blended synchronous learning: Engaging remote and face-to-face learners in rich-media real-time collaborative activities. *Australasian Journal of Educational Technology*, 30(3), doi: 10.14742/ajet.1697.

Branch, R.M. & Dousay, T.A. (2015). *Survey of instructional design models*, 5th edn. Bloomington, IN: Association for Educational Communications & Technology.

Brewer, M., Flavell, H., Harris, C., Davis, M. & Bathgate, K. (2014). Ensuring health graduates employability in a changing world: Developing interpersonal practice capabilities using a framework to inform curricula. *Journal of Teaching and Learning for Graduate Employability*, 5(1), 29–46.

Brighton, R., Mackay, M., Brown, R.A., Jans, C. & Antoniou, C. (2017). Introduction of undergraduate nursing students to an objective structured clinical examination. *Journal of Nursing Education*, 56(4), 231–4.

Bromley, P. (2017). From competence to capability. *Australian Nursing and Midwifery Journal*, 25(2), 34.

——— (2018). Contextualising capability: How we identify and recognise capability in registered nurses undertaking the Post Graduate Certificate in Neonatal Intensive Care. Unpublished professional doctoral thesis, University of Tasmania.

Caldwell, L. & Grobbel, C.C. (2013). The importance of reflective practice in nursing. *International Journal of Caring Sciences*, 6(3), 319–26.

Coetzee, M. (2014). Measuring student graduateness: Reliability and construct validity of the Graduate Skills and Attributes Scale. *Higher Education Research & Development*, 33(5), 887–902.

Dweck, C. (2006). *Mindset: The new psychology of success*. New York: Random House.

El-Mowafy, A., Kuhn, M. & Snow, T. (2013). Blended learning in higher education: Current and future challenges in surveying education. *Issues in Educational Research*, 23(2), 132–50.

Fernando, A., Attoe, C., Jaye, P., Cross, S., Pathan, J. & Wessely, S. (2017). Improving interprofessional approaches to physical and psychiatric comorbidities through simulation. *Clinical Simulation in Nursing*, 13(4), 186–93.

Foundation for Young Australians (2016). *The New Work Mindset*. Retrieved from https://www.fya.org.au/wp-content/uploads/2016/11/The-New-Work-Mindset.pdf.

Freeman, S., Eddy, S.L., McDonough, M., Smith, M.K., Okoroafor, N., Jordt, H. & Wenderoth, M.P. (2014). Active learning increases student performance in science, engineering, and mathematics. *Proceedings of the National Academy of Sciences*, 111(23), 8410–15.

Halasa, S., Abusalim, N., Rayyan, M., Constantino, R.E., Nassar, O., Amre, H., Sharab, M. & Qadri, I. (2020). Comparing student achievement in traditional learning with a combination of blended and flipped learning. *Nursing Open*, 7(4), 1129–38.

Healthcare Information and Management Systems Society (HIMSS) (2014). Health informatics defined. Retrieved from http://www.himss org/health-informatics-defined.

Hodges, C., Moore, S., Lockee, E., Trust, T. & Bond, A. (2020). The difference between emergency remote teaching and online learning. *Educause Review*, 27 March. Retrieved from https://er.educause.edu/articles/2020/3/the-difference-between-emergency-remote-teaching-and-online-learning.

Hrastinski, S. (2019). What do we mean by blended learning? *TechTrends*, 63, 564–9.

Husmann, P.R. & O'Loughlin, V.D. (2019). Another nail in the coffin for learning styles? Disparities among undergraduate anatomy students' study strategies, class performance, and reported VARK learning styles. *Anatomical Sciences Education*, 12, 6–19.

Jackson, D., Hickman, L.D., Power, T., Disler, R., Potgieter, I., Deek, H. & Davidson, P.M. (2014). Small group learning: Graduate health students' views of challenges and benefits. *Contemporary Nurse*, 48(1), 117–28.

Kasraie, N. & Alahmad, A. (2014). Investigating the reasons institutions of higher education in the USA and Canada utilize blended learning. *Mevlana International Journal of Education*, 4(1), 67–81.

Khazan, O. (2018). The myth of learning styles. *The Atlantic*, 11 April. Retrieved from https://www.theatlantic.com/science/archive/2018/04/the-myth-of-learning-styles/557687/

Kononowicz, A.A., Woodham, L., Georg, C., Edelbring, S., Stathakarou, N., Davies, D., Masiello, I., Tudor Car, L., Car, J. & Zary, N. (2016). Virtual patient simulations for health professional education. *Cochrane Database of Systematic Reviews*, 5, art. no.: CD012194. Retrieved from http://onlinelibrary.wiley.com/doi/10.1002/14651858.CD012194/epdf.

Leidl, D.M., Ritchie, L. & Moslemi, N. (2020). Blended learning in undergraduate nursing education – a scoping review. *Nurse Education Today*, 86, 104318.

Levett-Jones, T. (ed.) (2018). *Clinical reasoning: Learning to think like a nurse*, 2nd edn. Melbourne: Pearson.

McVicar, A., Andrew, S. & Kemble, R. (2015). The 'bioscience problem' for nursing students: An integrative review of published evaluations of Year 1 bioscience, and proposed directions for curriculum development. *Nurse Education Today*, 35(3), 500–9.

Means, B., Toyama, Y., Murphy, R., Bakia, M. & Jones, K. (2009). *Evaluation of evidence-based practices in online learning: A meta-analysis and review of online learning studies*. Washington, DC: US Department of Education, Office of Planning, Evaluation and Policy Development. Retrieved from https://www2.ed.gov/rschstat/eval/tech/evidence-based-practices/finalreport.pdf.

Morin, K.H. (2020). Nursing education after COVID-19: Same or different? *Journal of Clinical Nursing*, 29(17–18), 3117–19.

Nicol, J. & Dosser, I. (2016). Understanding reflective practice. *Nursing Standard*, 30(36), 34–40.

Nursing and Midwifery Board of Australia (NMBA) (2016). *Registered Nurse Standards for Practice*. Retrieved from https://www.nursingmidwiferyboard.gov.au/codes-guidelines-statements/professional-standards.aspx.

O'Connell, J., Gardner, G. & Coyer, F. (2014). Beyond competencies: Using a capability framework in developing practice standards for advanced practice nursing. *Journal of Advanced Nursing*, 70(12), 2728–35.

Okaz, A. (2015). Integrating blended learning in higher education. *Procedia – Social and Behavioral Sciences*, 186, 600–3.

Schwartz, S. (2019). *Educating the nurse of the future: Report of the independent review of nursing education*. Canberra: Australian Government Department of Health.

Scott, G., Chang, E. & Grebennikov, L. (2010). Using successful graduates to improve the quality of undergraduate nursing programs. *Journal of Teaching and Learning for Graduate Employability*, 1(1), 26–44.

Stephenson, J. & Yorke, M. (eds) (2012). *Capability and quality in higher education*. London: Routledge.

Talbert, R. (2017). Defining flipped learning: Four mistakes and a suggested standard. Professional blog, 27 June. Retrieved from http://rtalbert.org/how-to-define-flipped-learning.

Taylor, V., Ashelford, S., Fell, P. & Goacher, P.J. (2015). Biosciences in nurse education: Is the curriculum fit for practice? Lecturers' views and recommendations from across the UK. *Journal of Clinical Nursing*, 24(19–20), 2797–806.

Wilcox, J., Miller-Cribbs, J., Kientz, E., Carlson, J. & DeShea, L. (2017). Impact of simulation on student attitudes about interprofessional collaboration. *Clinical Simulation in Nursing*, 13(8), 390–7.

Willetts, G. (2015). From Nightingale nurses to modern profession: Nursing in Australia. Henry Parkes Oration, Tenterfield, New South Wales. Retrieved from https://parkesfoundation.files.wordpress.com/2015/09/hporation2015.pdf.

Wilson, A. & Wilson, M. (2011). *What I wish I knew about nursing: Real advice from real nurses on how to deeply care for patients while still caring for yourself*. Sydney: Marty Wilson.

Wong, F.M.F. (2018). A phenomenological study: Perspectives of student learning through small group work between undergraduate nursing students and educators. *Nurse Education Today*, 68, 153–8.

Preparing for success

Lolita Wikander and Judith Lyons

3

LEARNING OBJECTIVES

At the completion of this chapter, you should be able to:

1 Identify and access available forms of academic support.
2 Use the online study environment to your academic advantage.
3 Explore effective, self-directed and lifelong learning strategies.
4 Discriminate between and use various methods of collaborative learning and peer support.

Introduction

In this chapter you will learn how to plan your study around your commitments. You will be encouraged to build on your strengths and improve in areas that may hold you back. You will learn how to find time to study and be kind to your future self. This chapter gives you an idea of the different kinds of academic support you may be able to access and provides some hints for using the online study environment to your advantage.

Critical reflection forms the basis of reflective practice in nursing and an effective way to engage in self-directed learning to assist you in developing strategies for lifelong learning. Learning in the university context is often self-directed, and the skills developed in your nursing education will help to ensure you have acquired the attributes needed to continue learning after graduation and while you gain experience as a nurse. Self-directed learning means being active and constructive in your learning process. This entails being clear about what your learning goals are and choosing how you will achieve them. It also involves deciding what strategies you will adopt in your own learning, as well as what the educators require you to do for successful completion of your courses.

The section on reflection and self-directed learning provides you with strategies for deep learning, which is learning for understanding – as opposed to surface learning such as cramming to pass a test. If you employ deep learning strategies, this learning will form the basis of your knowledge and skills, and you will be able to build on and apply it in new contexts. You are a partner in the learning process, and this chapter provides you with strategies to enhance your study and to be successful in your learning endeavours.

You will discover that you can learn from your teachers and educators as well as from your peers and networks. You will be provided with hints for making formal and informal peer support and group work function effectively for you. Finally, you will be given suggestions for using social media to help feel connected while simultaneously avoiding the common pitfalls in your journey to becoming the best nurse you can be.

Tips, tricks and techniques for successful learning

Every student comes to university with unique strengths and challenges. It is your job as a student to confront your challenges and achieve your maximum potential.

Student attrition and success are closely related to the mode of study and the student's attributes. Attrition in online units, for example, is generally higher than it is in face-to-face units (Greenland & Moore 2014, Garratt-Reed, Roberts & Heritage 2016). Those in the online cohort of students tend to be older, are more likely to be in full-time employment and have more family obligations than face-to-face students (Ortagus 2016). These obligations, in turn, can compete with the time a student has available to dedicate to their studies.

If you have family and work commitments in addition to your studies, then it is important to carefully consider the effects these responsibilities may have on your academic success. Think about how much time you realistically have available and adjust your study commitment accordingly. If you have family or work commitments, assume you will have less rather than more time, and commit only to what you can do without depending on others. Unanticipated help may improve your marks, whereas the absence of anticipated help may result in a late submission or a failed exam.

Have a strategy

New students will soon learn that there is a pattern to most teaching periods. They will most likely spend the first few weeks finding their way around, getting to know people and making sense of the learning environment. The pace will then pick up and students may struggle to keep up as the workload increases. If a student is feeling overwhelmed, they may cut corners, focus only on the assignments and fail to regularly access learning materials and scheduled learning activities. Academic stress can be alleviated by scheduling sufficient time to accomplish academic tasks (Marrs & Sigler 2012).

Use the early weeks to start working on your assignments. Make sure you have a good understanding of the question and requirements. Start by searching the library databases and gather your resources for written assignments. Identify any areas of weakness and work on addressing these now. If you do not know how to correctly cite a reference or how to search for journal articles, contact the university library to find out what support is available. Make use of a diary and electronic reminders to ensure you have a realistic study plan in place to avoid a last-minute rush to complete assessments.

Get support

Many universities offer free tutorial assistance for students. This can be online support, peer support or other forms of tutoring. Have a draft or outline ready well in advance of accessing this type of assessment help. International students and Aboriginal and Torres Strait Islander students may be able to access additional support. There are often safeguards in place to assist students with disabilities or who are experiencing extenuating circumstances. Communicate with your teachers and available student support services. Make sure you have the support you need to succeed in your studies.

CASE STUDY

Utilise services and communicate with your lecturers

Sanjita's marriage broke down in the second year of her nursing degree. Her husband was frustrated by the amount of time she was spending on her studies, and she felt that she was receiving little support. Sanjita continued to be solely responsible for the care of their young child. She was a good student but she struggled to keep up with her new circumstances. She failed an assignment for the first time ever and received a Pass Conceded (PC) grade for the unit overall. She remembered her lecturer calling her to a meeting to ask why her grades had suddenly dropped. Sanjita was too proud to explain so she told him she would accept the PC grade. Reflecting on this, she now knows she should have communicated earlier with her lecturer and let him know what was going on. The system has safeguards for situations like this. Sanjita could have received assistance and special consideration, but at the time she was too embarrassed to ask for help.

QUESTION

What are some of the support services at your university that Sanjita could have accessed? If Sanjita had accessed some of these support services, how might the outcome have been different?

Focus on the important things

Students are likely to perform better academically if they attend their lectures and tutorials (Nyatanga & Mukorera 2017). The equivalent for online students is to attend their online lectures and access the learning materials. The benefit of having online resources is that they are often recorded and can be accessed repeatedly; they are also often available in advance. If the learning modules are available in advance, you can use the early weeks to get ahead. This will take off some of the pressure when you get busy. Recorded lectures and content give you the flexibility to organise your study around competing commitments. While getting a head start on the unit content and assignments can be an advantage, it is often a good idea not to submit assignments too early. Important information relating to assignments may become available as the submission date nears.

While there are benefits to studying online, there are also drawbacks. One example of an online teaching tool that can be either a drain on student time or of great benefit is the unit discussion board. A well-designed and well-managed discussion board, for example, has the potential to provide you with clarification on issues of common concern and can help you feel more connected to other students. A poorly designed discussion board, however, may add little academic value. An example is a discussion board in which students have to introduce themselves. If a unit has a small number of students this may be fine but if the unit has hundreds of students and you try to read all the introductions – or, worse, reply to them – this may take hours. This time may be better spent familiarising yourself with the assessment requirements or reading though the first module of work.

Find time

Time is a valuable commodity, and time management is an essential skill for students to acquire. Good time-management skills will ensure that students can achieve to the best of their abilities (Ghiasvand et al. 2017), reduce stress (Grissom, Loeb & Mitani 2015) and enjoy a balanced life (Kaya et al. 2012). There are also many useful time-management apps available and information that students can seek out to help them develop their time-management skills.

Prepare

Some students claim that they can leave the writing of an assignment to the night before and still pass. If this is true, then there is a good chance that they have successfully completed previous study. In comparison, an elite athlete who has not trained for months could easily compete in a fun run without preparation. However, to get to the elite status, they have previously put in significant time and effort. This previous training will enable them to do incredible things even a long time after they stop training. Students who are new to academia often need to work a lot harder than experienced students, as they are still developing the necessary academic skills (Gopee & Deane 2013). Once students have the necessary skills, they will be able to draw on them for future academic endeavours. Like the elite athlete, it is important to aim for excellence rather than just crossing the finish line.

Recover

Thinking of the example of the elite athlete, what do they need to ensure they remain at that level? In addition to spending many hours improving their technique and speed, the athlete needs time to recover. They will need sleep, healthy food, fluids and active recovery such as stretching and mobility work. Recovery is planned – just like their training. Students need to look after themselves in a similar way. They need to make sure they have enough time to eat healthy food (George et al. 2008), exercise (Mullender-Wijnsma et al. 2015) and sleep (Baert et al. 2015). Strategies for rest and recovery need to be factored into a good study plan, along with the due dates for assignments and exams.

REFLECTION 3.1

Be kind to your future self. You will get busier and busier as the semester progresses. Think about what you can do right now to help your future self. This may be learning how to structure an assignment, gathering your resources or getting ahead in your readings. Similar behaviours and strategies will serve you well throughout your future professional life.

Take a sheet of paper and write down your strengths. These are all the things you have working in your favour. What you have written down is what you need to go back to if you are struggling. Your strengths could be your motivation to become an excellent nurse and your ability to stick to things even if you sometimes fail, or skills and resilience gained through your life experiences.

Take a second sheet of paper and write down your weaknesses, or things that are likely to limit you or hold you back. Next to each of these, write down strategies you might use to mitigate these weaknesses or limitations. For example, if you have identified referencing as a weakness, then plan to attend a library presentation on

Short-answer question
Multiple-choice question

> referencing by the end of Week 2 and send a sample of your in-text referencing and reference list to your librarian for feedback before submitting your assignment for assessment. Do as much of this developmental work as you can in the first couple of weeks of the semester before you get too busy.

Reflection and self-directed learning

critical reflection questioning and reflecting on possibilities, implications and applications, as well as the consequences of what you are learning

self-directed learning an active, constructive process whereby self-initiated cognition, motivation and behaviours are used to manage and achieve learning outcomes. It is being responsible for your own learning in your own time, which requires self-motivation, self-discipline and resilience.

Critical reflection employed in **self-directed learning** leads to the development of lifelong learning capabilities and contributes to self-professional development. Often, the terms 'critical reflection' and 'reflection' are used interchangeably. Critical reflection represents another level of reflection, beyond what you may or may not cover in a reflective process such as journal writing. Critical reflection is an extension of critical thinking and involves asking probing questions during the process of reflecting in, on and for future actions. Using structured critical reflection when studying will help you identify your strengths, how you learn and how you can develop self-directed learning capabilities you can use in your nursing practice. For example, self-directed learning is the responsibility and accountability the student places on their learning. A student who receives an unsatisfactory grade could look back to see what they did and need to do to improve the grade next time, while a critical reflection leads the student to explore what contributed to their unsatisfactory performance, understand what was required, examine what they did to tackle the task, develop strategies to perform better next time and to implement and evaluate these strategies.

Self-directed learning attributes are essential to nursing education and practice as nurses need to continue learning and to engage in self-development and professional development to maintain their nursing registration. Reflection and reflective processes are discussed in detail in Chapter 9, so this chapter focuses on self-directed learning concepts.

Learning is a partnership, and the flipside of the learning and teaching process. Educators facilitate learning; the aim of teaching is to make student learning possible (Ramsden 2003). Student learners, as partners in the learning and teaching process, take ownership and are responsible and accountable for their learning, through teacher-directed and self-directed learning activities. Researchers including Angelo (2012), Boyer and colleagues (2014) and Slater and Cusick (2017) have shown that students who have developed self-directed learning skills and who know how to learn and manage their learning will achieve academic success.

At university you are expected to regulate and direct your own study, and to become an independent learner. You may have a distinct preference for how you learn or you may have a variety of ways in which you learn best. A visual learner prefers learning through images, diagrams and videos. An auditory learner has a preference for processing learning by listening. This may involve attending lectures or listening to recordings and podcasts. The read/write (linguistic) learner prefers to read and write notes while learning. Another style of learning is kinaesthetic, which is learning by doing, and this is important in learning nursing skills.

You may be a learner who prefers one or a combination of these styles but, as discussed in Chapter 2, try to avoid categorising yourself as a particular kind of learner. Instead, consider the ways in which you can adapt and tailor your own learning strategies and habits towards these strengths, and even more importantly, how you can build your capacity for the other learning styles and approaches you are likely to encounter. This will be particularly important if you prefer working on your own or as part of a team, as many learning and assessment tasks for nursing students are group-based learning tasks used to develop attributes that are crucial to working collaboratively within a healthcare setting.

REFLECTION 3.2

Consider your own learning preferences.

- Do you know how you prefer to learn?
- How do you process your learning – for example, by visualising what you learned when you reflect or recall what you have been studying?
- How might you build your capacity for other learning styles?

Learning at university

Learning at university may be different from your previous experiences of learning. It is not teacher-directed, as you are now an equal partner in the learning process and need to assume responsibility for your own learning. Learning how to learn in the university context is a critical survival strategy. Self-directed learning, also known as 'self-regulated learning', is learning initiated by the student without direct supervision by teachers. All nursing programs in Australia are accredited by the Australian Nursing and Midwifery Accreditation Council (ANMAC) and are considered equivalent to other higher education degree programs that adhere to the Australian Qualifications Framework (AQFC 2015). The Australian Qualifications Framework sets its standards for, and expectations of, students' contribution to learning through the volume and depth of learning in the program and the application of credit points to the study workload. For example, at any given university a unit or course of study is considered equal to approximately 10 hours of study per week, or 150 hours of study over the semester, which is required to achieve the learning outcomes. Therefore, for every hour of learning that is teacher-directed through active learning sessions, lectures or tutorials, and online and laboratory learning, the student needs to spend approximately three hours of student-directed learning to achieve the volume and depth of learning required for academic success.

Self-directed learning is an active, constructive process whereby self-initiated cognition, motivation and behaviours are used to manage and achieve learning outcomes (Morris, 2019, 2020; Slater et al. 2017; Alharbi 2018; Lemmetty & Collin 2020). Students can adopt surface, deep or strategic approaches to learning, according to Biggs and Tang (2011). *Surface learning* is when students rote-learn, or cram for examinations, or learn facts and figures without fully understanding the content.

Surface learning is easily forgotten, as it resides in short-term memory. *Deep learning* is learning for understanding, in ways that enable learners to link ideas and concepts though inductive and deductive, higher-order thinking skills. Deep learners can perform technical tasks, having understood the underlying knowledge and skills required to be competent in performing these skills. Deep learners can understand the cause-and-effect process and can apply and link theory to professional practice. Deep learning resides in long-term memory and can be recalled to build further learning. Deep learning enables the transfer of what is learned to any new context, which is extremely important in nursing, to consolidate learning and become a lifelong learner. The strategic approach to learning is when learners adopt both surface and deep learning approaches by prioritising what learning will take place and how it will occur.

Short-answer question

> ## REFLECTION 3.3
>
> - Are you a self-directed learner or do you like being told exactly what you have to learn?
> - Think of a learning situation. Reflect on what approach you took to complete the task and why you chose that approach.
> - What strategies could you have used to improve the learning experience and outcome?

Strategies for deep self-directed learning

Self-directed learning strategies that promote deep learning in traditional classrooms, online environments or blended modes can be achieved by seven principles of learning (Chickering & Ehrmann 1996).

Set realistic and meaningful learning goals

Goal-setting and planning for learning sequence and time are key strategies in self-regulated student learning. Set small, meaningful goals that are achievable; these will assist and motivate you to undertake the learning task and build confidence in your learning. It will also prevent procrastination, which can be a deterrent to your learning or completing of tasks.

Self-evaluate and monitor the progress and quality of your work at regular intervals by checking over the work to make sure it is correct and on track to achieve the goals. Seek help from your lecturers, student support officers and librarians to overcome academic challenges.

Overcome academic challenges

Be aware of your prior knowledge, attitudes, beliefs, preconceptions and values.

New learning is consolidated if it is associated with what you already know, which then can be used as a building block to scaffold your learning. The attitude, beliefs and values students bring to learning or a given task will frame their understanding and learning of that task. Be aware that other students' and clients' values and beliefs may not be similar to yours, so be open and accepting of other people's values, beliefs and perspectives.

Learn how to learn effectively

Learning requires knowing how to learn. This requires awareness, management and control of your thoughts through cognition and metacognition. Cognition is the ability to understand, and involves mental faculties and processes such as memory, learning, problem-solving, evaluating, decision-making and reasoning. Metacognition is the awareness and understanding of cognitive processes – for example, knowing how to learn for deeper understanding will ensure that what you have learned is stored in long-term memory, so you can draw on it to build your future learning and confidence in learning. Organise and rearrange your ideas and learning material by highlighting the main points in the topic or learning task. Ways to help you understand the topics include developing visual concept maps and mind maps that group similar ideas, show links and connections, and provide ordered structuring of processes. Development of higher-order thinking skills such as critical thinking, clinical reasoning, reflective thinking and creative problem-solving will help you to become a lifelong learner, enabling you to learn and transfer your learning to new contexts (see Chapter 9).

Engage in authentic learning tasks that connect to real-world applications

Learning is enhanced when students organise and transform the learning materials so that they make sense to them. For example, nursing students often enjoy nursing-specific subjects that develop the knowledge and skills they can use in nursing practice. The use of mnemonics helps students to remember and rehearse their learning tasks – for instance, 'ISBAR' refers to the interprofessional handover practice of client care: Introduction, Situation, Background, Assessment and Recommendation (Kitney et al. 2020, Mannix et al. 2017). It is also helpful to take notes, review the notes and elaborate on them by consolidating new and existing information to help embed the new material.

Understand criteria, standards and methods of assessing

Assessment drives learning (Hawe & Dixon 2017, Ballen et al. 2017) While purposeful assessment can drive teaching and learning activities, students often focus on the assessment tasks instead of the learning tasks. Assessment, according to Crisp (2012), can be diagnostic assessment to show what you do not know and what you need to learn. Assessment can also be formative in learning, summative as assessment of learning or integrative assessment for learning and of learning (Crisp 2012). Assessing the achievement of learning outcomes can be difficult, so ensure you are clear about the requirements of assessment tasks and how they will be assessed. A good measure is to examine the assessment criteria and standards, which often are presented as assessment rubrics or marking guides. This will help you to frame your assessment task and ensure it is relevant, and that all required information is included in the assignment. Being an effective learner requires the ability to identify errors and mistakes in your work, so pay attention to the feedback provided on your learning activities and assessment tasks when they are returned to you.

Collaborate in learning

Collaborative learning is covered later in the chapter. Peer learning involves cooperating with other learners in the learning or assessment tasks to help you learn (Effeney, Carroll & Bahr 2013). When working with others, the aim is to be an effective team member and contributor to the team. Sharing ideas, discussing and taking the lead are strategies to assist you in working effectively as part of a team. Collaboration is different from *collusion* with others, which is regarded as cheating and viewed as academic misconduct in assessment.

Invest time and engage in academic learning

To be successful in learning, students must spend time learning tasks. Regulate the effort you put into tasks, as last-minute efforts will not provide the results or rewards you may be anticipating. Manage your time carefully; time management is a critical competency in nursing. Managing time means planning your study time and tasks (Effeney, Carroll & Bahr 2013). Pace your learning to reduce stress, as this is crucial to success – especially if you are studying online or in a flexible mode.

Collaborative learning and peer support

During their studies, most students will learn not only from their teachers, but also from their formal and informal peer networks (Gopee & Deane 2013). Nursing students come from a variety of backgrounds, and some may even have experience as healthcare professionals in their home countries or in other roles or disciplines. Others may have worked as assistants in nursing or cared for an ill relative. Through structured and unstructured interactions in the classroom, students help each other to solve problems and complete projects.

Outside the classroom, students interact with facilitators, preceptors, clients, friends and family members with knowledge to share. Students can learn from interacting with all these people.

Working as a team or in a group

Working together as a team or in a group is an essential nursing skill. Teamwork in the clinical setting is a powerful process that has the potential to improve client care (Schmutz, Meier & Manser 2019). During your study, you will experience working in a group. Group work has many benefits but it also presents challenges. Participating in group work in the classroom, in a simulated setting or online can help you learn how to work through challenges, and achieve better outcomes and solutions than you can produce on your own (Fredrickson 2015).

If working in a group, ensure you do your best to contribute and keep the group on track. If there are problems with group members or in the way the group is functioning, discuss these openly. If the problems become protracted or are hard to resolve, seek advice and guidance from teachers or facilitators. Non-assessed group work during class time is an excellent way to learn about different perspectives and to gain new insights.

Online collaborative groups are becoming popular as the uptake of online learning increases (Xu, Du & Fan 2013). Online group work may create new challenges, as the actions and activities of your fellow students may not be easily visible (An, Kim & Kim 2008). Access to reliable technology may present further challenges, and it is a good idea to communicate with your group by other means (e.g. email or phone) if your ability to participate online is being hampered.

Short-answer question

Study groups

A useful self-selected form of group work is the study group. These may evolve from contacts made during class time. Study groups often naturally develop in face-to-face teaching environments but may be more difficult to cultivate in the online environment (Purarjomandlangrudi, Chen & Nguyen 2016). However, collaborative meeting tools, which are often embedded in online learning environments (e.g. Zoom, Microsoft Classrooms/Teams, Moodle), can help to overcome the isolation of studying remotely.

Social media

If you are studying online and want to connect with other students – and if this is not facilitated through the online interface – then social media may be an option. There is a good chance that a fellow student has set up a social media group for the unit. Social media groups are becoming the online equivalent of chatting after class. Students might use these forums to ask their peers questions related to the unit of study (Tower et al. 2015). This is fine if the answers are accurate but problems can arise when the students in the group misinform others. Ask your teachers about important questions, such as those relating to assignments.

Social media group members can be supportive and helpful. They can provide peer contact and help each other feel connected. On occasion, however, social media can be used inappropriately or to generate unnecessary stress among members, or can distract people from study (Flanigan & Babchuk 2015). If this is the case, then students need to be able to identify what is happening and develop strategies to deal with the situation. Most universities have social media policies to guide students' conduct when interacting in these forums. For health professionals, it is extremely important to behave professionally and ethically in all forums, including on social media, and to ensure they comply with relevant codes of conduct, codes of ethics and practice standards. This is particularly important as students should not use social media forums to discuss their clinical placement experiences, to ensure client confidentiality. The professional and ethical use of social media is discussed further in Chapter 14.

Peer tutors

Informal peer support can be complemented by formal peer support. Peer tutoring or mentoring programs may be available at some universities. They are a great way to confidently navigate the university environment and may increase the chance that students remain enrolled and successfully complete their course (Bryer 2012).

Multiple-choice question
Video: Teamwork tips

NURSING PERSPECTIVE

In my university experience so far, I have had to complete many group assignments. As someone who aspires to high grades and is capable of them, I often find it challenging to work in a group setting where I have to rely on others. In previous groups I've worked with students who have had different academic capabilities or aspirations than me. I don't always enjoy group assignments, as it can be difficult when there are language barriers, when my team members see group work as a social opportunity, or when we cannot coordinate time to work on the assignment in between our other study and employment commitments.

While I have an extensive history of working well within a team outside of study, having my university grade depend on the academic achievements of others creates a unique pressure. Our tutors always remind us that group work teaches us important skills that we will use in our clinical placements and after we graduate, so I do my best to think of group assignments as a multidisciplinary health team project. This helps me consider how we can work together to best utilise our own strengths and help each other to learn and develop as student nurses.

REFLECTION 3.4

- What makes or breaks teamwork?
- What facilitates good teamwork?
- Why is it important to work well in a team?

SUMMARY

- You should now have a better idea of what you can realistically take on and how you might schedule your study around your commitments. Areas you need to strengthen should be clear, and you should have a plan to access the help you need. Your plan should include time for rest, healthy eating and exercise, and should identify the best use of your time.
- Being critical and reflective while you are learning is important for the development of self-directed learning strategies. You are responsible for your learning and for completing the tasks set by your lecturers and teachers. You are an equal partner in the learning process, so continue to refine your self-directed learning skills throughout the years of your degree program. Acquiring this attribute will give you the study skills to continue learning after you graduate and to develop yourself, both as a nurse and as a professional. The strategies for deep learning and for understanding the content will be enhanced though self-directed learning in which you set meaningful goals that are achievable. You will also need to be aware of your preconceived ideas about what you are expected to do while learning. A way to support your learning endeavour is to understand your attitude to learning and change if necessary, and to be positive and value what you are doing to help you learn. Learning how to learn is just as important as the outcome. If you

were not successful or if you did not get the grades you expected, use critical reflection skills to work out what you might have done differently and what you will do next time. Always ask questions of yourself and others to help you learn. Learning with others and collaborating will help you to self-evaluate your learning needs. Choose tasks that focus on achieving your goals and help you to complete your assessment tasks. Frame your assessment as learning tasks and spend time on learning. Do not expect to excel if you do not spend time on your learning and assessment.

- After going through the final part of this chapter, you should have a better understanding of how to best use group work and peer support. The different types of group work and peer support should be clear, and you should be able to use each to your advantage.

REVIEW QUESTIONS

Suggested responses

1　What are some of the strategies you could use to better manage your time?
2　Give examples of deep learning strategies that you will use in your self-directed learning.
3　How will you overcome stress, anxiety and surface learning in your nursing program?
4　How will you collaborate with others to facilitate your learning?
5　What is the difference between collaboration and collusion?

RESEARCH TOPIC

What strategies can you use to transition into university study and be successful in your nursing studies?

FURTHER READING

Alharbi, H.A. (2018). Readiness for self-directed learning: How bridging and traditional nursing students differs? *Nurse Education Today*, 61, 231–4.
Baik, C., Naylor, R. & Arkoudis, S. (2015). The first year experience in Australian universities: Findings from two decades, 1994–2014. Available from https://melbourne-cshe.unimelb.edu.au/__data/assets/pdf_file/0016/1513123/FYE-2014-FULL-report-FINAL-web.pdf.
Berkeley Student Learning Center (2018). Study and success strategies. Available from https://slc.berkeley.edu/study-and-success-strategies.
Dearnley, C., Rhodes, C., Roberts, P., Williams, P. & Prenton, S. (2018). Team based learning in nursing and midwifery higher education: A systematic review of the evidence for change. *Nurse Education Today*, 60, 75–83.
Hillman, K. (2005). *The first year experience: The transition from secondary school to university and TAFE in Australia*. Sydney: ACER. Available from https://research.acer.edu.au/lsay_research/44.

REFERENCES

Alharbi, H.A. (2018). Readiness for self-directed learning: How bridging and traditional nursing students differs? *Nurse Education Today*, 61, 231–4.
An, H., Kim, S. & Kim, B. (2008). Teacher perspectives on online collaborative learning: Factors perceived as facilitating and impeding successful online group work. *Contemporary Issues in Technology and Teacher Education*, 8(1), 65–83.

Angelo, T. (2012). Designing subjects for learning: Practical, research-based principles and guidelines. In L. Hunt & D. Chalmers (eds), *University teaching in focus: A learning-centred approach*. London: Routledge, pp. 93–111.

Australian Qualifications Framework Council (AQFC) (2015). *Australian Qualifications Framework*, 2nd edn. Retrieved from http://www.aqf.edu.au.

Baert, S., Omey, E., Verhaest, D. & Vermeir, A. (2015). Mister Sandman, bring me good marks! On the relationship between sleep quality and academic achievement. *Social Science and Medicine*, 130, 91–8.

Ballen, C.J., Wieman, C., Salehi, S., Searle, J.B. & Zamudio, K.R. (2017). Enhancing diversity in undergraduate science: Self-efficacy drives performance gains with active learning. *CBE—Life Sciences Education*, 16(4), ar56.

Biggs, J.B. & Tang, C. (2011). *Teaching for quality learning at university: What the student does*. Maidenhead: McGraw-Hill Education.

Boyer, S.L., Edmondson, D.R., Artis, A.B. & Fleming, D. (2014). Self-directed learning: A tool for lifelong learning. *Journal of Marketing Education*, 36(1), 20–32.

Bryer, J. (2012). Peer tutoring program for academic success of returning nursing students. *Journal of the New York State Nurses Association*, 43(1), 20–2.

Chickering, A.W. & Ehrmann, S.C. (1996). Implementing the seven principles: Technology as lever. *AAHE Bulletin*, October, 3–6.

Crisp, G. (2012). Integrative assessment: Reframing assessment practice for current and future learning. *Assessment and Evaluation in Higher Education*, 37(1), 33–43.

Effeney, G., Carroll, A. & Bahr, N. (2013). Self-regulated learning: Key strategies and their sources in a sample of adolescent males. *Australian Journal of Educational and Developmental Psychology*, 13, 58–74.

Flanigan, A.E. & Babchuck, W.A. (2015). Social media as academic quicksand: A phenomenological study of student experiences in and out of the classroom. *ScienceDirect*, 44, 40–5.

Fredrickson, J. (2015). Online learning and student engagement: Assessing the impact of a collaborative writing requirement. *Academy of Educational Leadership Journal*, 19(3),127–40.

Garratt-Reed, D., Roberts, L.D. & Heritage, B. (2016). Grades, student satisfaction and retention in online and face-to-face introductory psychology units: A test of equivalency theory. *Frontiers in Psychology*, 7(673), 1–10.

George, D., Dixon, S., Stansal, E., Lund Gelb, S. & Pheri, T. (2008). Time diary and questionnaire assessment of factors associated with academic and personal success among university undergraduates. *Journal of American College Health*, 56(6), 706–15.

Ghiasvand, A.M., Naderi, M., Tafreshi, M.Z., Ahmadi, F. & Hosseini, M. (2017). Relationship between time management skills and anxiety and academic motivation of nursing students in Tehran. *Electronic Physician*, 9(1), 3678–84.

Gopee, N. & Deane, M. (2013). Strategies for successful academic writing: Institutional and non-institutional support for students. *Nurse Education Today*, 33, 1624–31.

Greenland, S. & Moore, C. (2014). Patterns of student enrolment and attrition in Australian open access online education: A preliminary case study. *Open Praxis*, 6(2), 45–54.

Grissom, J.A., Loeb, S. & Mitani, H. (2015). Principal time management skills: Explaining patterns in principals' time use, job stress, and perceived effectiveness. *Journal of Educational Administration*, 53(6), 773–93.

Hawe, E. & Dixon, H. (2017). Assessment for learning: A catalyst for student self-regulation. *Assessment & Evaluation in Higher Education*, 42(8), 1181–92.

Kaya, H., Kaya, N., Palloa, A.O. & Kucuk, L. (2012). Assessing time-management skills in terms of age, gender, and anxiety levels: A study on nursing and midwifery students in Turkey. *Nurse Education in Practice*, 12(5), 284–5.

Kitney, P., Tam, R., Bramley, D. & Simons, K. (2020). Handover using ISBAR principles in two perioperative sites: A quality improvement project. *Journal of Perioperative Nursing*, 33(4), 7.

Lemmetty, S. & Collin, K. (2020). Self-directed learning as a practice of workplace learning: Interpretative repertoires of self-directed learning in ICT work. *Vocations and Learning*, 13(1), 47–70.

Mannix, T., Parry, Y. & Roderick, A. (2017). Improving clinical handover in a paediatric ward: Implications for nursing management. *Journal of Nursing Management*, 25(3), 215–22.

Marrs, H. & Sigler, E. (2012). Male academic performance in college: The possible role of study strategies. *Psychology of Men and Masculinity*, 13(1), 227–41.

Morris, T.H. (2019). Self-directed learning: A fundamental competence in a rapidly changing world. *International Review of Education*, 65(4), 633–53

——— (2020). Creativity through self-directed learning: Three distinct dimensions of teacher support. *International Journal of Lifelong Education*, 39(2), 168–78.

Mullender-Wijnsma, M.J., Hartman, E.W., de Greeff, J.W., Bosker, R.J., Doolaard, S. & Visscher, C. (2015). Moderate-to-vigorous physically active academic lessons and academic engagement in children with and without a social disadvantage: A within subject experimental design. *BMC Public Health*, 15(404), 1–9.

Nyatanga, P. & Mukorera, S. (2017). Effects of lecture attendance, aptitude, individual heterogeneity and pedagogic intervention on student performance: A probability model approach. *Innovations in Education and Teaching International*, 26(2), 195–205.

Ortagus, J. (2016). From the periphery to prominence: An examination of the changing profile of online students in American higher education. *Internet and Higher Education*, 32, 47–57.

Purarjomandlangrudi, A., Chen, D. & Nguyen, A. (2016). Investigating the drivers of student interaction and engagement in online courses A study of state-of-the-art. *Informatics in Education*, 15(2), 269–86.

Ramsden, P. (2003). *Learning to teach in higher education*, 2nd edn. London: Routledge.

Schmutz, J.B., Meier, L.L. & Manser, T. (2019). How effective is teamwork really? The relationship between teamwork and performance in healthcare teams: a systematic review and meta-analysis. *BMI Open*, 9, doi: 10.1136/bmjopen-2018-028280.

Slater, C.E. & Cusick, A. (2017). Factors related to self-directed learning readiness of students in health professional programs: A scoping review. *Nurse Education Today*, 52, 28–33.

Slater, C.E., Cusick, A. & Louie, J C. (2017). Explaining variance in self-directed learning readiness of first year students in health professional programs. *BMC Medical Education*, 17(1), 1–10.

Tower, M., Blacklock, E., Watson, B., Heffernan, C. & Tronoff, G. (2015). Using social media as a strategy to address 'sophomore slump' in second year nursing students: A qualitative study. *Nurse Education Today*, 35(11), 1130–4.

Xu, J., Du, J. & Fan, X. (2013). 'Finding our time': Predicting students' time management in online collaborative group work. *Computers and Education*, 69, 139–47.

4 Health systems and models in Australia

Diana Guzys and Kathleen Tori

LEARNING OBJECTIVES

At the completion of this chapter, you should be able to:

1 Explain health and illness from biomedical and sociological perspectives.
2 Describe the healthcare continuum, from promoting health to care of the sick.
3 Discuss the Australian healthcare system – policies, priorities and funding.
4 Outline the role of nurses in the Australian healthcare system.

Introduction

Health systems are the products of social, cultural and political pressures that influence how problems and their solutions are conceptualised and enacted (Haslam et al. 2018, Kawachi & Subramanian 2018). The changing nature of illness and technology, as well as community demographics and expectations, have resulted in the evolution of a complex arrangement of delivery and financing health care in the Australian context. Healthcare delivery is shared between different levels of government and the private and public sectors. The federal and state governments, along with private health insurers and individuals themselves, fund or pay for healthcare services (Calder et al. 2019). The government-funded 'public system' is sometimes referred to as a 'welfare state model' of health care. 'Welfare state' refers to a system in which the government takes responsibility for providing healthcare services and funds them through the collection of taxes (Dixit & Sambasivan 2018). Such a system aims to protect the health and wellbeing of all citizens, particularly those who are in financial or social need. Other aspects of a welfare-state approach include providing social benefits payments such as aged and disability pensions, unemployment benefits, or subsidising housing, education and medications. Privately provided services, which are funded by private health insurers and private individuals, may be described as a 'market model'. Australia's healthcare system is supported by a mixture of these, which is referred to as a 'hybrid model' (Dixit & Sambasivan 2018).

In the public part of a hybrid model, governments formulate health policy, and collect and distribute tax revenue on the basis of political and ideological positions on priorities, cost, accessibility, quality and delivery of health care. Socially progressive governments are more likely to engage in direct government intervention and funding, whereas conservative governments tend to favour a market-driven agenda (McDonald & Duckett 2017). Despite these ideological differences, continuation of the hybrid model in the Australian healthcare system is supported by the major political parties. Health policy decisions are broadly based on the ways in which we interpret health and illness; specifically whether health is perceived as wellbeing or the absence of disease (Haslam et al. 2018).

You may be familiar with the World Health Organization's (WHO) definition of health, which was incorporated in the Constitution of the WHO in 1946: 'Health is a state of complete physical, mental and social well-being and not merely the absence of disease or infirmity.' Despite this decades-old definition, many people, governments and health services continue to think about health in terms of deficit, taking a 'sick care' view of health rather than focusing on wellness. In this chapter, we examine different models of health and discuss the principles and philosophy of primary health care in relation to the concept of health. We explore the concept of health and illness as culturally constructed experiences, which means these concepts are perceived differently by individuals because of varying social and professional understandings. Acknowledging and recognising these differences reinforces the need for nurses to practise our profession from a person-centred perspective.

Throughout this chapter, a range of healthcare services are considered, as the healthcare continuum is explored. We provide a brief overview of the various components of the Australian healthcare system and explain the fundamental aspects

of Australia's 'universal' healthcare coverage, as provided by Medicare. The concepts of primary, secondary and tertiary care are introduced and differentiated from primary, secondary and tertiary levels of health care. The chapter concludes with a discussion of the contribution of nurses and nursing to our healthcare system and to keeping Australians healthy.

Models of health

A model of health simply describes the framework, or lens, through which the key features of how health and, frequently, illness are thought about or conceived. Several models have been developed, which promote variations that emphasise the specific aspects and priorities of those advocating for them. Each model has critics.

The biomedical model of health

The biomedical model of health, sometimes simply referred to as the medical model of health, was developed during the eighteenth and nineteenth centuries. Advances in science during a time when infectious diseases were common causes of death promoted the belief that a better understanding of human biology and science would eradicate illness. Disease is the central feature of the medical model, and the absence of disease is used to indicate health (Garner 2016). In this model of health, the focus is on 'fixing' or treating a health deficit to restore normal function (Farre & Rapley 2017). Fuller (2017) describes this as the 'old medical model', which features treatments that rely on biomedical, mechanistic reasoning. However, in contemporary health care, chronic diseases and multimorbidity (having more than one chronic condition) are the reality. The 'new medical model' focuses on cure, prevention and management of biological disease(s), engaging the logic of evidence-based practice, which is frequently undertaken through the use of clinical guidelines (Fuller 2017).

The social model of health

social determinants of health conditions and circumstances influencing health and shaped by the distribution of money, power and resources

Disability rights activists and advocates are credited with highlighting the limitations of the traditional medical model of health, thereby contributing to the development of the social model of health. The work of Sir Michael Marmot (Wilkinson & Marmot 2003) demonstrated the effects of the **social determinants of health** and strengthened our recognition of how social, cultural, political and environmental factors influence health and wellbeing. People's life circumstances, such as their economic position, social exclusion and social supports, work and unemployment, stress, gender, early life development and experiences, indigeneity and ethnicity, create inequalities in health status and outcomes. The most disadvantaged groups in a society are more likely to have greater exposure to health-damaging risk factors and are found to have the poorest health (Guzys, 2020; Marmot et al. 2012). An imaginary line of advantage or disadvantage, referred to as the **social gradient**, is commonly used to explain how an individual, group or community may move in either direction as life circumstances change. This concept is represented in Figure 4.1.

social gradient an imaginary line representing the cumulative effects of advantage or disadvantage, caused by life circumstances

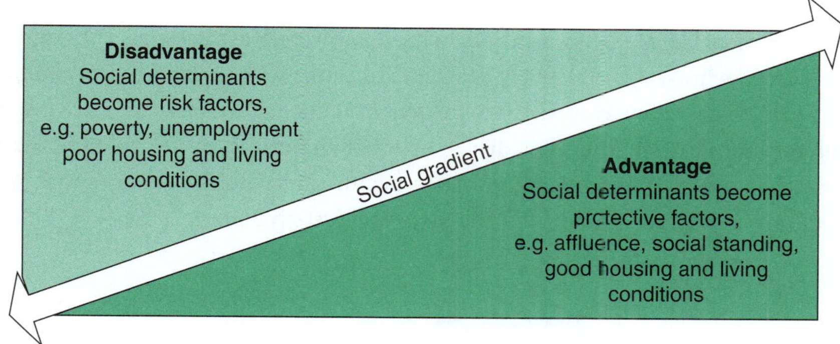

Figure 4.1   The social gradient

Source: Guzys (2020, p. 7).

The biopsychosocial model of health

This model was developed in recognition that health results from the broader and often interwoven influence of biology, psychology and sociology. The ideology underpinning the biopsychosocial model aimed to reverse what some saw as the disempowerment and dehumanisation of clients by impersonal, biomedically oriented technicians (Wade & Halligan 2017). In the biomedical model, anything that could not be objectively verified or explained at the cellular or molecular level was either ignored or devalued. It has been argued that the biopsychosocial model has led to **person-centred care** through recognition of the person within the body as well as their personal context, which influences their experience of health and ill-health as a result of their personality, attitudes, expectations, stage of life and stage of their illness (Farre & Rapley 2017; Wade & Halligan 2017).

The eco-biopsychosocial model of health

The emphasis in this model of health is on the recognition of the increasing influence of the environment on human health and wellbeing (Peel, Maxwell & McGrath 2019). The consequences of the depletion of natural resources, soil and water degradation, air pollution, climate change, food shortages, human conflict and population movement are associated with discrimination, poverty and poor health (Talbot & Verrinder 2018). Interrelated stressors include overpopulation, systemic environmental impacts of economic activities, urbanisation and the spread of consumerism.

person-centred care health care that ensures a 'collaborative and respectful partnership built on mutual trust and understanding through good communication (Nursing and Midwifery Board of Australia 2016, p. 6)', whereby each person is treated as an individual, their dignity is protected and they are empowered to make choices

Short-answer questions

The healthcare continuum

The healthcare continuum describes services that exist to support and maintain health (Figure 4.2). At the wellness end of the continuum are services that engage with people who are well, with the aim of keeping them well. Such services promote healthy behaviours and work towards creating a healthy environment. Some people who work in roles that contribute to wellness may not be recognised as healthcare professionals at all,

such as urban planners who work to ensure that there are sufficient green spaces in the built environment, or geologists working to keep our waterways flowing. The continuum includes those who work to actively prevent ill-health, such as health promoters who engage in health education campaigns to prevent or reduce substance use or driving under the influence of alcohol and other drugs, or other unhealthy or health-compromising behaviours. However, most people associate health care with the services that we use once we start to feel unwell and enter the 'sick care' system (Guzys 2020).

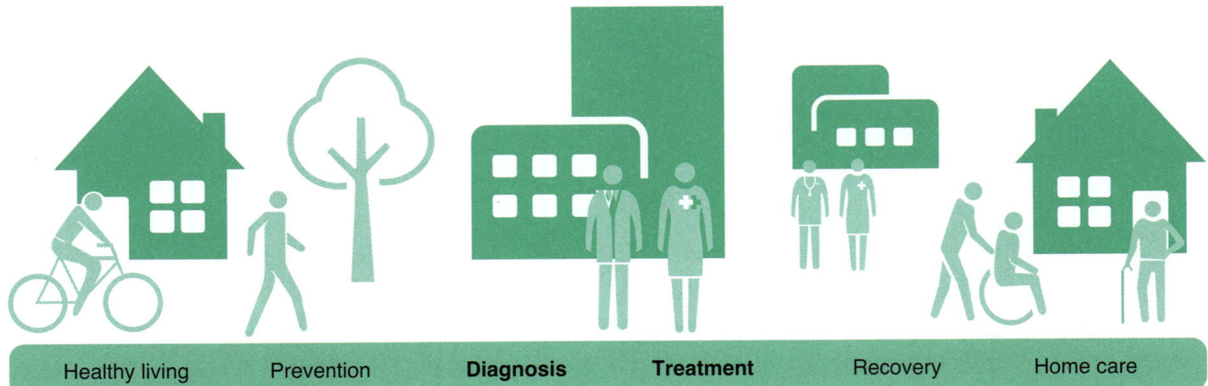

Figure 4.2   The healthcare continuum

Source: Adapted from Travis (1975, p. 654).

Levels of health care

As the complexity of health care increases, so does the level of health care provided. This is described using language we are familiar with in terms of education: primary, secondary and tertiary.

Primary care

Primary care is the term used to describe the first point of contact people have with the Australian health care system, usually accessed when a person is unwell. The term 'primary care' also describes the level of care required at this point of service.

Secondary care

Health services provided by medical specialists and other health professionals who do not have first contact with clients are considered secondary care. This includes 'acute care', which is considered short-term treatment of a serious injury or period of illness – usually relatively urgent. Secondary health care can also refer to the provision of continuing services that are not necessarily provided in hospitals, such as psychiatry, physiotherapy, speech therapy and occupational therapy.

Tertiary care

Tertiary care refers to highly specialised health care, most commonly provided for inpatients and on referral from a primary or secondary health professional. This may involve particularly complex medical or surgical procedures.

To add to the potential confusion associated with the terminology used for levels of care, it is important to bear in mind that similar terms are used to describe the levels of *complexity* in care provided by healthcare organisations and services. Hospitals that provide specialist services for complex health issues are frequently referred to as tertiary hospitals. These are commonly located in major cities and regional centres. Hospitals and services providing less specialised or less complex care may be described as secondary or primary services.

The Australian healthcare system

The Australian healthcare system consists of a range of healthcare services and programs provided and funded by various levels of government and private providers. In fact, the Australian healthcare system could be described as the composite of multiple systems, such as state healthcare systems, private and public healthcare systems, and hospital and public healthcare systems, to mention just a few. Hospitals and the delivery of acute care are the most commonly identified components of any healthcare system; however, many other components of care, such as general medical practice, pharmacy, allied health care, aged and residential care, dentistry, community health care, health promotion and public health, contribute to the broader health system.

The national government has the greatest capacity to raise revenue to support the funding of healthcare services through taxation. This money is distributed to the states and territories through a negotiated funding arrangement, to enable the state and territory governments to provide public health and healthcare services. The funding of health care in Australia has a complex history, which reflects changes in political ideologies and changes to the political party in power at the time (McDonald & Duckett 2017). Similar to other developed countries, the Australian healthcare system has associated strengths and challenges (Cashin 2015). The system needs to remain responsive to demographic changes, such as an ageing population and the increasing complexity of chronic disease and its associated comorbidities (Calder et al. 2019, Woods & Murfet 2015). Cashin (2015) argues, however, that **medical dominance** of the healthcare system is one of the greatest challenges in responding to the changing health needs of Australians, as restrictions to rebates for clients undergoing care from other practitioners are currently limited.

medical dominance the professional autonomy of doctors and the collective influence of medical associations over the economics of health services, administrative decision-making and other health disciplines

Medicare

Before 1974, Australia's healthcare system relied mainly on people having private insurance, with some funding from government for charitable hospitals. Many older hospitals were built and run with funds raised by the community. In 1974, the first national universal health insurance scheme, known as Medibank, was introduced. This was financed through taxation and was operated until a change of government in 1976 (Hall 2015). From 1976 until 1984, there was a short return to the former healthcare system, which relied predominantly on people having private health insurance, with some government subsidies to cover care of the uninsured public. Following a further change to the national government in 1984, **Medicare** was established. This provided national universal health insurance funded entirely through taxation until 1996. From

Medicare the provision of medical services, including free or low-cost treatment in all public hospitals, subsidised by the federal government

that time until 2013, the policy relating to the funding of the Australian healthcare system was based on a mix of national universal health insurance along with publicly subsidised private health insurance. As of 2013, means testing for private insurance and an age incentive to take out private health insurance were added to this arrangement (Hall 2015). Medicare enables access to a range of medical services, either for free or at lower cost to the client, and includes medical, specialist, optometry, some dental and allied healthcare services. Medicare benefits do not extend to medical treatments acquired overseas; however, some countries do have reciprocal healthcare agreements for Australian citizens (Department of Human Services 2017).

Healthcare services for citizens and permanent residents in Australia are funded through Medicare. This provides free treatment in all public hospitals, subsidised medical services and pharmaceutical subsidies for all prescription medicines listed on the **Pharmaceutical Benefits Scheme (PBS)**. The PBS lists government-subsidised medications, updated monthly, which are available to all Australians who hold a Medicare card (PBS 2021). Overseas visitors from countries such as the United Kingdom, Ireland, Sweden and Finland, to name a few, are also eligible to access the PBS if they hold a Reciprocal Health Care Agreement (RHCA) card. Essentially, the PBS provides affordable access to timely and reliable medications necessary to treat most medical conditions, with new ones added regularly (PBS 2021). The majority of medicines are dispensed by community pharmacists and are used by clients in the home, with specialised medicines requiring medical supervision or supervised administration, such as chemotherapy, being only accessible at specialised medical services, usually hospitals (PBS 2021).

Pharmaceutical Benefits Scheme (PBS) the provision of specific medications that are approved and listed to be dispensed at a subsidised price set by the federal government

Connecting with practice:
Medicare
Multiple-choice question

Public hospitals

Australia has more than 1300 public and private hospitals (AIHW 2021). Both public and private hospitals are important to the operation of Australia's healthcare system, collectively providing almost 30.9 million days of client care in the 2018–19 data-collection period (AIHW 2021). According to the Australian Institute of Health and Welfare (AIHW), 'All hospitals receive funding from governments, individuals and insurers' (p. v). Public hospitals are managed by state and territory governments, and private hospitals are owned and operated by private, for-profit and not-for-profit organisations (AIHW 2021). Universal coverage through Medicare ensures free public hospital care, although waiting lists apply to non-emergency care (AIHW 2021; Cashin 2015). Private health insurance facilitates access to a medical specialist of choice and reduces waiting times for non-emergency care, which usually is provided in private hospitals with a partial gap payment (AIHW 2016).

Medical services

Most medical services funded through the federal government are provided by general practitioners (GPs). Around one-fifth of national health funding is spent on medical services (Duckett & Willcox 2011). The federal government funds set payments for a range of medical services through the Medicare scheme, with individuals paying the remainder of the fee above the scheduled amount charged by doctors (Dixit & Sambasivan 2018). Ideally, low-income families are protected from the requirement to pay the gap between the scheduled fee and what is charged for the service, when issued with a means-tested Health Care Card (Epstein et al. 2020; McDonald & Duckett 2017). In reality, there is no requirement for GPs to 'bulk bill' anyone, and even those with a Health Care Card may incur 'gap' payments.

Most GP practices are operated as small businesses (Hall 2015; Willis, Reynolds & Keleher 2016). For more than 80 per cent of Australians – particularly those who live in urban areas where a large number of GPs compete for business – there are no out-of-pocket expenses when visiting a doctor (Hall 2015). The practice of charging clients the standard government-prescribed fee for a service – referred to as 'bulk billing' – encourages a sufficient volume of clients to be seen to maintain a viable business. Exceptions are sometimes made for services provided for children. In rural and remote areas, where there is more likely to be a shortage of GPs, only clients receiving government welfare payments, children and people from low-income groups are likely to be offered bulk-billing services. The additional out-of-pocket cost for clients attending these services is set by the service providers.

More recently, rebates for professional health services listed on the Medicare Benefits Schedule have been introduced for tele-health consultations, multidisciplinary case conferences and some services provided by allied health professionals – for example, psychologists, physiotherapists and speech pathologists (Hall 2015).

Pharmacy

Many medications are subsidised by the federal government through the PBS, following a rigorous process of cost–benefit analysis prior to being listed (Epp, Parkinson & Hawse 2020; Willis et al. 2016). The PBS is a scheme that provides subsidised prescription medications to Australian residents. Commencing in a limited mode in 1948, with free medicines for pensioners and a listing of 'lifesaving and disease-preventing medications', the PBS has expanded to encompass the cost of medicines for most medical conditions (PBS 2021). The aim of the PBS is to provide affordable, timely and reliable access to necessary medicines for Australians. The PBS is part of the Australian government's broader National Medicines Policy (PBS 2021).

Connecting with practice: PBS

Models of health care

There are many models of health care that provide a wide range of services, from public health and preventative services to primary health care, emergency health services, hospital-based treatment in public and/or private facilities, rehabilitation and palliative care (AIHW 2016).

Acute care

The dominant feature of acute care services is their use of the medical model of health, with intervention, prevention of further illness or injury, and restoration of function as the main goals of practice. Acute care includes services that aim to treat psychiatric illnesses, not only physical health issues. Although predominantly working from a medical model, this does not exclude recognition of the social model of health; however, it is not central to practice. Services that work from an acute care model include the majority of hospital services and emergency health services such as paramedicine.

Primary care

For most clients, a primary care clinician will be their first point of contact in the Australian health system, which they access when unwell. These services also principally work from a medical model of health. Primary care provides initial care to individuals, incorporating diagnosis, treatment, and primary, secondary and tertiary disease prevention, as well as opportunistic health education (Willis et al. 2016). Primary care is sometimes described as the 'medical end' of the primary healthcare spectrum. Primary care service providers include GPs, pharmacists, nurses and allied health practitioners.

The burden of disease in Australia no longer results primarily from infectious diseases and injury. The current model of healthcare delivery continues the biomedical model, with the focus on disease management rather than the prevention of disease and enhanced management of **chronic conditions**. Australians are living longer, yet more commonly with multiple chronic conditions, which are beginning earlier in life (Australian Health Ministers' Advisory Council 2017). Health reforms are necessary to develop a system that will respond effectively to the management of chronic conditions. The prevention of chronic conditions and better coordination of care from a range of healthcare providers are necessary for a sustainable healthcare system.

> **chronic conditions** 'a broad range of chronic and complex health conditions' (AIHW 2021), including mental illness, trauma, disability and genetic disorders

Primary health care

Primary health care emphasises care that addresses the underlying social, economic and political causes of poor health while attending to healthcare needs (Sanders et al. 2011). A greater emphasis on working from a social model of health is a feature of primary health care. Health promotion and preventative services are a feature, and practice activities focus on positively influencing the health of groups, communities and populations. Primary healthcare practice can be undertaken in various healthcare settings when understood as a philosophy of practice, rather than solely as an area of practice. This concept is reflected in the primary healthcare patchwork presented in Figure 4.3.

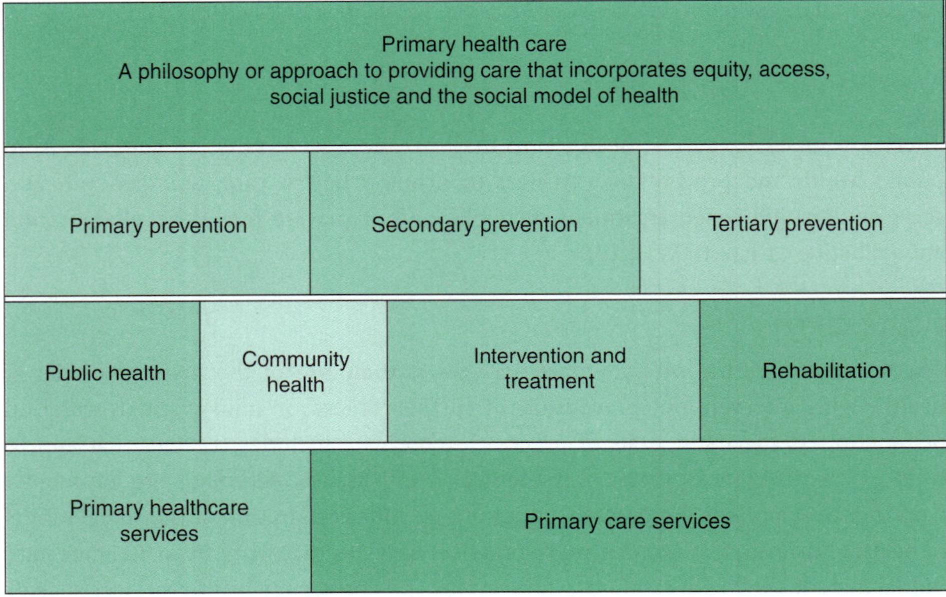

Figure 4.3   The primary healthcare patchwork

Source: Guzys (2020, p. 12).

Public health

Public health takes a population approach rather than focusing on delivery of care to an individual. The aim of public health is to create conditions under which people can be healthy, improve their health and prevent sickness or injury (Baum 2016). This may involve immunising children and adults to prevent the spread of disease, setting safety standards to protect workers or advocating for laws that promote the use of seatbelts or restrict smoking in public places (Baum 2016). The COVID-19 pandemic has resulted in wider public recognition of the work of the public healthcare system in tracking the spread of disease outbreaks, providing health advice to minimise risk and improve prevention of illness, and undertaking health communication.

The public health workforce is multidisciplinary and incorporates professionals with backgrounds in epidemiology, social sciences, medicine, nursing, environmental health, health promotion, public policy, health communication, health economics and health service management. Increasingly, the focus of public health and the population health workforce has been to undertake research and programs aimed at addressing the social determinants of health (Willis et al. 2016).

All three levels of government – federal, state and territory, and local – have public health responsibilities. The primary responsibilities of the federal government involve the funding of family planning services, food safety, supply of blood and blood products, setting national health priorities, and national health-promotion campaigns. Since the advent of the COVID-19 pandemic the responsibilities for monitoring and managing infectious and communicable diseases outbreaks, including epidemiological surveillance, immunisation and vaccination programs, have been shared between federal and state/territory governments. Other public health responsibilities include emergency responses, health promotion, school and dental health, dangerous drugs and poisons, and the funding of maternal and child health, which is frequently administered by local government (Willis et al. 2016). Local government tends to focus on the built environment, such as reducing environmental hazards, waste disposal, land-use planning, roads, footpaths and drainage, recreational development, and food premises, production and selling.

Short-answer question
Multiple-choice questions

Consumer expectations

Consumer expectations of the healthcare system have changed over the past few decades. Changing disease epidemiology, an ageing society, workforce changes, alternative modes of health delivery and advances in technology have seen a shift in emphasis from treatment-focused care to a wellness focus (Humphreys & Wakerman 2008). Accompanying these changes has been a shift in the locus of control for health care from the health practitioner to the consumer. Greater transparency for healthcare actions and increasing professional accountability on behalf of those professions that deliver the care is now the norm. The consumer has the right to high-quality, safe, equitable, timely and accessible health care that is client-centred, or person-centred (Jennings, Lowe & Tori 2017). However, despite the importance of understanding consumer expectations for quality health care, there is often a mismatch between expectations and delivery, particularly in rural and remote primary care (Jennings, Lowe & Tori 2021). Noting that the mismatch is an untheorised concept (Roder-DeWan et al. 2019), consumer expectations and quality of care warrant further research.

Person-centred care (PCC) is multidimensional – it acknowledges the person's expectations, beliefs and values regarding wellbeing and promotes greater flexibility in the provision of health care (Delaney 2018). Unlike traditional, older models of care, which focused on treating a client's diseased state, PCC focuses on the quality of care that each person receives (Lewis 2015). PCC, which is growing in prominence, involves the inclusion of the client in planning their health care, empowering them to make informed decisions; it is based on mutual respect and consideration.

The benefits of PCC is shared collaboration in decision-making, enhanced communication and improved concordance between healthcare providers and the client's adherence to treatment regimens (Delaney 2018). Within the person-centred model of health the client is viewed as an active rather than passive participant in their healthcare plans, with the emphasis on the promotion of wellness rather than only on cure (Delaney 2018; Fix et al. 2017).

The Picker Institute's Eight Principles of Patient-centred Care constitute one well-known model, and define the primary dimensions of client-centred care as:

1 respect for clients' preferences
2 coordination and integration of care
3 information and education
4 physical comfort
5 emotional support
6 involvement of family and friends
7 continuity and transition
8 access to care (Picker Institute n.d.).

Multiple-choice questions

Connecting with practice:
Patient-centred care
Video: Empathy
Multiple-choice question

CASE STUDY

Person-centred palliative care

Mr Brown was a 46-year-old farmer from a small rural community who had lived on his family's farm for most of his life. He was a father of two, a son and a daughter, and had recently been diagnosed with a terminal illness. He was now in the final stages of care. Mr Brown was being cared for in a large regional hospital, nearly two hours' drive from his home town, his family and friends, which was not in keeping with his wishes of wanting to die at home. Mr Brown found the placement in the regional palliative care ward to be an isolating experience, with no one he knew around him, and he believed no one understood what he needed at this stage. He had a heavy symptom burden, requiring constant care and pain relief, and felt that the nurses were 'too busy' for him and that 'they had other things to do rather than bother with [him]'.

A friend of the family referred Mr Brown to a rural nurse practitioner (NP) from the same community, who arranged for a liaison visit with Mr Brown and his family, to see what, if any, improvements could be made in his care. After speaking with the client and his family, the NP arranged for a case management meeting with the palliative team caring for Mr Brown. Following discussions, and with Mr Brown being fully informed of the actual and potential consequences a late move could have on his condition, a transfer to his place of residence on the farm was arranged. There, Mr Brown received the appropriate PCC with supports for administration of medication, at-home palliative care, counselling services for his family, social worker involvement and regular follow-up visits from the NP. Mr Brown passed away at home, in accordance with his wishes, surrounded by his family, friends and beloved animals.

QUESTION

Do you think the nurses in the regional hospital demonstrated PCC?

REFLECTION 4.1

Reflecting on the content above, consider the following questions:

- How was PCC demonstrated in the case study?
- How and in what way will you ensure PCC for future recipients of your nursing care?

Nurses and nursing in the Australian healthcare system

The nursing profession is the largest healthcare provider in the Australian healthcare system. Nurses are integral to the healthcare system. Nursing as a profession encompasses the prevention of ill-health, the promotion of health and care of people who are physically and mentally ill as well as people of all ages who are living with a disability (International Council of Nurses 2017). Nurses comprise over 40 per cent of the healthcare workforce in Australia, with the majority being registered nurses. There are 409 205 nurses nationally (including registered midwives) – 72 105 enrolled nurses and 2069 **nurse practitioners** (NMBA 2020a). There are 5962 nurses, either registered or endorsed to practice, who are not actively employed in the provision of nursing care in the 2020 registrant data (NMBA 2020a). Interestingly, there are 266 nurses who remain registered at either the enrolled nurse level of nursing (23) or the registered nurse level (242), along with one midwife, at or above the age of 80 years (NMBA 2020a). However, despite the longevity that nursing as a profession offers, workforce projections indicate that demand for nurses will significantly exceed supply, with shortfalls estimated to be 85 000 by 2025 and 123 000 by 2030 (Health Workforce Australia 2014). Australia is not unique in these predicted nurse shortages, with shortfalls being experienced

nurse practitioner a registered nurse endorsed as a NP by the NMBA. The NP practices at an advanced level, meets and complies with the nurse practitioner standards for practice, has direct clinical contact and practices within their scope under the legislatively protected title 'nurse practitioner' under the National Law (NMBA 2020c).

worldwide across the public and private sectors (Parliament of Australia 2020). This will affect not only the delivery of health services, with maldistribution of nursing across different practice settings and geographical locations, but may also affect access to, and the quality of, healthcare services.

Nursing takes place in a number of practice environments, including 'hospitals, rural and remote nursing posts, Indigenous communities, schools, prisons, residential aged care facilities, the armed forces, universities, TAFE colleges, mental health facilities, statutory authorities, general practice offices, businesses, professional organisations and people's homes' (ANMF 2016). Working collaboratively as part of a team, or independently, nurses provide professional and holistic nursing care that incorporates the promotion of good health, prevention of illness and direct care for people who are ill, disabled or dying (ANMF 2016).

In Australia, there are two distinct levels of regulated nursing: Registered Nurse (RN) and Enrolled Nurses (EN), both protected titles under the National Law (NMBA 2020a). Within these levels are other identified tiers, which require endorsement to expand nursing practice to an advanced level, such as RNs who hold specialist postgraduate qualifications and may be eligible to seek endorsement as Nursing Practitioners (NP) (ANMF 2016). Within these levels are other non-protected titles such as Clinical Nurse Specialist (CNS), Medication Endorsed Enrolled Nurse (EEN), Clinical Initiative Nurses (CIN), Transitional Nurse Practitioner (TNP) etc. As such, the nomenclature used within the profession of nursing to denote levels, clinical skills and other hierarchical information can at times be quite confusing (Tori 2016). Added to the recognised levels of nursing are the unregulated, and not protected, titles under the National Law of Assistants in Nursing (AINs) or Patient Care Attendants (PCAs) who, while technically are not nurses in the true sense of the word, perform personal care under the direction and supervision of a RN. While the unregulated group of healthcare providers may not be governed by the Health Practitioner Regulation National Law (NMBA 2020c) they may have a TAFE qualification, such as a Certificate III in Aged Care. The group of unregulated caregivers accounts for up to 85 000 of the health service workforce, providing care predominantly in the residential aged-care sector, both public and private (ANMF 2016).

Registered nurses are responsible for assessing, planning, implementing and evaluating care. As regulated health practitioners, nurses are responsible and accountable for their own practice to the regulatory board and to those for whom they provide care (NMBA 2016). The professional accountability and associated competence and proficiency of any practitioner are paramount, regardless of their discipline (Tori 2016). All nursing roles incorporate PCC that is evidence-based and focused on supportive, formative, restorative, preventative and curative elements of healthcare provision (NMBA 2016). Working collaboratively with other healthcare providers, nurses enter into therapeutic and professional relationships with families, groups and communities (NMBA 2016) to facilitate PCC based on self-determined needs and choices.

Advanced practice nursing

Advanced practice nursing (APN) within the Australian context identifies the additional legislated functions that are outside the contemporary RN scope of practice (NMBA 2020b). In the words of Kathleen Tori, 'Nursing is a dynamic profession … and its roles and practices are continually evolving to meet changing nursing care-delivery requirements' (Tori 2016). There is an increased demand for nurses with enhanced skills who have the ability to manage more acutely ill, diverse and complex clients (Gray 2016). A plethora of new advanced nursing roles have been introduced into the Australian healthcare system, such as the clinical nurse consultant (CNC), the rural and isolated practice endorsed registered nurse (RIPERN) and NPs. Disrupting the traditional understandings about nurses' roles and responsibilities, the introduction of APN roles has been viewed as ambiguous with regard to actual scope of practice and models of care. Seeking to clarify what is meant by the term 'advanced practice nursing', the Australian College of Nursing (ACN) released a white paper in 2019, which offers the following definition:

> Advanced practice nursing is the experience, education and knowledge to practice at the full capacity of the registered nurse practice scope. It is neither a title nor a role: It is a level of clinical practice that involves cognitive and practical integration of knowledge and skills from the clinical, health systems, education and research domains of nursing. The nurse practising at this level is a leader in nursing and health care. Advanced practice nursing is enabled through education at master's level. (ACN 2019, p. 19)

The NP role is an advanced role that has been recognised in the Australian healthcare system for more than two decades (ACNP 2020). With the role aligned to the nursing philosophy of care, it offers an alternative healthcare option for consumers (Tori 2020). To date, the role has been found to be cost-effective, safe and instrumental in ensuring that health care is timely, accessible and of a high quality (Scanlon et al. 2018, Clifford et al. 2020).

Originally introduced to address service gaps in health care in underserviced and marginalised communities, the Australian NP role is predominantly specialist rather than generalist in its focus, and as such the majority of the NP role can be found in the acute-care hospital sector (Currie et al. 2020). In 2020 there were 2069 NPs endorsed to practise in Australia (NMBA 2020a).

NP practice is differentiated from other levels of nursing practice, as it integrates the education, leadership, research, management, consultation and clinical decision-making that are inherent in an advanced nursing role (Jennings et al. 2016). NPs have significant clinical experience, underpinned by advanced education, and have the ability to perform duties and roles in situations that are more specialised than those traditionally seen in the nursing profession.

These advanced practice roles build upon the platform of an RN (NMBA 2020c) and see the NP as managing episodes of care in either an independent or collaborative manner, across a variety of healthcare environments and in a

number of specialty practice areas. As such, the scope of practice for endorsed NPs includes initiating pathology and diagnostic imaging investigations, prescribing medications and referring clients to other healthcare practitioners (Chiarella et al. 2020).

REFLECTION 4.2

Reflecting on the content in this section, consider the following questions:

- What role do you think advanced practice nurses have in the provision of health care?
- How do you think advanced practice nurses contribute to client care, leadership, research and mentoring of the nursing workforce?
- How and in what way do you think advanced practice nurses can augment health service access and care, particularly in rural and remote areas?

NURSING PERSPECTIVE

Having had the privilege of being a nurse for over 30 years, there have been many areas in which I have practised. I have moved through all stages of the nursing continuum, from an EN to RN, then NP and now in the twilight of my career I am a nursing academic and have recently completed a PhD. Additionally, I have practised in both the more conventional clinical environments such as emergency departments and critical care environments in large regional hospitals, and in small rural health facilities, and I have spent many years in the Department of Defence (Army) as a Medic and as a commissioned Nursing Officer.

With each progression along the nursing continuum, there have been significant changes to my personal and legislative scope of practice, depending on the context in which I was practising, level of education, policy and organisational requirements. Each role enabled a different level of care that I could offer my clients. For example, as an enrolled nurse I could not – at that stage – administer medications, and now I can prescribe those same medications. Yet, the overall objective has remained the same: to meet the care requirements of my clients in the best possible manner and to improve the health outcomes of those who rely on me to provide safe, competent and confident nursing care. Even today, when my role is predominantly that of an academic, the client, or consumer of the health care, is still uppermost in my mind, be it whether I am teaching nursing students or conducting health-focused research. Would I have done anything differently? No, I value making a difference for my clients and enjoy making their experiences of the healthcare system a positive one.

SUMMARY

- Health and illness are culturally constructed experiences, which can be influenced by diverse biomedical and sociological factors in the Australian context. There are several models of health, including the biomedical, the social, the biopsychosocial and the eco-biopsychosocial models. There are also several models of health care that cover a wide range of services, including acute care, primary care, primary health care and public health care. It is important to be aware of all of these models to understand the complex concepts of health and illness.
- The healthcare continuum describes services that exist to support and maintain health. At the wellness end of the continuum are services that engage with people who are well, with the aim of keeping them well. The continuum includes those who work to actively prevent ill-health, such as health promoters who engage in health education campaigns to prevent or reduce harmful substance use and driving under the influence of alcohol and other drugs, or other unhealthy or health-compromising behaviours. When people begin to feel unwell, they engage with the other end of the continuum, which many associate with the traditional healthcare system.
- The Australian healthcare system consists of a range of healthcare services and programs provided and funded by various levels of government and private providers. The vast majority of government funding for the healthcare system is spent on public hospitals and medical services, which can be seen as medical dominance. Medicare is the national universal health insurance scheme, providing free treatments and subsidies for all citizens and permanent residents. However, as the burden of disease results mostly from chronic diseases in the contemporary context, it is likely that healthcare priorities will have to change to cater for this shift.
- Nurses comprise over 40 per cent of the healthcare workforce and are integral to Australia's healthcare system. Nursing roles include prevention, health promotion and care of people who are physically and mentally ill and people of all ages who are living with disability.

REVIEW QUESTIONS

1. What is your understanding of the key differences between the models of health explored in this chapter?
2. Is there a relationship between the models of health and the models of health care?
3. Reviewing the levels of health care, what are the predominant differences?
4. Which level of government is responsible for funding public hospitals?
5. How is the nurse practitioner role different from the registered nurse role?

Suggested responses

RESEARCH TOPIC

Refer to the 'Challenge of chronic conditions' section of the National Strategic Framework for Chronic Conditions (Australian Health Ministers Advisory Council 2017). How do you believe this will influence nursing practice in the next five to ten years?

FURTHER READING

Australian College of Nursing (ACN) (2019). A new horizon for health services: Optimizing advanced practice nursing – a white paper. Canberra: ACN. Available from https://www.acn.edu.au/wp-content/uploads/white-paper-optimising-advanced-practice-nursing.pdf.

Fisher, M., Baum, F.E., MacDougall, C., Newman, L. & McDermott, D. (2016). To what extent do Australian health policy documents address social determinants of health and health equity? *Journal of Social Policy*, 45(3), 545–64.

Guzys, D. (2020). Community and primary healthcare. In D. Guzys, R. Brown, E. Halcomb & D. Whitehead (eds), *An introduction to community and primary healthcare*, 3rd edn. Melbourne: Cambridge University Press, pp. 3–20.

Halcomb, E.J., Salamonson, Y., Davidson, P.M., Kaur, R. & Young, S.A. (2014). The evolution of nursing in Australian general practice: A comparative analysis of workforce surveys ten years on. *BMC Family Practice*, 15(1), 52.

Korda, R.J., Paige, E., Yiengprugsawan, V., Latz, I. & Friel, S. (2014). Income-related inequalities in chronic conditions, physical functioning and psychological distress among older people in Australia: Cross-sectional findings from the 45 and up study. *BMC Public Health*, 14(1), 741.

Powell Davies, G., Harris, M., Perkins, D., Roland, M., Williams, A., Larsen, K. & McDonald, J. (2017). *Coordination of care within primary healthcare and with other sectors: A systematic review*. Canberra: Australian Primary Healthcare Research Institute (APHCRI).

Ross, H., Tod, A.M. & Clarke, A. (2015). Understanding and achieving person-centred care: The nurse perspective. *Journal of Clinical Nursing*, 24(9–10), 1223–33.

Sav, A., King, M.A., Whitty, J.A., Kendall, E., McMillan, S.S., Kelly, F. … & Wheeler, A.J. (2015). Burden of treatment for chronic illness: A concept analysis and review of the literature. *Health Expectations*, 18(3), 312–24.

Tori, K. (2020). Nurse practitioners. In D. Guzys, R. Brown, E. Halcomb & D. Whitehead (eds), *An introduction to community and primary healthcare*, 3rd edn. Melbourne: Cambridge University Press, pp. 421–31.

REFERENCES

Australian College of Nurse Practitioners (ACNP) (2020). What is a Nurse Practitioner? Retrieved from https://www.acnp.org.au/aboutnursepractitioners.

Australian College of Nursing (ACN) (2019). A new horizon for health services: Optimizing advanced practice nursing – a white paper. Canberra: ACN. Retrieved from https://www.acn.edu.au/wp-content/uploads/white-paper-optimising-advanced-practice-nursing.pdf.

Australian Health Ministers' Advisory Council (2017). National Strategic Framework for Chronic Conditions. Canberra: Commonwealth Government.

Australian Institute of Health and Welfare (AIHW) (2016). *Australia's health 2016*. Canberra: Commonwealth Government. Retrieved from https://www.aihw.gov.au/reports-data.

——— (2021). *Australia's health 2020*. Canberra: Commonwealth Government.

Australian Nursing and Midwifery Federation (ANMF) (2016). A comprehensive analysis of nurses' and midwives' wages. *Nurses & Midwives' Paycheck*, 15(4).

Baum, F. (2016). *The new public health*, 4th edn. Oxford: Oxford University Press.

Calder, R., Dunkin, R., Rochford, C. & Nichols, T. (2019). *Australian health services: too complex to navigate: a review of the national reviews of Australia's health service arrangements*. Australian Health Policy Collaboration, Policy Issues Paper No. 1 2019, AHPC.

Cashin, A. (2015). The challenge of nurse innovation in the Australian context of universal healthcare. *Collegian*, 22, 319–24.

Chiarella, M., Currie, J. & Wand, T. (2020). Liability and collaborative arrangements for nurse practitioner practice in Australia. *Australian Health Review*, 44, 172–7.

Clifford, S., Lutze, M., Maw, M. & Jennings, N. (2020). Establishing value from contemporary nurse practitioners' perceptions of the role: A preliminary study into purpose, support and priorities. *Collegian*, 27, 97–101.

Currie, J., Carter, M.A., Lutze, M. & Edwards, L. (2020) Preparing Australian nurse practitioners to meet health care demand. *The Journal for Nurse Practitioners*, 16(8), 629–33.

Delaney, L. (2018) Patient-centred care as an approach to improving health care in Australia. *Collegian*, 25(1), 119–23.

Department of Human Services (2017). Medicare. Retrieved from http://www.humanservices.gov.au/individuals/medicare.

Dixit, S.K. & Sambasivan, M. (2018). A review of the Australian healthcare system: A policy perspective. *SAGE Open Medicine*, 6, 1–4.

Duckett, S. & Willcox, S. (2011). *The Australian healthcare system*, 4th edn. Melbourne: Oxford University Press.

Epp, J., Parkinson, B. & Hawse, S. (2020) Health system sustainability: The Pharmaceutical Benefits Scheme in Australia. In L. Wood, L. Tan, Y. Breyer & S. Hawse (eds), *Industry and higher education*. Singapore: Springer.

Epstein, D.S., Barton, C., Mazza, D., Woode, M.E. & Mortimer, D. (2020). Patient chosen gap payments in primary care: Predictions of patient acceptability, uptake and willingness to pay from a discrete choice experiment. *Social Science & Medicine*, 263, art. 113284.

Farre, A. & Rapley, T. (2017). The new old (and old new) medical model: Four decades navigating the biomedical and psychosocial understandings of health and illness. *Healthcare*, 5(4), 88.

Fix, G.M., Lukas, C., Bolton, R.E., Hill., J.N., Mueller, N., LaVela, S.L. & Bokhour, B.G. (2017). Patient-centred care is a way of doing things: How healthcare employees conceptualize patient-centred care. *Health Expectations*, 21(1), 300–7.

Fuller, J. (2017). The new medical model: A renewed challenge for biomedicine. *Canadian Medical Association Journal*, 189(17), E640–1.

Garner, A.S. (2016). Thinking developmentally: The next evolution in models of health. *Journal of Developmental and Behavioral Pediatrics*, 37(7), 579–84.

Gray, A. (2016). Advanced or advancing nursing practice: What is the future direction for nursing? *British Journal of Nursing*, 25(1), 8–13.

Guzys, D. (2020). Community and primary healthcare. In D. Guzys, R. Brown, E. Halcomb & D. Whitehead (eds), *An introduction to community and primary healthcare*, 3rd edn. Melbourne: Cambridge University Press, pp. 3–20.

Hall, J. (2015). Australian healthcare: The challenge of reform in a fragmented system. *New England Journal of Medicine*, 3763(6), 493–7.

Haslam, S.A., McMahon, C., Cruwys, T., Haslam, C., Jetten, J. & Steffens, N.K. (2018). Social cure, what social cure? The propensity to underestimate the importance of social factors for health. *Social Science & Medicine*, 198, 14–21.

Health Workforce Australia (HWA) (2014). *Australia's future health workforce: Nurses*. Canberra: Commonwealth Government.

Humphreys, J. & Wakerman, J. (2008). *Primary healthcare in rural and remote Australia: Achieving equity of access and outcomes through national reform – a discussion paper*. Canberra: National Health and Hospitals Reform Commission.

International Council of Nurses. (2017). Definition of nursing. Retrieved from http://www.icn.ch/who-we-are/icn-definition-of-nursing.

Jennings, N., Lowe, G. & Tori, K.E. (2017). Revisiting innovation: Nurse practitioner solutions. Paper presented to the Western Alliance Health Research Symposium, Geelong.

——— (2021). Nurse practitioner locums: A plausible solution for health care access for rural communities. *Australian Journal of Primary Health*, 27(1), 1–5.

Jennings, N., Lutze, M., Clifford, S. & Maw, M. (2016). How do we capture the emergency nurse practitioner's contribution to value in health service delivery? *Australian Health Review*, 41, 89–90.

Kawachi, I. & Subramanian, S.V. (2018). Social epidemiology for the 21st century. *Social Science & Medicine*, 196, 240–5.

Lewis, J. (2015). Patient-centered care (PCC) and nursing: A case study. Retrieved from https://www.linkedin.com/pulse/patient-centered-care-pcc-nursing-case-study-joshua-lewis.

Marmot, M., Allen, J., Bell, R., Bloomer, E. & Goldblatt, P. (2012). WHO European review of social determinants of health and the health divide. *The Lancet*, 380(9846), 1011–29.

McDonald, F. & Duckett, S. (2017). Regulation, private health insurance, and the Australian health system. *McGill Journal of Law & Health*, S31, 11.

Nursing and Midwifery Board of Australia (NMBA) (2016). *Registered Nurse Standards for Practice*. Retrieved from http://www.nursingmidwiferyboard.gov.au/Codes-Guidelines-Statements/Professional-standards/registered-nurse-standards-for-practice.aspx.

——— (2020a). Registrant data: 30 June 2020. Retrieved from https://www.nursingmidwiferyboard.gov.au/About/Statistics.aspx.

——— (2020b). Advanced nursing practice and specialty areas within nursing. Fact sheet. Retrieved from https://www.nursingmidwiferyboard.gov.au/Codes-Guidelines-Statements/FAQ/fact-sheet-advanced-nursing-practice-and-specialty-areas.aspx.

——— (2020c). *Nurse Practitioner Standards for Practice*. Retrieved from https://www.nursingmidwiferyboard.gov.au/codes-guidelines-statements/professional-standards/nurse-practitioner-standards-of-practice.aspx.

Parliament of Australia (2020). Parliamentary Business: Nurse shortages and the impact on health services. Retrieved from https://www.aph.gov.au/parliamentary_business/committees/senate/community_affairs/completed_inquiries/2002-04/nursing/report/c02.

Peel, N., Maxwell, H. & McGrath, R. (2019). Leisure and health: conjoined and contested concepts. *Annals of Leisure Research*, 3, 295–309.

Pharmaceutical Benefits Scheme (PBS) (2021). About the PBS. Retrieved from http://www.pbs.gov.au/info/about-the-pbs.

Picker Institute (n.d.). Principles of patient-centred care. Retrieved from https://www.picker.org/impact-report-2019-2020/?gclid=EAIaIQobChMIzufi_cKn8gIVWTErCh2RNAjSEAAYASAAEgIo8vD_BwE.

Roder-DeWan, S., Gage, A.D., Hirschhorn, L.R., Twum-Danso, N.A.Y., Liljestrand, J., Asante-Shongwe, K., Rodriguez, V., Yahya, T. & Kruk, M.E. (2019). Expectations of healthcare quality: A cross-sectional study of internet users in 12 low- and middle-income countries. *PLOS Medicine*, 16(8), doi: 10.1371/journal.pmed.1002879.

Sanders, D., Baum, F.E., Benos, A. & Legge, D. (2011). Revitalising primary healthcare requires an equitable global economic system – now more than ever. *Journal of Epidemiology and Community Health*, 65(8), 661–5.

Scanlon, A., Murphy, M., Tori, K. & Poghosyan, L. (2018). Nurse practitioner's organizational practice environment. *Journal of Nurse Practitioners*, 14(5), 414–18.

Talbot, L. & Verrinder, G. (2018). *Promoting health: The primary health care approach*, 6th edn. Marrickville, NSW: Elsevier.

Travis, J. (1975). Key concept #1: The illness-wellness continuum. *The Wellspring*. Retrieved from http://www.thewellspring.com/wellspring/introduction-to-wellness/357/key-concept-1-the-illnesswellness-continuum.cfm.html.

Tori, K.E. (2016). The role of the emergency nurse practitioner: An ethnographic study. PhD Thesis, La Trobe University, Bendigo.

——— (2020). Nurse practitioners. In D. Guzys, R. Brown, E. Halcomb & D. Whitehead (eds), *An introduction to community and primary healthcare*, 3rd edn. Melbourne: Cambridge University Press, pp. 421–31.

Wade, D.T. & Halligan, P.W. (2017). The biopsychosocial model of illness: A model whose time has come. *Clinical Rehabilitation*, 31(8), 995–1004.

Wilkinson, R.G. & Marmot, M. (2003). *Social determinants of health: The solid facts*, 2nd edn. Geneva: World Health Organization.

Willis, E., Reynolds, L. & Keleher, H. (2016). *Understanding the Australian healthcare system*, 3rd edn. Sydney: Elsevier.

Woods, M. & Murfet, G. (2015). Australian nurse practitioner practice: Value adding through clinical reflexivity. *Nursing Research and Practice*, 2015, art. 829593.

World Health Organization (1946, 2020). *Constitution, 49th edn*. New York: World Health Organization. Retrieved from https://apps.who.int/gb/bd/pdf_files/BD_49th-en.pdf.

Health care in Australia

Nick Arnott and Melanie Eslick

LEARNING OBJECTIVES

At the completion of this chapter, you should be able to:

1 Explain the models and perspectives that influence and shape health care in Australia.
2 Describe Australia's dynamic and evolving healthcare landscape.
3 Discuss the issues and trends affecting health care now and into the future.

Introduction

As highlighted in Chapter 4, health care in Australia is delivered through a large, diverse and complex system (or set of systems) that is constantly evolving and changing. The system is often considered to be in a state of perpetual reform (change), with frequent restructuring of healthcare priorities and how services are organised, funded and governed (Reynolds, Willis & Rudge 2020).

Within this dynamic system and reform agenda, a chapter on contemporary health care can describe how things currently stand, but these existing roles and services need to be considered in the context of the frequent changes as noted. Even similarly named roles and services can differ markedly in design and implementation, based on local needs and priorities, and the varying strategic, policy and operating contexts of different organisations and systems.

We begin the chapter by briefly revisiting some of the key concepts from Chapter 4 and examining the current health landscape (the 'lay of the land'). We then turn our attention to some of the current and emerging issues, trends and opportunities in health care, and explore how these might influence and shape the ways in which health, social and community services are designed, prioritised and delivered in Australia.

Definitions and models

It is generally accepted that health is holistic and multifaceted, emphasising 'a state of complete physical, mental and social wellbeing, and not merely the absence of disease or infirmity' (WHO 1946; see Chapter 4). In Chapter 4 we introduced several models of health and wellbeing, each of these stemming from two contrasting perspectives: the 'medical' (or biomedical) perspective and the 'social' perspective.

The biomedical model of health

The biomedical model views health from a 'deficit', or problem (illness, disease and infirmity), perspective. It focuses on early detection, diagnosis and intervention to 'treat, fix or cure' these problems, using medical and scientific technologies at the individual level. Biological 'disease' or injury is the central feature of this perspective, with the absence of disease being considered the key indicator of 'health'. Despite being challenged for several key limitations, the biomedical model underpins much of what we think about, or see, as 'health care' in Australia – hospitals, general practice, allied health and emergency care – and has a dominant influence on most major healthcare policies, services and funding or expenditure decisions (Guzys 2021; Haslam et al. 2018).

The social model of health

The social model views health as a positive and holistic concept (rather than the 'ill-health or deficit' perspective of the biomedical model), with an emphasis on 'wellness' or someone's physical, social, cultural, intellectual, emotional, spiritual and environmental wellbeing (Clendon & Munns 2019; Keleher 2020a). Rather than focusing on treatment or 'sick care', a social health approach emphasises equity, justice, health promotion and the prevention of illness, which we discuss later in this chapter.

How do these models and perspectives shape health care as we know it?

These models reflect different understandings of health and wellbeing, and it is these understandings or interpretations that then influence the ways in which healthcare systems and services are designed and delivered (Reynolds et al. 2020).

For example, on the one hand the medical profession is closely (and theoretically) aligned to the biomedical model. In most developed countries, including Australia, the medical profession holds great power and influence, which has contributed to a system that continues to be dominated by hospitals and 'Big Pharma' (giant multinational producers of medicines) and is designed to treat or cure 'biological' problems.

On the other hand, advocates of the social model (which also includes parts of the medical profession) argue that health and wellbeing are influenced and shaped by a range of individual, societal and socio-economic factors or determinants. These 'determinants of health' refer to the social, cultural, economic, political and environmental conditions in which people live, grow, work and age, as well as the biological factors and health behaviours that are part of an individual's lifestyle and genetic make-up (Guzys 2021; Keleher 2020a). There is also growing recognition that determinants of health include the structural and policy drivers of these social environments and conditions, including the availability of and access to necessary services, supports and resources (Clendon & Munns 2019).

This 'social health' perspective has contributed to greater investment in policy and action on the determinants of health, through various public and primary healthcare endeavours, based on social justice, prevention and health promotion.

As nurses and health professionals, we need to be aware of these different perspectives on health and wellbeing, and what it means for individuals, families and communities to be 'ill' or 'well'. For example, in Australia, Aboriginal and Torres Strait Islander peoples have definitions or understandings that reflect the importance of social, emotional, spiritual and cultural wellbeing of individuals and whole communities, along with their physical environment (land/Country), dignity, self-esteem and justice (National Aboriginal Health Strategy Working Party, cited by Clendon & Munns 2019, p. 5). This awareness guides how we think, act and make decisions in practice. It not only ensures that our practice is aligned with the philosophy and expectations of the roles we hold and the systems and settings in which we work, but also supports our engagement in person-centred, empathetic, respectful and culturally safe relationships (also see Chapter 10) with our clients, their support networks and our colleagues (McCormack & McCance 2016; Stein-Parbury 2018).

The current healthcare landscape (the 'lay of the land')

Figure 5.1 provides a snapshot of Australia's health landscape. It captures many of the factors, determinants and considerations that influence and inform the breadth of health and community services that we see, engage with and work within at the national, state and/or local levels.

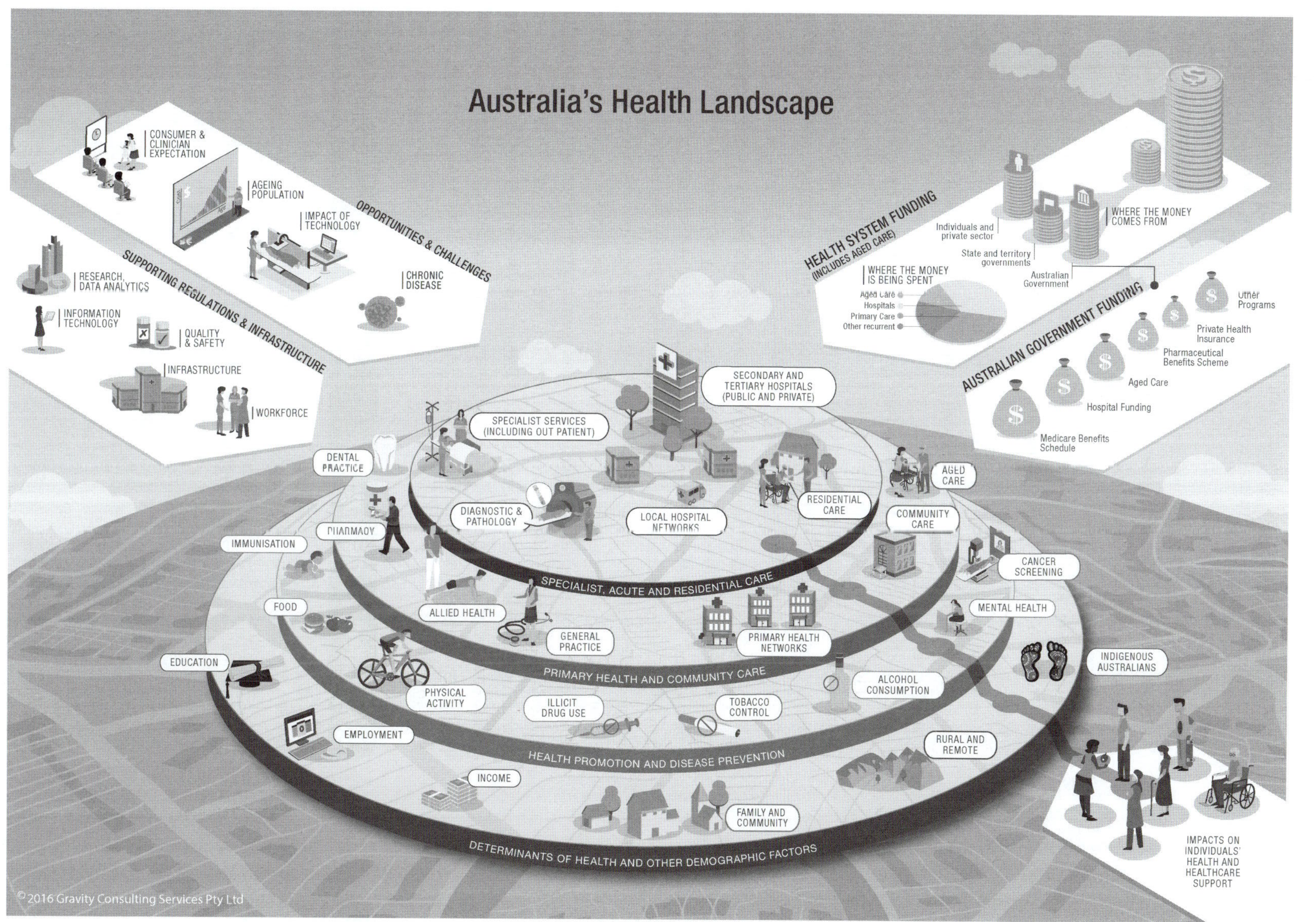

Figure 5.1 Australia's health landscape infographic

Source: Department of Health (2017).

We explore some of these factors or influences in this section to gain an understanding of the current 'lay of the land' for health care in Australia.

According to Figure 5.1, Australia's health landscape has four tiers, each influencing healthcare systems and services in various ways (Department of Health 2017):

- The first and largest tier comprises 'determinants of health and other demographic factors'. This includes education, employment, income, family and community, rural and remote communities, and Aboriginal and Torres Strait Islander peoples.
- The second tier is 'health promotion and disease prevention'. This includes immunisation, food (supply or security) and nutrition, physical activity, illicit drug use, tobacco control, alcohol consumption, mental health and cancer (and other disease) screening.
- The third tier is 'primary and community care'. This includes general practice, dental services, pharmacy, allied health, primary health networks and community aged care.
- The fourth and smallest tier comprises 'specialist, acute and residential care'. This includes public and private hospitals, specialist services (including outpatients), diagnostic and pathology services, and residential care. Although depicted as the smallest tier, these services receive the greatest policy attention and the biggest proportion of healthcare funding in Australia.

While this provides a useful visual representation of health care in Australia, it should not be viewed as a 'fixed' concept. As we have already highlighted, health care is dynamic, and we are likely to see a great deal of crossover and interaction between many of the factors, determinants and services depicted here. For example, emotional and psychological issues can arise in all health settings and contexts (influenced by many of the determinants identified in tier one), and every nurse needs to be prepared to recognise and assist with their management and prevention, including the promotion of mental wellbeing for ourselves and others (Schwartz 2019). Depicting mental health in the 'health promotion and disease prevention' tier seems appropriate in this regard, but we also know, of course, that the management of 'mental illness' and specific psychopathologies may require specialist acute or residential care, as depicted in the fourth tier.

NURSING PERSPECTIVE

I have been a nurse for only a few short years. In that time I have been involved in so many incredible and intense moments. I have performed life-support in remote communities where there is no doctor. I have palliated people in their homes. I have been present for births, traumas and deaths, and everything in between. I have removed maggots from wounds and attended jellyfish stings and crocodile bites. I am so proud to be a nurse and a future midwife. I am proud to be able to hold hands with people when they are vulnerable or afraid on their hardest days. I have loved every single one of my clients and am not ashamed to have cried tears for them or to have hugged them when they have overcome so much. I love my job and all that it has given me.

REFLECTION 5.1

What 'type' of health care do you have in mind for your own future nursing practice? In what healthcare setting or service do you expect or hope to be working?

In Chapter 4 we considered different types or models of health care that arise from the biomedical and social models of health discussed earlier – acute care, primary care, primary health care and public health. Let us briefly review these and show how they broadly align with the different tiers outlined in Figure 5.1.

Acute care

The dominant feature of acute-care services is their alignment with the biomedical model of health, with intervention (medical and surgical), treatment, secondary prevention (prevention of further illness, injury, escalation or complications) and the restoration of function as the main goals of practice. Acute care can include services to treat both physical and psychiatric illnesses. Acute care includes the majority of services provided in and by hospitals, some specialist clinics and public dental services, and most emergency health and paramedicine services (AIHW 2016; Hirshon et al. 2013).

NURSING PERSPECTIVE

I work as a registered nurse in an oncology day unit. It's a different type of 'ward'. Our clients come in for their treatment, sit in a cubicle in their outside clothes and then go home when it is done. They may come for chemotherapy, immunotherapy, blood and/or plasma transfusions, or other medications – cancer treatments come in many forms. Many of our clients are immunocompromised but they are generally quite well. On any given day I might see up to eight clients, treating a few concurrently. Before the COVID-19 pandemic they often brought family members or carers with them. Since most are undergoing a series of treatments, we get to know them, and their loved ones, very well. Although they have cancer, and some are participants in clinical trials, they are generally well and, in cancer care, the day unit is a cheery place to work.

My role is to greet my client, weigh them, ask questions about how they are feeling and their response to previous treatments, take bloods for pathology testing, administer the medications or treatments, and then send them home with a date for their next appointment and any referral information.

My colleagues and I were really worried when COVID-19 cases started to increase and it became clear that there would be a lockdown. We did not know what to expect for our clients, many of whom have weekly treatment. They are all vulnerable, and what I saw when it all started was that they were all afraid – not only of the virus, but also that they may have to put a hold on their (in many cases, lifesaving and life-extending) treatments for an unknown length of time. However, the hospital snapped into action, and I was so proud. In the outpatients (chemotherapy) ward we already use full personal protective equipment (PPE), so there was little change in that regard, and we had no problems with stock. The hospital created an entirely new entrance for vulnerable clients (cancer or renal clients and some other immunocompromised or immunosuppressed clients), so they would not be exposed to the wider client population. The specialists continued to practise and offered phone or video consultations where possible, instead of face-to-face. We had extra multidisciplinary team meetings to discuss each client and whether their treatment could be delayed or, in some cases, switched to oral medications. Our nursing team rallied and continued to work with a smaller cohort of clients; we phoned our regular clients to check on them every week.

With many of our clients, there comes a time when they stop coming to our unit for treatment. Their disease may have progressed, or they may be ill due to comorbidities and become inpatients instead. Some progress to palliative care, a special, small unit where they receive comfort care when they have no further treatment options. I feel privileged to work with these clients – they are so motivated to thrive and to live their best lives while they can. I cannot imagine working outside of cancer care now.

Primary care

Primary care is a term that is often used interchangeably with primary health care (see next section), but while aligned or even part of a primary healthcare continuum there are some distinctions between the two. Working principally from the biomedical model of health, primary care services are often the first point of contact that many people have with the Australian health system; they provide services focused on treatment, rehabilitation and primary 'medical' care, mainly delivered by doctors, nurses and allied health practitioners. Primary care is usually provided from a clinic, or medical or allied health practice, mostly as a one-off or short-term (episodic) consultation, but sometimes as continuing care for chronic conditions or rehabilitation (Keleher 2020a).

Early diagnosis, timely and effective treatment, as well as screening, prevention and disease management, are the core priorities for most primary care services; however, opportunistic health education and promotion may also occur. General practice is a key example of primary care in the Australian context but it may also include pharmacy and various nursing and allied health services (Reynolds et al. 2020).

According to the Australian Primary Health Care Nurses Association (APNA 2021), general practice nursing is one of the fastest-growing areas in health care and may involve many areas of nursing practice for diverse client groups, including acute clinical care, chronic disease management, mental health support, child and family health, aged care, and health promotion and prevention activities such as health education, screening and immunisation.

Primary health care

On the back of a globally endorsed goal of 'Health for All', the First International Conference on Primary Health Care was held in September 1978 at Alma-Ata in the former USSR. This conference culminated in the signing of the Alma-Ata Declaration, which reaffirmed health as a fundamental human right, and endorsed comprehensive primary health care (PHC) as a new and alternative approach to conventional biomedical models and practices (Keleher 2020a; WHO & UNICEF 1978).

Underpinned by principles of social justice, equity and community participation, PHC places greater emphasis on the social model of health, aiming to address the underlying social, economic, political and environmental determinants of poor health while still attending or contributing to specific healthcare needs (as in 'primary care' above). Health promotion and preventative services are features of PHC, with activities focusing on positively influencing the health and wellbeing of groups, communities and populations, not just individuals (Clendon & Munns 2019; WHO 2021). PHC is a whole-of-society approach that involves multisectoral policy and action to address the broader determinants of health, reduce health inequities and disadvantage, and empower individuals, families and communities to take charge of their own health (Keleher 2020a; WHO 2021).

Video: 'My nursing future'
Video: 'What is primary health care?'
Short-answer question

Public health

The broad aim of **public health** is to create conditions that protect and improve the health of populations, with a focus on preventing avoidable disease, injury, disability and death, while also promoting a healthy and sustainable environment for current and future generations (Baum 2016; Keleher 2020b; PHAA 2018). Unlike acute and many primary care services, which focus on individual diagnosis and treatment of disease, illness or injuries once they have occurred, public health works to prevent people from getting sick or injured in the first place (Baum 2016; Keleher 2020b).

Interdisciplinary in nature, public health draws knowledge from a variety of fields including biology, sociology, medicine, business, epidemiology, health economics, psychology, biostatistics and community development. Brought together by the commitment to improve the public's health, public health researchers, practitioners and educators work collaboratively to provide innovative solutions to health barriers and inequalities at the local, national and international levels (PHAA 2018, p. 1). These solutions or strategies include the implementation of health education, promotion and prevention programs and campaigns (including vaccinations); health screening and surveillance (testing, tracking and monitoring the spread of disease outbreaks); recommendations for public health legislation or policies; and the conduct of research on communicable diseases and contemporary prevention strategies (Baum 2016; Keleher 2020b; Liamputtong 2019).

Public health measures generally target entire populations or specific groups, defined by geographical location, age, ethnicity, sex or risk factors, but they may also involve services to individuals such as testing, screening and vaccinations, behavioural counselling, or health education and advice. While only a small number of nurses may work in designated public health roles or services, many of these strategies represent 'core business' for nurses in a range of different roles and settings.

public health 'the art and science of preventing disease, prolonging life and promoting health through the organised efforts of society' (WHO, cited in Public Health Association of Australia 2018, p. 1)

Video: 'What is public health?'

The profile and visibility of public health have increased significantly in recent years, particularly in the area of 'health protection', which involves:

- ensuring the safety and quality of food, water, air and the general environment;
- preventing the transmission of communicable diseases; and
- managing disease outbreaks, natural and/or environmental disasters, and other actual or potential mass-casualty events (NHS Borders 2021).

Concerns such as climate change, immunisation, food-borne infection, seasonal influenza, healthcare-associated infections and communicable diseases have been increasingly in the public eye, none more so than the COVID-19 pandemic. While many public health measures relating to COVID-19 have been coordinated at the state, territory or local level, the Australian Health Protection Principal Committee (AHPPC), which is chaired by the Australian Chief Medical Officer and comprises all state and territory Chief Health Officers, is responsible for providing information, advice and recommendations on health protection matters and national health emergencies (AHPPC 2021). You can visit the AHPPC website to learn more about Australia's response to the pandemic, with statements on issues such as vaccination, physical distancing, testing and tracing, border control and quarantine, PPE, the wearing of masks by members of the public and protocols for schools, workplaces and aged-care settings.

Short-answer question

NURSING PERSPECTIVE

I work as a registered nurse (RN) in a screening service for a government agency. When COVID-19 cases began to emerge in Australia we had to make the difficult decision to shut down our mobile screening service. We did not know for how long. Our team was redeployed to undertake close-contact tracing. This is not the 'detective work' of contact tracing undertaken by specialists working in public health units. Rather, we phoned the 'close contacts' of people diagnosed with COVID-19: people who had been exposed to the positive cases and who therefore had to self-isolate for 14 days. We were given access to a database and scripts, depending on who we were calling – everyone from airline crew to cruise ship passengers, to residential aged-care staff. Our role was to check whether they were symptomatic or needed support, and that they were indeed staying home as instructed. Of course, we had to stay on top of the daily news reports and changing public health orders. There were lots of parallels with clinical nursing – client education, an uplifting chat, notes! Some days I spoke to 70 people in a single shift. We were pleased to play a role in managing the pandemic for our community but also felt lucky that we were not facing the risks of working in a clinical environment, like so many of our friends and colleagues. I would recommend this role, but also hope we will never be in this situation again.

Issues and trends affecting contemporary nursing and health care

The Department of Health (2017), along with other industry researchers and reviewers (e.g. Daley et al. 2018; Productivity Commission 2015; PwC 2019), has identified a range of factors that contribute to, and influence, our dynamic and changing health landscape (see Figure 5.1). These include:

- social and biological determinants of health and wellbeing, and a shift in focus from 'sick care' to 'wellness and prevention';
- opportunities and challenges, including consumer expectations (right care, place and time), the ageing population (and workforce), changing technologies and chronic disease;
- supporting regulations and infrastructure, including research and data, information technology, quality and safety, infrastructure (including a shift from institutional to community settings), and workforce requirements and trends; and
- health system expenditure and resource priorities.

With regard to nursing, many of these factors and trends were reaffirmed in the recent independent review of nursing education in Australia (Schwartz 2019). This review was underpinned by the central question: *Is the current preparation of nurses sufficient to meet the present and, more importantly, the future health needs of all Australians?* This focus on the future was considered particularly important. Australians are living longer but many older people live with the burden of complex and chronic conditions (and comorbidities) such as arthritis, diabetes and dementia (Schwartz 2019). Nursing, at all levels, must also reflect national health priorities, and one of the most urgent is mental health, including building the knowledge, skills and resilience required to protect the wellbeing of our clients, our communities and ourselves (Schwartz 2019). Many nurses currently practising in (and educationally prepared for) hospitals and acute care will be increasingly required to deliver care in the community. And the nurses of the future will also have to implement a range of advanced technologies and expand their focus on health promotion and the prevention of illness (Schwartz 2019). Increasing public debate and first-hand experiences of climate change, extreme weather events, bushfires, floods and infectious disease outbreaks (e.g. COVID-19) have also placed a spotlight on 'environmental health' issues.

Let's take a closer look at these issues and trends and explore what they might mean for health care now and into the future.

Ageing and aged care

With one of the longest life expectancies in the world, older Australians make up a steadily increasing proportion of our total population. According to the Australian Bureau of Statistics (ABS), the proportion of people aged 65 years and over in the total population is projected to increase from 15 per cent in 2017 to between 21 per cent and 23 per cent in 2066 (ABS 2017).

While this demographic change is supported by the data, it would be contentious and inappropriate to simply view 'ageing' as a health issue or 'aged care' as being synonymous with health care (Sadana & Michel 2019). However, it is generally accepted that, as people age, they experience a decline in their physical and cognitive health, which can affect their ability to live independently and to care for themselves (Aged Care Royal Commission 2019). Research commissioned by the federation of nine Councils on the Ageing (COTA) across Australia found that health was the key factor that influenced older Australians' perceptions of their quality of life. When asked what they were most concerned or worried about at this point in their life, a third (top

response) of older Australians mentioned health issues. The top reason people gave for a poor (0–4 out of 10) quality of life rating was 'health problems', while 'good health' was the top reason given for a very high (9–10) quality of life rating (COTA 2018; ABS 2017).

As the population ages and life expectancy increases, the burden of disease is shifting from acute illness to complex and chronic conditions, often involving multiple comorbidities (AIHW 2020; Schwartz 2019). This may signal a need for long-term health care such as medical, nursing and personal care services that can help with activities of daily living, the management of chronic conditions and complex medication regimens (Aged Care Royal Commission 2019). Many older Australians have also expressed particular concern about losing their cognitive capacity, their identity, independence and social connections as they age, and fear that this loss of control over one's own circumstances may lead to life in a nursing home or a lingering death in hospital (Aged Care Royal Commission 2019). This speaks to the importance of **healthy ageing** (ageing well) and **ageing in place**, and the need for social supports that emphasise action on the social determinants of health and inequity through prevention, health promotion and support for self-management, and that empower older people to have greater choice and control over the services they require to sustain their independence and participation in community life (Aged Care Sector Committee 2017; Michel 2019; WHO 2016).

healthy ageing the process of developing and maintaining the social and functional ability required to enable wellbeing in older age

ageing in place the preference for ageing (and receiving any necessary care) in one's home and community in order to maintain independence and social connectivity

Most Australians who reach older age will require some form of care and support, whether from family members and friends or from the formal care system (Aged Care Royal Commission 2019). Australia's aged-care system involves a continuum of care, from low-level to intensive support, delivered through a mix of health, social and residential services, across three main types:

- home support – providing entry-level assistance with everyday living activities for older Australians in their own homes, with a focus on supporting independence and social participation;
- home care – providing different levels of care for older people, from basic care, which includes personal care for tasks such as bathing, dressing, eating, and toileting, to more complex needs such as nursing and medical care, chronic disease management and allied health support (e.g. physiotherapy, dietetics and dentistry); and
- residential care – providing care and accommodation for people who can no longer live independently in their own homes (Aged Care Royal Commission 2019; Jeyaratnam & Jackson-Webb 2019).

In addition to these home and residential care options, there are also other programs and services to address specific needs and circumstances, including equipment and home modifications, transitional care, short-term restorative care, respite care and targeted services for specific population groups, such as the National Aboriginal and Torres Strait Islander Flexible Aged Care Program (Aged Care Royal Commission 2019).

For several decades, continuing waves of reform and numerous reviews have attempted to improve the quality, performance and sustainability of the aged-care system and its capacity to grow and meet changing demographics, demands and care expectations (Aged Care Royal Commission 2019). Despite such initiatives, public confidence in the quality of aged care and the effectiveness of the regulatory framework has continued to fall (particularly with regard to residential aged care), leading the Australian government to establish a Royal Commission into Aged Care Quality and Safety (the Aged Care Royal Commission).

After almost three years of hearings, submissions and deliberations, the Aged Care Royal Commission handed down its final report in March 2021. The Commissioners noted that the extent of substandard and unsafe care in Australia's aged-care system reflected both poor quality on the part of some aged-care providers and fundamental systemic flaws in the way the system has been designed, governed and funded (Aged Care Royal Commission 2021). Calling for fundamental reform of the aged-care system, the report set out 148 wide-ranging recommendations, including several relating specifically to ageing well, access to health care, and the roles and responsibilities, quality standards and employment arrangements (e.g. mandated ratios, skill-mix, and reduced casualisation) for RNs. Enrolled Nurses, Nurse Practitioners, Assistants in Nursing and Personal Care Workers. At the time of writing, we are yet to see a formal policy response to these recommendations but it has been encouraging to see the vital role of nurses in providing quality care and support for older Australians being recognised and promoted in this report.

Mental health care

To understand the principles and priorities of contemporary mental healthcare, we need to briefly consider the evolution of such services over time. Interestingly, in the early years of colonisation, mental illness was not even regarded as a 'health' issue, with those deemed to be 'mentally ill' (often referred to as 'lunatics' and 'inmates') being managed within the penal system without any medical input or oversight (Henderson & Roberts 2020).

This custodial system involved the 'institutionalisation' of people who were deemed to be mentally ill in asylums (sometimes called 'lunatic asylums'), which used detention and deprivation of liberty to 'punish' these people and reduce the assumed risk they posed to the wider community (Vrklevski, Eljiz & Greenfield 2017). Apart from a shift to medical control in the 1880s, this was the prevailing model up to the mid-1900s. The number of 'psychiatric patients' grew dramatically over that time, leading to the building of more asylums across the country (Henderson & Roberts 2020).

While the term psychiatric 'hospital' was increasingly used to describe these asylums, they had little resemblance to what we see or consider a hospital to be today. Unlike the contemporary focus on short-term or episodic acute and specialist care, many people in asylums remained there for years (often for the reminder of their life following the diagnosis or 'certification' of mental illness).

In the 1950s, various government reports and rising community insight and agitation triggered moves towards **deinstitutionalisation**. This was based on a belief that mental illness could be prevented (or better 'managed') through early intervention and community support, and a recognition that long-term institutionalisation had a negative effect on mental health outcomes (Henderson & Roberts 2020).

deinstitutionalisation the moving of individuals from institutional care to care in the community, and the reform or modification of an institution to remove or disguise its institutional character

Deinstitutionalisation involved the establishment of a range of community services such as community mental health centres, community housing and outpatient care for people newly diagnosed or acutely ill. It also involved the movement of older people, people with alcohol and other drug problems, and those with intellectual or cognitive disabilities into separate services and settings, and the relocation of 'inpatient care' (for acute, chronic and complex mental illness) from psychiatric hospitals to mental health units in general hospitals. State governments also invested in the development of psychological services and supports for children and young people based on the understanding that mental illness and related behaviour can be prevented or reduced through early intervention and support when (and where) these issues and behaviours first occur (Henderson & Roberts 2020).

A key feature of contemporary mental health care is the emphasis on 'health' rather than 'ill-health' (illness). According to the WHO there is 'no health without mental health' and mental health is more than just the absence of mental disorders or psychiatric symptoms (WHO 2018). In its Mental Health Action Plan 2013–2020, the WHO (2013) defined mental health as:

> a state of well-being in which the individual realises his or her own abilities, can cope with the normal stresses of life, can work productively and fruitfully, and is able to make a contribution to his or her community (p. 6).

While reform of the system needs to recognise and respond to the fact that an individual's capacity to cope and function can be diminished to varying degrees and at various times (which may or may not include diagnosis of mental illness), much of the policy and service landscape is now oriented towards the promotion, maintenance and/or restoration of 'mental health and wellbeing' (WHO 2018).

Since the 1990s, reforms in the Australian mental health system have been guided by a series of national mental health strategies, policies and plans. The early versions of these centred on the key goals of deinstitutionalisation, as highlighted earlier. Later versions focused on prevention and early intervention, the development of service partnerships, establishing improved mechanisms for consumer and carer participation, and strengthening research and evaluation. The latest reforms have shifted the focus to 'recovery oriented' services, mental health promotion and social inclusion, with an emphasis on building personal resilience and meaningful relationships with others, promoting access to suitable housing, education and employment opportunities, peer and social support, and community engagement and participation (AIHW 2021; Henderson & Roberts 2020). There is also greater emphasis on the integration and coordination of community mental health care, with the federally funded Primary Health Networks playing a key role in this regard.

As outlined above, mental health systems have experienced a global shift in recent decades from institutional care to community and consumer-centred models and approaches. There is now greater consumer and carer involvement in the design, control and management of mental health services (WHO 2013), including the transition of some people living with chronic, complex and/or long-term mental health problems (psychosocial disability) to individualised planning, funding and support arrangements under the National Disability Insurance Scheme (NDIS).

In Australia, the contemporary framework for mental health services is a complex mixture of public and private systems, with funding and service responsibilities shared between the federal, state and territory governments, non-government organisations (NGOs), religious and charitable organisations, and the private sector, including for-profit primary care and allied health services and private hospital services (AIHW 2021; Department of Parliamentary Services 2019). A range of mental health services are delivered in Australia, including inpatient services in public and private hospitals, emergency response services, residential mental health services (rehabilitation, treatment or extended-care), and community mental health services (often provided by NGOs), which support independent living, engagement in education and employment, and a range of mental health and wellbeing information, promotion and self-care programs (AIHW 2021).

Mental health is an integral part of the holistic care provided by nurses. While some may view this as a specialist area of nursing practice (which of course it can be), specialist mental health nurses are not the only health professionals who encounter people with mental health problems (Schwartz 2019). Nurses encounter people with mental health needs in all clinical settings, from primary care and community health through to medical and surgical settings, emergency departments, residential care facilities, workplaces and prisons (O'Brien 2021). Since the COVID-19 pandemic arrived in Australia in early 2020, there has been growing concern and evidence about the effect of the virus and control measures such as 'physical distancing' on the mental health of Australians, including that of frontline nurses and healthcare workers (AIHW 2021; Maben & Bridges 2020). Likewise, nursing environments themselves can be stressful, with many reports of aggression from clients and bullying from colleagues (Schwartz 2019). These issues make self-care and the promotion of mental health, wellbeing and resilience essential priorities for all nurses (Maben & Bridges; Schwartz 2019).

Of course, people with mental health problems often have other health concerns as well. According to the National Mental Health Commission (2016), 'four out of every five people living with mental illness have a co-existing physical illness'. Compared to the general population, people living with mental illness are 65 per cent more likely to smoke, and between two and six times more likely to develop cardiovascular disease, respiratory disease, diabetes, osteoporosis and dental problems. Moreover, 'people with co-existing mental and physical illness are twice as likely as people with only one physical or mental illness, and eight times more likely than people with no physical or mental illness, to struggle with regular functional activities' (National Mental Health Commission 2016).

Because of their focus on the whole person, and the likelihood of encountering such issues in a range of healthcare settings and contexts, nurses are especially well placed to help people with both psychological and physical needs through treatment, education, health promotion, prevention and self-management strategies (Schwartz 2019).

Prevention and health promotion

Prevention and health promotion are core priorities of public health and build on the vision and principles of PHC (as discussed earlier) by providing a framework for action on the social determinants of health and for empowering individuals and communities to have greater control and self-reliance over their own health and wellbeing.

Preventative health (prevention)

Prevention is essentially about looking at 'upstream' risk factors and determinants for ill-health, with the aim of removing or modifying these to eliminate, reduce or delay the occurrence of health problems 'downstream'.

In Chapter 4 we introduced the idea of primary, secondary and tertiary 'levels of care'. Preventative measures can also be provided at these three levels. Primary prevention focuses on prevention of actual disease or injury. This may include, for example, immunisation programs, anti-smoking campaigns, seatbelt laws, drink-driving campaigns, and nutrition or physical activity programs. Secondary prevention aims to reduce the damage caused by an existing injury or disease. Examples might include the provision of wound care and prophylactic antibiotics to reduce the chances of infection, or substitution or diversional strategies (e.g. nicotine gum or patches, physical activity, breathing exercises) to help quit or reduce smoking. Tertiary prevention aims to minimise disability or long-term damage or disadvantage that might follow a disease or injury through the provision of medical care, rehabilitation and self-management strategies. For example, a person living with diabetes might monitor their own blood-glucose levels at home and then modify their diet and medications according to a predetermined self-management plan (Liamputtong 2019). The key message here is that prevention is not only applicable 'before the event' but can also be applied with individuals or groups to reduce the consequences or progression of an existing health issue.

In Australia, health prevention activities have long played a part in improving the health of the population (AIHW 2016). Some prevention activities target all people in a given population (e.g. fluoridation of water, sewerage systems), while others target particular groups based on age or other risk factors (e.g. breast or prostate cancer screening for different age-groups and genders), or even individuals who may have secondary or tertiary prevention strategies included in their chronic disease self-management plans (AIHW 2016). A recent example might be strategies such as sanitation (e.g. hand hygiene and mask-wearing), quarantine, vaccinations and community or workplace safeguards (e.g. physical distancing and lockdowns) implemented during the COVID-19 pandemic.

Short-answer question

Health promotion

health promotion the process of enabling people to increase control over, and to improve, their health

Health promotion embraces the view that health is a state of complete physical, mental and social wellbeing. It recognises that health is a fundamental human right, essential for a long and happy life, and something we all strive for (VicHealth 2021). According to the Victorian Health Promotion Foundation (VicHealth 2021), health promotion is a set of actions that foster good health and wellbeing. It involves working in partnership with individuals, communities, organisations and policymakers on actions that:

- inform people of what they can do to stay healthy;
- empower and enable people to exercise greater control over their own health and to make better health choices and decisions; and
- address the things in the community that influence health and wellbeing the most, thereby promoting health and preventing ill-health of individuals, groups and communities.

Health promotion action may be geared towards the population as a whole or at individuals in their everyday lives.

The Ottawa Charter for Health Promotion

The Ottawa Charter is a clear statement of action for health promotion that is widely used to guide health promotion practice. The Ottawa Charter came out of the first International Conference on Health Promotion, held in Ottawa, Canada in November 1986. The conference aimed to establish an action framework for achieving the primary healthcare goal of 'health for all' (WHO 1986).

The Ottawa Charter sets out five action areas that are considered essential for health promotion success:

- build healthy public policy;
- create supportive environments;
- strengthen community action;
- develop personal skills; and
- reorient health services (WHO 1986).

While evidence strongly supports a multi-pronged and multisectoral approach across all five action areas (especially when the aim is large-scale population change), this is unlikely to fit with the practice context or role of most nurses. Even so, every nurse can (and should) incorporate health promotion into their practice. This could include providing health education for a client (building their health literacy) as a strategy for 'developing personal skills', or advocating for the redesign of the clinical setting to make it more accessible or friendly for children, families or people with dementia, for example as a strategy to 'create supportive environments'.

Video: 'Understanding health promotion'

Multiple-choice question

> ## REFLECTION 5.2
>
> What are some of the health promotion, or prevention strategies or actions you would like to incorporate in your own practice or workplace?

Technology in health care

Central to many of the trends, opportunities and priorities in health care is the growing and changing role of technology.

Nursing and health care in the digital age

> Digital initiatives in health have the potential to affect every aspect of care delivery, delivering significant results in assisting patients to make smarter choices, improving the utilisation of time and resources, assisting in the coordination of services across the care continuum, enhancing real-time communication, supporting continuous patient monitoring, expanding access to evidence-based resources and increasing the time available for patient interaction at the point of care (Bichel-Findlay 2019, p. 14).

e-Health and **health informatics** are terms or concepts that are often used in reference to digital health.

Connecting with practice: Health technology

e-health an 'umbrella term' for the range of technologies that are used to support, enable and promote health care, health management and health information

health informatics the term used to describe the design, development, adoption and application of information technology-based innovations in healthcare service delivery, management and planning

Video: e-Health

Today, many Australians use digital technology to monitor their own health and to engage with health information, services and professionals (often remotely) (AIHW 2018). For example, they might wear a fitness device to record how much exercise they do, use a smartphone to keep track of what they eat, or collect and transmit health information and data to a health professional in 'real time' (AIHW 2018).

For individuals, this technology can help to track and control their own health information and inform self-management decisions (Infrastructure Australia 2019). For service providers, it can support continuity of care, strengthen interactions and information-sharing between providers and clients, support real-time and remote monitoring of clients' health-related activities and status (thereby promoting independence) and improve the quality, safety and efficiency of services (Department of Health 2021; Infrastructure Australia 2019).

The power and potential of digital technology in health care is reflected in the following statistics (Department of Health 2021, AIHW 2018):

- 86 per cent of households have internet access
- 88 per cent of people aged 18–75 years own or have access to a smartphone
- 78 per cent of adults use the internet to find health-related information
- 96 per cent of general practitioners (GPs) use computers for clinical purposes
- by April 2020, there were more than 22.75 million personally controlled electronic health records (My Health Record) in Australia.

Tele-health

One example of e-health is tele-health. Originally describing the use of video-conferencing to facilitate consultation at a distance, tele-health has evolved over time and the term is now used more generally to describe 'any technology-mediated communication that facilitates clinical care' (Coiera 2015, p. 343). Tele-health may involve the transmission of voice, data, images and information, which reduces the need for healthcare recipients and professionals to travel or be physically present. This has been especially beneficial in improving healthcare access and equity for people living in regional, rural and remote areas. More recently, tele-health has become a mainstream option for delivering physically distant health care during a pandemic. It can encompass diagnosis, treatment, monitoring, education, health promotion and self-management aspects of health care (Department of Health 2021).

Multiple-choice question

m-Health

m-Health is a term used for health care supported by mobile devices such as smartphones, tablets and laptop computers. These may be used by nurses to access healthcare information and evidence, record clinical health data in the community or at the bedside, and for real-time monitoring of clients (Cummings, Macdonald & Arnott 2021). m-Health also includes the use of wearable sensing devices and mobile apps to track or monitor clients' activity, diet, mood, vital signs, blood-glucose levels and other clinical data, which can often be transmitted to health professionals in real time or uploaded at a later consultation to support treatment decisions and client education (Cummings et al. 2021). Many m-health devices also include built-in artificial intelligence (AI), which can detect and report early signs of deterioration or complications.

The increased attention on health promotion and self-management has seen an explosion of health and fitness apps for personal use. There are literally thousands of these apps currently available, from fitness monitors to diet and exercise planning, brain games and stress-busting techniques; there's an app for just about everything to help people achieve their personal health goals (or so the marketers say). Of course, the quality and efficacy of such apps needs to be a key consideration. Fortunately, a variety of reviews, studies and trials have been undertaken to help guide consumers on the best options available in a range of categories.

Connecting with practice: Healthy living apps

Electronic health records

In Australia, one of the government's digital health priorities has been the introduction of a personally controlled electronic health record (EHR), known as My Health Record. This platform stores a person's health information and records, which the person and their authorised healthcare providers can then access securely online from any device connected to the internet, to assist them to make decisions and plan any necessary care (Department of Health 2021, Cummings et al. 2021, AIHW 2018). Clients can give permission for health professionals anywhere in the country to access their relevant history. Healthcare providers can upload information to the record to supplement information added by the client or other health professionals. A key feature of My Health Record is the option for clients to record information about their own health and wellbeing, which can be shared with healthcare providers as required, supporting clients to be active participants in their own care, including self-management (Cummings et al. 2021).

By April 2020:

Multiple-choice question

- There were more than 22.75 million My Health Records.
- Around 91 per cent of pharmacies, 92 per cent of GPs and 94 per cent of hospital services were registered to use the My Health Record System.
- There were more than 65 million clinical documents, over 128 million medicine documents and more than 304 000 documents provided by record-holders themselves contained in My Health Records (Department of Health 2021).

Videos: My Health Record

But not all technology is 'digital'

A range of assistive devices and technologies can assist people in their daily lives to optimise functioning, promote safety and improve access, mobility and independence.

Assistive technology can, of course, include digital innovations such as 'smart homes' (home automation and environmental control systems) and specialised computers and communication aids, but this is not always the case. Other assistive technologies include modified vehicles, wheelchairs, bathboards, knives with built-up handles and simple products that assist people with everyday tasks such as opening a jar or bottle, turning a tap or opening a door.

Many other technological innovations are emerging in health care, including robotics, 3D printing, virtual reality and gamification. At the end of this chapter we encourage you to do some further research on how these technologies might influence nursing practice and client outcomes in the future.

Connecting with practice: Independent Living Centres Australia

Environmental health

The WHO (2020) estimates that healthier environments (avoiding known environmental risks) could prevent almost one-quarter of the burden of disease – around 13 million deaths each year – globally. **Environmental health** is not just about climate change; it encompasses clean air, safe water, food security, sanitation, safe workplaces, safe use of chemicals, health-supporting built environments (including hospitals and residential facilities), waste management, infection prevention and control, and measures that sustain and preserve biodiversity. All of these factors influence health outcomes and challenge health equity (WHO 2020).

Climate change

Climate change is occurring at an unprecedented rate. This significantly affects social and environmental determinants of health, which in turn influence individual and population health outcomes. Since 2015, the world has experienced the five hottest years on record. Extremes in weather, including exposure to storms, droughts and bushfires, compromise human health and may affect work capacity and infrastructure (Cook 2018). Health is affected through direct mechanisms, such as extreme weather events and temperature-related incidents, and indirect mechanisms, such as air pollution, water quality and rising sea levels (ICN 2018).

Natural disasters and respiratory health

Air pollution is linked to many diseases, including asthma, chronic obstructive pulmonary disease (COPD), bronchitis, pneumonia and cardiovascular disease (Barria 2019). In Australia, for example, we feel the regular effects of summer bushfires, and cases of thunderstorm asthma, where meteorological factors combine with high allergen loads in the air to trigger bronchospasm in susceptible people, were recently seen and reported. Barria (2019) proposed that in cases of natural disaster nurses have a role in four phases: mitigation, preparation, response and recovery. Mitigation includes health promotion activities and professional and public education regarding health risk factors. In the preparation phase, nurses can help people understand what to do to protect their health and stay safe during the disaster; for example, how to best prevent smoke inhalation during a bushfire. Nurse responses to disasters will vary depending on their practice roles and workplaces, and their own personal circumstances. Recovery occurs at the personal and community levels, and may involve nursing activities such as education, advocacy and support for self-management.

Food insecurity

Food insecurity is the lack of consistent access to enough quality and variety of food for an active, healthy life. While socio-economic factors may contribute to this, a range of environmental determinants can lead to food insecurity (for example, unfavourable environmental conditions or drought, flood or fire events impacting food crops). This can lead to poor health outcomes, including stress, depression, anxiety and chronic health conditions such as hypertension, hypercholesterolaemia and type 2 diabetes (Grenier & Wynn 2018). Negative health outcomes may arise from poor nutrition, inability to meet requirements of diet-dependent conditions such as diabetes, non-adherence to treatment or medication regimens, stress and isolation (Spitzer, Shenk & Mabli 2020).

environmental health involves aspects of public health concerned with the factors, circumstances and conditions in the environment or our surroundings that influence health and wellbeing)

climate change a change in climate attributed directly or indirectly to human activity that alters the composition of the global atmosphere and that is, in addition to natural climate variability, observed over comparable time periods (UN 1992)

Short-answer question

CASE STUDY

The Rush Surplus Project

The Rush Surplus Project is a nurse-led initiative in the United States that decreases hospital food waste by donating unused hospital cafeteria food to local shelters, for distribution to food-insecure individuals. It provides around 700 meals per month, benefiting around 8400 people per year, and saving nearly 4000 kilograms of food from going to landfill.

There is a Rush Surplus Project Guidebook available for nurses interested in piloting a similar program elsewhere. Considerations include:

- What are your local health department rules?
- What local data is available to prompt a food surplus project?
- Who is the target population?
- Is there system-level support for the program?
- Who will be involved, and what internal and external resources can help?
- How will you measure and evaluate success?

QUESTIONS

1 How could you go about getting a program such as this set up in your workplace (or university)?

2 What might need to be considered or adapted to make this a success in your setting?

Infectious diseases

New, emerging and re-emerging infectious diseases are increasing around the world. These infectious diseases can be foodborne, airborne or vector-borne (transmitted by mosquitoes, fleas and ticks) (McArthur 2019). Some are zoonotic diseases, which are transmitted from animals to humans through direct contact or through food, water and the environment. For example, COVID-19 is a novel zoonotic disease caused by the virus SARS-CoV-2. It is still unclear how this virus moved from animals to humans, although the incidence of zoonoses is increasing as humans live in closer contact with animals and/or encounter animals in new geographic regions (McArthur 2019). Demographic change, global trade, global travel and climate change are all cited as drivers of infectious disease outbreaks. This may be further influenced further by increased population density, forestry and agricultural expansion (habitat loss bringing some animals into closer proximity to humans), environmental stress, environmental contamination and changing vector habitats – warmer temperatures allowing mosquitoes to move to new areas, for example (McArthur 2019).

Multiple-choice question

I'm an RN and I recently completed an accredited certificate in immunisation to prepare for some public health work in administering the COVID-19 vaccine. The vaccine roll-out is occurring in stages and I am currently working with priority groups in a large public hospital, vaccinating frontline health workers, and some residential aged-care facilities, vaccinating residents and staff. As the roll-out expands to the broader population, I have been advised that I may be deployed to a community pharmacy, a 'mass-vaccination' centre/hub, or even a school or university. I am enjoying working in different places and with different people for such a positive outcome!

So, what can nurses do?

Nurses see many of the challenges that communities and clients face as a consequence of current and future environmental threats. As stakeholders, nurses have the power to influence changes that can lead to more positive environmental health outcomes (Cook 2018).

Research on nurses' perceptions of environmental health and its application to nursing reveals a growing awareness and interest in related issues, but also challenges faced by the profession, and barriers to finding opportunities to influence and apply change (Hanley & Jakubec 2019). Relating environmental health to particular practice contexts or settings can be difficult. Some may see this as being the domain of others (e.g. public health nurses), and many nurses do not know how (or have the support) to apply change in their own workplaces (Kalogirou et al. 2020).

A variety of resources are available to assist with your engagement in environmental health. Two policies of the Australian Nursing & Midwifery Federation (ANMF), *Climate change* (2018a) and *Health and the environment* (2018b), provide guidance for nurses, midwives and assistants in nursing to participate in debate, identify opportunities in their workplaces to shape policy, conduct relevant research, be educated about current and future effects of climate change on public health, and implement and showcase nursing initiatives that address climate change and healthy environments. In addition, the ICN has a position statement calling on governments to finance climate-resilient health systems, including developing sustainable healthcare worker practices, and to invest in climate change and public health research, monitoring and surveillance (ICN 2018).

Short-answer question

You can also seek out information and opportunities through related professional associations and networks. This might include Australia's Climate and Health Alliance (CAHA 2021), which leads the Our Climate Our Health campaign for a national strategy on climate, health and wellbeing; the Alliance of Nurses for Healthy Environments; and the Global Green and Healthy Hospitals (GGHH) network, an international community of hospitals and health organisations working together to share best practices and find solutions for promoting environmental health and sustainability.

REFLECTION 5.3

What environmental health programs or initiatives would you like to see occur or be a part of at your university or workplace?

SUMMARY

- Understandings of health are influenced by different social, cultural, political and theoretical perspectives and experiences. Several models of health have been proposed (see Chapter 4) but they all essentially stem from two contrasting models: the biomedical model and the social model. The biomedical model views health from a deficit or disease perspective and focuses on diagnosis and intervention to treat, fix or cure these biological problems. The social model views health as a positive and holistic concept (wellness) and focuses on promoting health and preventing ill-health by acting upon the social, cultural and environmental determinants and conditions that positively influence and shape the wellbeing of individuals, communities and entire populations. It is important to be aware of these different perspectives on health and wellbeing. They not only influence different healthcare roles and ways of working, but also guide how nurses think, act and make decisions in practice and support their engagement in person-centred, empathetic, and respectful relationships with clients and their supporters.
- There are different types or models of health care that arise from the biomedical and social models of health – acute care, primary care, primary healthcare and public health. In Australia's current health landscape, these have been represented across four tiers (see Figure 5.1), each influencing healthcare services in various ways. The first two tiers are aligned with the social model of health, reflecting the broad range of social, cultural and environmental determinants that influence health and wellbeing, and emphasising health promotion and disease prevention, which are key priorities of PHC and public health approaches. The third tier is primary and community care. This includes elements of health promotion and social support but is dominated by general practice, pharmacy and allied health services, which mostly involve a biomedical approach to health care. The fourth tier involves biomedically oriented specialist and acute care delivered mainly through hospitals and residential services. Although depicted as the smallest tier, these services receive the greatest policy attention and the majority of healthcare funding in Australia.
- Based on changing demographics and service demands (e.g. an ageing population and workforce); national health priorities (e.g. mental health and chronic conditions); calls for improved quality, safety and efficiency of services (e.g. the Aged Care Royal Commission, COVID-safety protocols); and a shift in focus from 'sick care' to wellness and prevention; this chapter has explored ageing and aged care, mental health, health promotion and prevention, technology and environmental health as key issues, trends and priorities influencing nursing and health care now and into the future.

Suggested responses

REVIEW QUESTIONS

1 How do different models of health influence health care?
2 What are the key priorities in contemporary mental health reform?
3 What is the central premise of preventative health?
4 What are some of the reported benefits of nursing and health care in the 'digital age'?
5 Is 'environmental health' just about climate change?

RESEARCH TOPIC

Research some of the emerging technologies in health care – AI, virtual reality, robotics and 3D printing, for example. How do you think these technologies might influence nursing practice (benefits and limitations) and client outcomes over the next ten years?

FURTHER READING

Aged Care Royal Commission (2021). *Final report: care, dignity and respect. Volume 1 – Summary and recommendations*. Canberra: Australian Government. Available from https://agedcare.royalcommission.gov.au/publications/final-report-volume-1.

Australian Government (2020). Collection of environmental health publications. Available from https://www1.health.gov.au/internet/main/publishing.nsf/Content/health-pubhlth-publicat-environ.htm.

Australian Institute of Health and Welfare (AIHW) (2020). *Australia's health 2020: Digital health snapshot*. Available from https://www.aihw.gov.au/reports/australias-health/digital-health.

World Health Organization (WHO) (2018). *Mental health: Strengthening our response*. Available from https://www.who.int/news-room/fact-sheets/detail/mental-health-strengthening-our-response.

REFERENCES

Aged Care Royal Commission (2019). *Navigating the maze: An overview of Australia's current aged care system*. Background Paper 1. Canberra: Australian Government. Retrieved from https://agedcare.royalcommission.gov.au/sites/default/files/2019-12/background-paper-1.pdf.

——— (2021). *Final report: Care, dignity and respect. Volume 1 – Summary and recommendations*. Canberra: Australian Government. Retrieved from https://agedcare.royalcommission.gov.au/publications/final-report-volume-1.

Aged Care Sector Committee (2017). *Aged Care Sector Statement of Principles*. Canberra: Australian Government Department of Health. Retrieved from https://www.health.gov.au/resources/publications/aged-care-sector-statement-of-principles.

Australian Bureau of Statistics (ABS) (2017). *Population projections in Australia, 2017 (base) – 2066*. Cat. no. 3222.0. Retrieved from http://www.abs.gov.au.

Australian Institute of Health and Welfare (AIHW) (2016). *Australia's health 2016: Health promotion and prevention*. Retrieved from https://www.aihw.gov.au/

getmedia/8913d477-33cc-4edd-8246-ef4ed1a0851d/ah16-6-1-prevention-health-promotion.pdf.aspx.

—— (2018). *Australia's health 2018: Digital health*. Retrieved from https://www.aihw.gov.au/getmedia/95830c0a-ee53-4f95-a6a4-860190e4bd66/aihw-aus-221-chapter-2-4.pdf.aspx.

—— (2020). *Chronic disease: Overview*. Retrieved from https://www.aihw.gov.au/reports-data/health-conditions-disability-deaths/chronic-disease/overview.

—— (2021). *Mental health services in Australia*. Retrieved from https://www.aihw.gov.au/reports/mental-health-services/mental-health-services-in-australia/report-contents/summary-of-mental-health-services-in-australia/overview-of-mental-health-services-in-australia.

Australian Nursing & Midwifery Federation (2018a). *ANMF policy: Climate change*. Retrieved from https://anmf.org.au/documents/policies/P_Climate_Change.pdf.

—— (2018b). *ANMF policy: Health and the environment*. Retrieved from https://anmf.org.au/documents/policies/P_Health_Environment.pdf.

Australian Primary Health Care Nurses Association (APNA) (2021). *General practice nursing*. Retrieved from https://www.apna.asn.au/profession/what-is-primary-health-care-nursing/general-practice-nursing

Barria, R.M. (2019). Wildfires as a public health problem: A setting for nursing in disasters. *Investigacion & Educacion En Enfermeria*, 37(3), 7–10.

Baum, F. (2016). *The new public health*, 4th edn. Oxford: Oxford University Press.

Bichel-Findlay, J. (2019). The nursing profession in a digital age. *The Hive*, 28(Summer 2019/20), 14–15.

Clendon, J. & Munns, A. (2019). *Community health and wellness: Principles of primary health care*, 6th edn. Sydney: Elsevier.

Climate and Health Alliance (2021). Global green and healthy hospitals. Retrieved from https://www.caha.org.au/globalgreen_healthyhospitals.

Coiera, E. (2015). *Guide to health informatics*, 3rd edn. Boca Raton, FL: CRC Press, Taylor & Francis.

Cook, C. (2018). Climate change and health: Nurses as drivers of climate action. *Interdisciplinary Journal of Partnership Studies*, 5(1).

Councils on the Ageing (COTA) (2018). *State of the (older) nation*. Retrieved from https://www.cota.org.au/policy/state-of-the-older-nation/.

Cummings, E., Macdonald, B. & Arnott, N. (2021). Putting the 'e' in health. In J. Crisp, C. Douglas, G. Rebeiro & D. Waters (eds), *Potter & Perry's fundamentals of nursing*, 6th edn. Sydney: Elsevier.

Daley, J., Duckett. S., Goss, P., Terrill, M., Wood, D., Wood, T. & Coates, B. (2018). *State orange book 2018: Policy priorities for states and territories*. Grattan Institute. Retrieved from https://grattan.edu.au/report/state-orange-book-2018.

Department of Health (2014). *Overview of environmental health*. Retrieved from https://www1.health.gov.au/internet/main/publishing.nsf/Content/health-pubhlth-strateg-envhlth-index.htm.

—— (2017). *Australia's health landscape infographic*. Retrieved from https://www.health.gov.au/resources/publications/australias-health-landscape-infographic.

—— (2021). *Health technology*. Retrieved from https://www.health.gov.au/health-topics/health-technology.

Department of Parliamentary Services (2019). *Mental health in Australia: A quick guide*. Retrieved from https://parlinfo.aph.gov.au/parlInfo/download/library/prspub/6497249/upload_binary/6497249.pdf.

Grenier, J. & Wynn, N. (2018). A nurse-led intervention to address food insecurity in Chicago. *Online Journal of Issues in Nursing*, 23(3), 1.

Guzys, D. (2021). Community and primary healthcare. In D. Guzys, R. Brown, E. Halcomb & D. Whitehead (eds), *An introduction to community and primary healthcare*, 3rd edn. Melbourne: Cambridge University Press, pp. 3–20.

Hanley, F. & Jakubec, S.L. (2019). Beyond the slogans: Understanding the ecological consciousness of nurses to advance ecological knowledge and practice. *Creative Nursing*, 25(3), 232–40.

Haslam, S.A., McMahon, C., Cruwys, T., Haslam, C., Jetten, J. & Steffens, N.K. (2018). Social cure, what social cure? The propensity to underestimate the importance of social factors for health. *Social Science & Medicine*, 198, 14–21.

Henderson, J. & Roberts, L. (2020). Organising care for the mentally ill in Australia. In L. Reynolds, E. Willis & T. Rudge (eds), *Understanding the Australian health care system*, 4th edn. Sydney: Elsevier.

Hirshon, J.M., Risko, N., Calvello, E.J.B., de Ramirez, S.S., Narayan, M., Theodosisa, C. & O'Neill, J. (2013). Health systems and services: The role of acute care. *Bulletin of the World health Organization*, 91, 386–8.

Infrastructure Australia (2019). *Australian Infrastructure Audit*. Retrieved from https://www.infrastructureaustralia.gov.au/sites/default/files/2019-08/Australian%20Infrastructure%20Audit%202019%20-%206.%20Social%20Infrastructure.pdf.

International Council of Nurses (2018). *Position statement: Nurses, climate change and health*. Retrieved from https://www.icn.ch/sites/default/files/inline-files/ICN%20PS%20Nurses%252c%20climate%20change%20and%20health%20FINAL%20.pdf.

Jeyaratnam, E. & Jackson-Webb, F. (2019). Confused about aged care in the home? These 10 charts explain how it works. *The Conversation*, 21 March. Retrieved from https://theconversation.com/confused-about-aged-care-in-the-home-these-10-charts-explain-how-it-works-113923.

Kalogirou, M.R., Dahlke, S., Davidson, S. & Yamamoto, S. (2020). Nurses' perspectives on climate change, health and nursing practice. *Journal of Clinical Nursing*, 29(23/24), 4759–68.

Keleher, H. (2020a). Primary health care in Australia. In L. Reynolds, E. Willis & T. Rudge (eds), *Understanding the Australian health care system*, 4th edn. Sydney: Elsevier.

——— (2020b). Public health in Australia. In L. Reynolds, E. Willis & T. Rudge (eds), *Understanding the Australian health care system*, 4th edn. Sydney: Elsevier.

Liamputtong, P. (ed.) (2019). *Public health: Local and global perspectives*, 2nd edn. Melbourne: Cambridge University Press.

Maben, J. & Bridges, J. (2020). COVID-19: Supporting nurses' psychological and mental health. *Journal of Clinical Nursing*, 29(15–16), 2742–50.

McArthur, D.B. (2019). Emerging infectious diseases. *The Nursing Clinics of North America*, 54(2), 297–311.

McCormack, B. & McCance, T. (2016). *Person-centred nursing and health care: Theory and practice*, 2nd edn. Oxford: Blackwell.

Michel, J.-P. (2019). *Prevention of chronic diseases and age-related disability*. New York: Springer.

National Mental Health Commission (2016). *Improving the physical health and wellbeing of people living with mental illness in Australia*. Retrieved from https://www.mentalhealthcommission.gov.au/getmedia/567c9dbe-3d53-4a0c-96ef-88428edf5064/Equally-Well-Consensus-Statement.

NHS Borders (2021). Health Protection Team. Retrieved from https://www.nhsborders.scot.nhs.uk/patients-and-visitors/our-services/general-services/health-protection-team.

O'Brien, A. (2021). Working in the mental health sector. In J. Crisp, C. Douglas, G. Rebeiro & D. Waters (eds), *Potter & Perry's fundamentals of nursing*, 6th edn. Sydney: Elsevier

Pricewaterhouse Coopers (PwC) (2019). *Reimagining healthcare in Australia: Budget 2018 – progress towards reform*. Retrieved from https://www.pwc.com.au/health/federal-budget-health-8aug18.pdf.

Productivity Commission (2015). *Efficiency in health*. Commission research paper. Canberra: Commonwealth of Australia. Retrieved from https://www.pc.gov.au/research/completed/efficiency-health/efficiency-health.pdf.

Public Health Association of Australia (PHAA) (2018). *What is public health?* Retrieved from https://www.phaa.net.au/documents/item/2757.

Reynolds, L., Willis, E. & Rudge, T. (2020). *Understanding the Australian health care system*, 4th edn. Sydney: Elsevier.

Sadana, R. & Michel, J.-P. (2019). Healthy ageing: What is it and how to describe it. In J.-P. Michel (ed.), *Prevention of chronic diseases and age-related disability*. New York: Springer.

Schwartz, S. (2019). *Educating the nurse of the future: Report of the independent review of nursing education*. Canberra: Australian Government.

Spitzer, A.K.-L., Shenk, M.P.R. & Mabli, J.G. (2020). Food insecurity is directly associated with the use of health services for adverse health events among older adults. *Journal of Nutrition*, 150(12), 3152–60.

Stein-Parbury, J. (2018). *Patient and person: Interpersonal skills in nursing*, 6th edn. Sydney: Elsevier.

United Nations (UN) (1992). *United National Convention on Climate Change (UNCCC)*. Geneva: UN.

Victorian Health Promotion Foundation (VicHealth) (2021). *Health Promotion*. Retrieved from https://www.vichealth.vic.gov.au/about/health-promotion#.

Vrklevski, L., Eljiz, K. & Greenfield, D. (2017). The evolution and devolution of mental health services in Australia. *Inquiries*, 9(10), 1–2.

World Health Organization (WHO) (1946). *Constitution*. New York: WHO. Retrieved from https://apps.who.int/gb/bd/PDF/bd47/EN/constitution-en.pdf?ua=1.

——— (1986). *The Ottawa Charter for Health Promotion*. Retrieved from https://www.who.int/teams/health-promotion/enhanced-wellbeing/first-global-conference.

——— (2013). *Mental health action plan: 2013–2020*. Geneva: WHO.

——— (2016). *Global strategy and action plan on ageing and health*. Retrieved from https://www.who.int/ageing/global-strategy/en/.

——— (2018). *Mental health: Strengthening our response*. Retrieved from https://www.who.int/news-room/fact-sheets/detail/mental-health-strengthening-our-response.

——— (2020). *WHO global strategy on health, environment and climate change: The transformation needed to improve lives and well-being sustainably through healthy environments*. Geneva: WHO.

——— (2021). *What is PHC?* Retrieved from https://www.who.int/activities/what-is-PHC.

WHO & UNICEF (1978). *Declaration of Alma-Ata*. Retrieved from https://www.who.int/publications/almaata_declaration_en.pdf.

PART 2

Becoming

6 The heart of nursing

Melanie Eslick, Lolita Wikander and Nick Arnott

With acknowledgement to Danielle Williams
for her contributions to the first edition.

LEARNING OBJECTIVES

At the completion of this chapter, you should be able to:

1 Discuss some of the common perspectives on nursing and how these inform or influence what you consider to be the 'heart of nursing'.
2 Describe your motivation for becoming a nurse and identify some career goals.
3 Reflect on what it means to be a nurse and your emerging sense of your own professional identity.
4 Explain the notions of caring, compassion and kindness that are central to the heart of nursing.

Introduction

What is the 'heart of nursing'? An answer to this question cannot be simply told or taught: it requires a process of discovery that emerges through one's learning, observations, interactions and experiences *of* and *in* this great profession. The heart of nursing is intrinsically linked to what you do as a nurse and why you do it, but it is also about *how* you do it – the ways in which you represent and enact the core values and intention of the profession.

People choose to enter and remain in a nursing career for a variety of reasons. While some of your views and beliefs are likely to be shared with other students and nurses, your reasons for wanting to be a nurse and what you consider to be at the heart of nursing will vary depending on your personal perspectives and experiences, and the external views and influences to which you are exposed along the way. This chapter begins by considering some of the common perspectives on nursing, noting how your own perspective is likely to change as you progress through your studies and into practice. We look at why people choose nursing, the different views and influences they are likely to encounter and the diverse range of roles and settings in which they may work. We then discuss how all of this informs what it means to be a nurse, and your own emerging sense of professional identity. The chapter concludes by exploring the notions of caring, compassion and kindness – concepts that we believe lie at the very heart of nursing, even though they are likely to be understood, applied and experienced differently in the context of each nurse's own practice.

Perspectives on nursing

> No, it's not glamorous, the hours are unsociable and it's hard, but at the same time it's a rewarding and exciting profession (Gracia 2016).

A person's perspective on nursing is determined by a variety of factors. In most parts of the world, nursing is a female-dominated profession, so perspectives on nursing are likely to be influenced to some extent by the way a given society views women (Lin et al. 2015). Other social, cultural or religious views may also influence these perspectives, along with the ways in which nurses are portrayed in popular culture and the media (Gill & Baker 2019). Of course, your own values, observations and experiences will probably have the most profound influence on the way you perceive and practise nursing, and on your personal ideas of what it means to be a nurse. The first section of this chapter considers some common perspectives of nursing, with links to other chapters where these ideas are explored in greater depth.

Short-answer question

The student perspective

As noted in Chapter 1, there is a good chance that the conception, definition or perspective of nursing you had when you first commenced your degree was influenced by your personal values and beliefs (see Chapter 10 for a discussion of the importance of self-awareness and emotional intelligence in nursing); any personal experiences you may have had with the healthcare system; the views or experiences of family members and friends; and depictions of nurses in the media (Gill & Baker 2019; McKenna, Brooks & Vanderheide 2017).

When you begin studying nursing, it is possible that your perspective has been informed, at least in part, by some of the scientific, technical or 'hands-on' aspects of nursing you may have observed or experienced. You are also likely to see nursing as a **caring** profession, and your desire to care for people in meaningful ways may have been a strong motivating factor in your decision to study nursing (McKenna et al. 2017). Caring means different things to different people, and thus you will care, or enact caring, differently in your own practice. Caring is a central phenomenon in nursing. We explore some of the theories and conceptualisations of caring later in this chapter to guide your own understanding and application of this important concept.

The final thing to note about your own perspective on nursing is that it is not a 'fixed' concept. As you progress through your degree program, your perspective will continue to evolve and change – perhaps subtly or possibly even profoundly – as you learn more about different roles and the profession, and as you observe and work alongside more experienced nurses in different roles and settings during your clinical placements. Your own professional identity as a nurse – how you perceive yourself in the profession (Browne et al. 2018) – may change over time, too. You can read more about professional identity later in this chapter.

The experienced nurse perspective

We cannot present a single or universal experienced nurse perspective here, as every nurse's background, experiences and practices are different. Just as your own perspective on nursing is likely to differ from those of other students, experienced nurses also have different perspectives, informed by their own career and experiences. Remember that your own views will also change as you progress from being a student to becoming a more experienced nurse. Learning is often described as a continuous or lifelong process, and nursing is a diverse and dynamic profession. Your perspective will continue to develop as your experience grows and you take on new roles, pursue new opportunities and work with different clients and colleagues. Your idea of caring and what it means to care will also evolve in response to different experiences, practice areas and client groups. For some, your perception of nursing, and your pathways within the profession, may closely mirror your early expectations. However, many graduates may come to realise that nursing is completely different from what they thought it would be, and their career may develop in directions they had never considered (or maybe were not even aware of) when they entered the profession. This is one of the things that makes nursing such an exciting and fulfilling career.

The public perspective

Members of the public are generally exposed to many of the same factors and influences as you are (direct experience, friends and family, media), so their perspectives of nursing and nurses are likely to be similar to your own when you commenced this degree. Some of these public images, stereotypes and perspectives are explored further in Chapter 8.

A person's (or society's) perspective on nursing may also be different depending on where they are from. Nursing is a global profession, and nursing has developed differently in different countries. It is important to remember that our colonial and convict history (Lewis 2014) as well as Florence Nightingale's legacy (Haynes 2020; Reinking 2020) have played a big part in how nursing is perceived and has evolved in Australia. However, this is not necessarily the developmental path nursing has taken in other parts of the world. For example, nursing in India has historically been regarded as a stigmatised and low-status profession, although this perspective is slowly changing due to the forces of globalisation (Timmons, Evans & Nair 2016).

REFLECTION 6.1

Do some research on the development of nursing in a country other than Australia, the United States, Canada or the United Kingdom (which all have similar systems to our own) to see how it is different from the development or evolution of nursing in Australia. Does the public perspective of nurses and nursing in your chosen country differ from the perspectives discussed in this chapter?

Traditional social and cultural values may also determine or influence how the public perceives the nursing profession (ten Hoeve, Jansen & Roodbol 2013). The way a society views women may be intrinsically linked to the way it views nurses (Lin et al. 2015). In their research, Lin and colleagues (2015) found that the religiously influenced patriarchy that existed in their study community often viewed (or degraded) women as being a secondary class in society. The findings from this study found that people (men and women) with this intrinsic religious or cultural orientation were more likely to consider nurses (who were mainly female) as having no great professional knowledge and to rate their professional skills as unreliable. Some of these traditional or cultural perceptions of nursing have been challenged in recent times as the wider public has been exposed, in person or through the media, to the dedication, knowledge and professionalism of nurses around the globe during the COVID-19 pandemic, often operating in situations and environments that present great risk to their own physical and mental wellbeing and that of their loved ones (Bennett, James & Kelly 2020). This led, in some countries, to public expressions of gratitude, like clapping and 'thank a nurse' campaigns. See Chapter 8 for further discussion of the images and stereotypes of nursing.

Why do you want to be a nurse?

Your answer to this question might include to earn money, travel, flexibility, to meet like-minded people or to pursue a particular specialisation, but the most common response is wanting to care for others and to make a positive difference in their lives (McKenna et al. 2017). Prospective nursing students may view nurses as kind, capable, busy and hardworking, but may weigh this against less-appealing factors such as unsociable working hours, arduous tasks, low salaries, limited opportunities for advancement or leadership, and the perception that nursing is a 'girl's job' (Rubbi et al. 2017; Gracia 2016). Although such deliberations are a normal part of career decision-making, these cursory, uninformed or predetermined views can strongly influence the perspective, motivation and attitude you bring to your studies and the way you engage with and represent the profession (Traynor & Butus 2016).

Video: 'What if you became a nurse?'

> ## REFLECTION 6.2
>
> It is important to consider why you want to become a nurse and what you hope to achieve. Who were the most influential people in your decision to study nursing, and what were the most decisive factors or perspectives that influenced this choice?

The diversity of roles and settings

While it may be the desire to care for others that attracts many students to nursing, an aspect that is likely to keep them in the profession is the variety and breadth of roles and opportunities. As a profession, nursing is diverse and flexible. Although you may come to nursing with a specific career pathway or specialisation in mind, you may end up surprised by the roles (clinical and/or non-clinical) you take on as you move through your career. It is important to remember that if at any stage you are struggling to find satisfaction in your work, perhaps you only need to change your role or your setting, rather than leaving nursing altogether.

Nursing is not just about caring: it is a highly skilled, knowledge-based profession, offering roles in clinical care, management, research and education. More recently, there has also been a growing focus on advanced practice and nurse practitioner roles, providing another set of perspectives and opportunities. A hospital may be the first setting that comes to mind when you think about your own future nursing practice, and this may be reinforced through clinical placements in hospitals as a student. However, nurses work in a variety of settings, some of which you will experience as you progress through your degree program, and you may be exposed to even more in your graduate-year roles and rotations. Of course, a specific role or setting does not represent the heart of nursing in and of itself but may influence the way you view nursing and how you think and act as a nurse.

Short-answer question
Connecting with practice:
Your nursing goals
Video: 'A tribute to nurses'

Professional identity

Your studies will introduce you to some of the core knowledge, expectations and realities of nursing, and will hopefully provide ideas about how you would like to shape your own practice. However, **professional identity** is not something you can simply accomplish or 'tick off'. It requires immersion or professional socialisation in the profession, and will emerge, evolve and change throughout your nursing career, based on critical thinking and reflection on the things you learn, do, observe and experience.

You may start out by identifying with the profession's perceived values and ideals (Wei et al. 2021) but, during your studies, your graduate year and each time you change

professional identity the acquisition and embodying of the knowledge, values, norms and ways of behaving of a professional group

jobs, you will also need to assimilate into accepted ways of thinking and behaving in each particular role and setting. This process may go smoothly with clear alignment to your existing views and expectations; however, sometimes the culture, behaviours and expectations in certain environments may conflict with or challenge your personal values or perspective. Thus, your professional identity will be constructed and deconstructed throughout your career in response to the interpersonal relationships and interactions you have with others, the different roles you take on and your unique interpretation of the experiences you have. Each of these experiences is likely to be a determining factor in how much you enjoy being a nurse.

As a student, it is very important that you can see yourself as a nurse and that you begin to formulate what that means and how you would like to go about your own practice (how to *be* and *act* as a nurse) (Browne et al. 2018). Remember, your nursing colleagues already have their own socialised perspective, and the public may have a predetermined idea of what a nurse should look like and how they should behave, so if you are different from these perceptions or expectations you may face additional challenges in discovering your 'place' and identity (Frogeli, Rudman & Gustavsson 2019). Interacting with like-minded role models and mentors can be beneficial as you progress through your education (and beyond), helping you to make sense of the experiences you have, and providing coaching and support for decision-making or improvements you may wish to pursue (Davey, Jackson & Henshall 2020; Talley, Talley & Collins-McNeil 2016). You may identify with one of your lecturers or tutors, a clinical preceptor, a practising nurse or even another student (perhaps someone in the year ahead). This interaction or role-modelling may be informal, but you might also consider looking into formal mentoring programs or opportunities (see Chapter 16). The more you can identify with the profession, the more likely you are to successfully make the transition from student nurse to registered nurse (RN) (Levett-Jones, Palmer & Wilson 2019).

NURSING PERSPECTIVE

My first placement as a graduate nurse was on a COVID-19 testing ward at a major hospital. I thought I was starting out in the emergency department but was told right before I started of the change in plan. I had no time to consider my professional identity or how I would present myself as a nurse – we were simply too busy establishing new and efficient systems to cope with the number of tests that needed to be done. To be honest, I was too busy following orders and trying to keep up to think about it very much. A couple of weeks into the placement, an experienced nurse made time to ask how I was feeling, and he gave me the best nursing advice I have received to date: 'Consider your nursing persona.' He explained that my nursing persona may be different to my actual personality; it's a way of being with and presenting myself, not just to clients, but also to colleagues. I had been expressing my enthusiasm a lot and apologising even more for all the things I felt unsure about, so I considered 'toning it down a bit'. I found I was less tired at the end of the long and busy shifts by talking less and listening more. My nursing persona is something I will consider with each rotation because it may change depending on the types of clients I care for, and the types of healthcare professionals I work with.

Multiple-choice question

REFLECTION 6.3

- How do you think this perspective, from a brand-new nurse, is different from the perspective of nurses portrayed in the media and by the general public?
- How can you, as a nursing student, use this insight to prepare yourself for your forthcoming clinical placements (see Chapter 14) and your first day on the job as a graduate nurse?

Your professional identity and capability will develop and change as you progress from novice to expert nurse. There are several nursing theorists you may find interesting if you are curious about how you become an 'expert' nurse. A good starting point is Benner's (1984) book, *From Novice to Expert: Excellence in clinical nursing practice*. Benner traces the development of a novice nurse to expert through five stages: novice, advanced beginner, competent, proficient and expert. At the end of your undergraduate nursing education, it is expected that you will be operating at the competent stage.

Caring, compassion and kindness

Caring

Despite the fact that nursing has changed dramatically since the Nightingale Home and Training School for Nurses opened at St Thomas's Hospital in London in the 1860s, *caring* continues to be acknowledged as the inner core or the essence of nursing (Tang et al. 2019; Andersson et al. 2015). As a phenomenon central to nursing, several theories and conceptions of caring have emerged. One well-known theory is Leininger's (1991) theory of cultural care, which describes care as 'the essence of nursing and the central, dominant, and unifying focus of nursing' (p. 35). Leininger purports that care and culture are inseparable; she definines culture as 'the learned, shared, and transmitted values, beliefs, norms, and life-ways of a particular group that guides their thinking, decisions, and actions in patterned ways' (1991, p. 47). Leininger stresses that nurses need to 'discover ways to provide culturally congruent care to people of different or similar cultures in order to maintain or regain their well-being, health or to face death in a culturally appropriate way' (1991, p. 39). This link between caring and cultural safety is particularly relevant to contemporary nursing in Australia, which is exposed to global issues and considerations more than ever, and takes place within diverse, multicultural and Indigenous communities.

Multiple-choice question

Another notable theory is Boykin and Schoenhofer's (1993) theory of nursing as caring, which argues that 'all persons are caring', and that 'caring is an essential feature and expression of being human' (see Chapter 7 for further discussion on the philosophical underpinnings of such ideas). Boykin and Schoenhofer (1993) define caring in nursing as:

Short-answer question

the intentional and authentic presence of the nurse with another ... where the nurse endeavours to come to know the other as a caring person and seeks to understand how that person might be supported, sustained, and strengthened in their unique process of living, caring and growing in caring (p. 25).

Perhaps two of the most enduring perspectives on caring in nursing are Jean Watson's (1979, 1985) theory of human care and Simone Roach's (1984) conceptualisation of caring, both of which are outlined in the following sections.

Watson's theory of human caring

In the 1970s, nurse theorist Jean Watson emphasised 'caring' as the focus of her nursing theory. Watson's still-evolving theory of caring built on Nightingale's earlier perspectives (see Chapter 8), incorporating broader philosophical and spiritual elements.

Watson's theory is based on seven assumptions about nursing caring:

- It is effectively demonstrated and practised interpersonally.
- It is made up of ten **caritas** factors or processes that satisfy various needs.
- It promotes health and growth.
- Caring responses accept the patient as they are, as well as what the patient may become.
- A caring environment offers the development of potential and allows the patient to choose the best action at any time.
- The science of caring is complementary to the science of curing.
- Its practice is central to nursing (Watson 1979).

caritas loving kindness, charity and virtue

Watson's clinical caritas processes, adapted from Watson (2008), are:

1 Practising loving-kindness and equanimity within a context of caring consciousness
2 Being authentically present and enabling, and sustaining the deep belief system and subjective life world of self and one-being-cared-for
3 Cultivating one's own spiritual practices and transpersonal self, and going beyond ego self
4 Developing and sustaining a helping-trusting, authentic caring relationship
5 Being present to, and supportive of, the expression of positive and negative feelings
6 Creatively using self and all ways of knowing as part of the caring process, engaging in artistry of caring-healing practices
7 Engaging in genuine teaching–learning experiences that attend to wholeness and meaning, while attempting to remain within the other's frame of reference
8 Creating healing environments at all levels, whereby wholeness, beauty, comfort, dignity and peace are potentiated
9 Assisting with basic needs, with an intentional caring consciousness that administers 'human care essentials', which potentiates alignment of mind–body– spirit, wholeness in all aspects of care
10 Opening and attending to mysterious dimensions of one's life–death; soul care for self and the one-being-cared-for; 'allowing and being open to miracles'.

Later, Watson (1996) drew on this list to develop a set of caring paradigm assumptions related specifically to nursing care, including that 'you must care for yourself before you can care for others' (p. 149).

Watson did not just propose theories relating to nursing care; she also created a range of instruments to help contextualise, apply and measure these processes or ideas, including the perceptions of nursing behaviour associated with caring processes; client perceptions of nurses' caring behaviours; nurses' caring attributes; and nurses' belief in their ability to be caring.

Incorporating Watson's theory into nursing education and practice can create better workplace satisfaction for nurses and better outcomes for their clients – helping nurses to provide better care for clients, and also for themselves (Durgun Ozan et al. 2020; Sterchi et al. 2019).

Sister Simone Roach

In the 1980s, nun and nurse theorist Sister Simone Roach (1984) proposed various theories, or conceptualisations, of caring in nursing. Roach's theories drew on existential philosophy, with the core premise being that caring is the human mode of being and is at the heart of what nurses do every day. According to Roach (1992), caring as the human mode of being involves:

- having the capacity or the power to care;
- calling forth this capacity;
- responding to being called to someone who, or something that, matters;
- actualising the capacity or the power to care; and
- the activity or performance of caring via specific caring behaviours.

Roach identified the '5Cs' of caring: compassion, competence, commitment, confidence and conscience. She later added a sixth: comportment. Roach (1984) asserted that caring is not unique to nursing, but it is unique *in* nursing, which is a 'helping discipline' (p. 12). Roach's theories started with the question, 'What is the nurse doing when caring?' The attributes revealed in answer to that question were then organised under the Cs, which are:

1 *Compassion* – living with awareness of our relationship with all living creatures; a quality of presence that enables us to share with others and make room for them
2 *Competence* – being equipped with knowledge, skills and experience to respond to professional responsibility
3 *Confidence* – a quality that fosters relationships
4 *Conscience* – a state of moral awareness; a compass directing our behaviours
5 *Commitment* – a convergence between our desires and obligations and a deliberate choice to act in accordance with them
6 *Comportment* – maintaining the harmony between beliefs about ourselves and others; where our clothes and language are symbols of communication in a caring presence (Roach 1984, 1992, 2002).

According to Roach (2002), compassion is necessary to humanise the 'cold and impersonal technology' used in health care; she also recognises that 'compassion without *competence* may be no more than a meaningless, if not harmful, intrusion into the life of a person … needing help' (p. 54, emphasis added). This acknowledges that nursing involves the sophisticated integration of art and science: the head and the heart.

Roach's ideas on caring and compassion have been embraced and adopted in various policies, codes and frameworks across the world. For example, Roach developed the first Canadian Nurses' Association Code of Ethics, and in 2012 the National Health Service (NHS) in the United Kingdom launched *Compassion in Practice: Nursing, Midwifery and Care Staff – Our Vision and Strategy*, which adapted Roach's 6Cs to a policy and action framework for all nurses, midwives and care staff and was rolled out in 2016 (NHS 2016).

Some of the ideas presented here may not immediately resonate or even make sense; however, your continuing engagement with, and reflection on, such theories is an important part of developing and nurturing your nursing knowledge and identity, and your own perspective on what it means to *be* and *act* as a nurse. We also suggest reading the studies by Andersson and colleagues (2015) and Tang and colleagues (2019), who examine RNs' own descriptions and conceptions of caring.

Compassion

Compassion is central to Roach's ideas about caring, and it is a characteristic that reflects the very heart of nursing.

What is compassion?

Compassion is 'sensitivity shown in order to understand another person's suffering, combined with a motivation and willingness to promote the wellbeing of that person by helping to find a solution to their situation' (Health Navigator New Zealand 2021; see also Tierney, Bivins & Seers 2019). It is a humane quality that requires an awareness of others' suffering and a desire to do something about it. It involves entering into the other person's experience 'through relational understanding and action' (Sinclair et al. 2016, p. 193), and acting in a way that is meaningful to them.

For nurses, this means recognising a client's vulnerability, listening, hearing what is and is not said, and responding in a respectful and client-centred way (Tehranineshat et al. 2019). Compassionate care can be provided in any setting, as long as you have knowledge of the client in that context. When you administer compassionate care, the challenge is to maintain objectivity while you make an emotional connection with your client (Post et al. 2014). Compassionate actions arise from empathy and are sometimes called acts of intelligent kindness (Campling 2015).

> **compassion** sensitivity to other people's pain, struggles or suffering; similar to empathy but accompanied by the motivation to 'take action' to help alleviate this suffering

Multiple-choice question

What does compassion mean to you?

Where do sympathy and empathy fit in?

Sometimes, compassion is confused with sympathy or empathy. All three concepts sit on the same continuum; however, we have chosen to emphasise compassion in this chapter, as it is the most pertinent to the *doing* (actual practice) of nursing. **Sympathy** is *feeling for* another person or feeling pity or sorrow towards the misfortune of another person – particularly if you feel that person is suffering unnecessarily (Jeffrey 2016). **Empathy**, on the other hand, involves *feeling with* another person, or perceiving and understanding their feelings or perspective (Kenny 2016). Compassion is different from sympathy and empathy in that it is proactive – it requires action to alleviate the other person's suffering (Soto-Rubio & Sinclair 2018). These concepts are discussed further in Chapter 10.

Interestingly, research has shown that, among nursing students, empathy declines as clinical experience increases (Cowin & Johnson 2015; Ward et al. 2012). Many

> **sympathy** feeling pity or sorrow towards the misfortune of another person, particularly if you feel that person is suffering unnecessarily

> **empathy** the ability to perceive and share in another person's reality

Video: Sympathy
versus empathy
Multiple-choice question

aspects of nursing work are inherently emotional and stressful, so this decline or disassociation with clients' experiences may be a subconscious protective or self-care mechanism on the part of the nurse. The dilemma here is that while self-care is necessary and important, empathy and compassion are essential for the provision of high-quality, person-centred care. Thus, it is imperative that you consciously cultivate and bring these concepts to the fore throughout your studies and beyond, to support your ability to feel and express empathy, and to act with compassion as a nurse.

Why is compassion important to nursing care?

Compassionate care benefits clients, nurses and the broader healthcare system. Clients receiving compassionate care adhere more closely to treatment protocols, heal or recover faster and report greater satisfaction with their care (Post 2011). They also experience less anxiety and stress, and participate more actively in preventative health measures (Post et al. 2014), thereby reducing the overall health burden and healthcare costs.

Clients value the compassionate care they receive, and so do their families, with research showing that compassionate care matters to them as much as physical care (Lown et al. 2017). This is evidenced by clients clearly remembering and describing examples of compassionate nursing care, and also noting where this was lacking or absent (Bramley & Matiti 2014). Clients treated in settings that promote compassionate care are more likely to recommend these services and to rate them more highly than those that do not (McClelland & Vogus 2014).

Importantly, compassion in the form of *self-compassion* also positively affects nurses' own wellbeing, health and resilience, as discussed later in this chapter.

NURSING PERSPECTIVE

How to be a compassionate nurse:

- Listen fully: hear the emotion, not just the words or the tone.
- Seek out commonalities with people, whether they are clients, families or loved ones, or other team members.
- Ask yourself: Why is my client acting this way? Why are they vulnerable? Remember, it is likely that you are in a more fortunate and secure position than your client.
- Suspend judgement of your client and their behaviour.
- Show genuine concern, putting aside your own emotions and focusing on the other person's needs.
- Show empathy by imagining yourself in your client's situation – but do not take your client's suffering on board as your own.
- Acknowledge your own emotions and share them if it is appropriate to do so. If your client has just died, it is okay to shed a tear in front of family members.
- Make sure you have good support, and maintain your own work–life balance outside of work.

- Practise self-compassion: Are you hard on yourself? Why? Could you be kinder to yourself?
- Realise you will never be a perfect nurse, and you will never be able to control everything. Forgive yourself if things sometimes go pear-shaped.
- Express gratitude – what are you thankful for, and why? Keep a daily gratitude diary.
- Meditate, reflect journal, exercise and eat well, and be sure to look after your own health.

Can you learn to be compassionate?

Compassion can be cultivated by engaging in compassion meditation or mindfulness meditation training (Mahon et al. 2017). In one study, young people listened to guided meditations during which they were asked to think of a time someone had suffered and then to practise wishing that the person's suffering could be relieved. The study examined activity and changes in the participants' brains and found that such changes were evident after only seven hours when participants looked at images showing human suffering. Over time, participants were able to regulate their emotional responses so that they could more actively engage with people's suffering (Weng et al. 2013). You can build your meditation and mindfulness practices through intentional effort and training (see Chapter 10 for various strategies and tools you can use for this).

Short-answer question

NURSING PERSPECTIVE

Starting out as a student or graduate nurse on a new ward can be stressful, so it is the perfect time to engage in self-care practices such as mediation and mindfulness. If you set out to be a compassionate nurse from the very start of your career, you will reduce the risk of compassion fatigue (discussed in the next section). Westwood (2010) sets out a few simple rules on how to choose compassion at work:

- Know what compassion means to you. How will you behave with clients and with colleagues?
- Show yourself compassion: be kind to yourself! Take your breaks. Find a quiet space for a breather if you need it. Focus on what you have done well. Remind yourself about what is good about your role and workplace.
- Act with compassion, whether or not you feel like doing so. Be deliberate about it and it will soon come naturally.
- Keep an eye out for other nurses who model compassion, and learn from them. Other nurses will see your compassion and follow your lead, too: this is how cultural change happens.
- If you are not feeling acknowledged or recognised, again be the change agent: start by giving others positive feedback or thanking them for their support or teamwork at the end of the day.
- Find others who want to change things, set some goals together and take action!

Compassion fatigue

Unfortunately, there are many barriers to compassionate care in nursing: unreasonable workloads, staff shortages, long working hours, negative workplace culture, poor role models and stress. You can think of compassion fatigue as a type of burnout. Compassion fatigue affects nurses who are emotionally exhausted and are often unable to make compassionate connections with clients because they have done so for too long (Hevezi 2016). They show signs of physical exhaustion and may depersonalise clients by, for instance, referring to them by their bed number or disease rather than their names. Lower-quality client care, client dissatisfaction, poor decisions and an increase in errors often occur as a result of burnout (Post et al. 2014).

Joinson (1992) first defined 'compassion fatigue' for nurses who had lost 'their ability to nurture' (p. 119). However, we now know that it extends beyond one's ability to show compassion towards clients; nurses with compassion fatigue also fail to engage compassion for their colleagues and, importantly, for themselves. Because of this, compassion fatigue negatively affects nurses' own health, their personal and professional relationships, their performance at work and their retention in the profession (Hofmeyer et al. 2018; Sinclair et al. 2017).

It is vitally important that as a novice nurse you learn to protect yourself from burnout.

First, try not 'buy into' any negative talk among other students or nurses in your workplace. Focus on your own behaviour and develop your own nursing persona.

Second, if you are struggling emotionally and feel exhausted, speak with your preceptor, educator, unit manager or a mentor, who can help you to make sense of your experience and to plan strategies to address the issue. It is not unusual to feel very tired or overwhelmed when you are on a steep learning curve. As a student, you may need to negotiate a period of leave or access the support services at your university to help develop self-care and coping strategies, and to achieve a better study and work–life balance. As a graduate, book some recreation leave if you can, consider reducing your hours and work with your supportive team members to develop strategies to build your resilience.

Finally, try to engage in mindfulness. Just as meditation and other techniques can help build compassion, they can also help to prevent compassion fatigue (Yu, Quia & Gui 2021).

NURSING PERSPECTIVE

I was a great student with a high grade point average. I did well on placements and had good references, all noting my compassionate manner. My best nursing 'skill' as a student was forming therapeutic relationships with clients, which I found easy. I was lucky to be placed for a full graduate (transition to practice) year in the area of nursing and the hospital I wanted. I did not have much time off between finishing university and starting my graduate year. I was enthusiastic and motivated, so I thought I would learn fast and settle into the ward pretty well.

Three weeks into my graduate year, I was feeling incredibly tired and shaky and, as a result, was learning new skills more slowly than I expected. I was truly tired to the bone. I would get home from my shift, sit on the couch with a cup of tea and fall asleep. This was happening every day. I had friends who were having similar experiences, and many of us were crying every day, too.

Three months in, and I was loving my job and the close client interaction, but I was still very tired and I started to get sick. I picked up every virus that went around and, as I was working with particularly vulnerable clients, it meant I had to take a lot of sick leave. Eventually my nurse unit manager chatted to me and recommended I see a counsellor at the Employee Assistance Program (EAP), as she could see I was struggling emotionally. Most workplaces have an EAP, which provides access to a counsellor, free of charge and completely anonymously. Seeing the counsellor was life-changing. She recommended some sleeping strategies and taught me mindfulness techniques, suggesting some meditation apps I could install on my phone as well. A month later, I was clear-headed and healthy, was experiencing increasing efficiency at work and, best of all, I no longer felt exhausted.

Since then, I have spoken with many of my graduate friends who had similar experiences. As grads we place more pressure on ourselves than our preceptors place on us. We often have expectations of ourselves that are too high and that do not correspond to our low levels of experience. Some of us are perfectionists, a trait that mindfulness and meditation can help us to 'unlearn'. Some have had successful prior careers and found starting from scratch a challenge. It was clear that many of us could have been kinder to ourselves in that first six months of practice. If I was a student now, I would be honing my self-compassion practices to build up resilience before my graduate year – and I am sure I would be a happier student nurse, too!

Self-compassion in nursing

Self-compassion is directing compassion to ourselves, just as we direct it to others. It is the inverse of the 'golden rule', which states that we should treat others as we wish to be treated ourselves. Self-compassion builds **resilience**, which is our ability to perceive and respond well to stressful situations. Resilient nurses administer higher-quality care and are more likely to stay in the profession than nurses with low levels of resilience (Hofmeyer et al. 2018). Self-compassion is vital for preventing compassion fatigue. It enables the caregiver to apprehend the suffering of others, and also to recognise their own feelings and needs, and the 'shared humanity' between the caregiver and care recipient (Wiklund & Wagner 2013, p. 180). Self-compassion provides benefits beyond improving your nursing: it also increases positive wellbeing, resilience, strength, motivation and health (Bluth & Neff 2018).

resilience the ability to perceive and respond well to stressful situations

Short-answer questions
Connecting with practice:
Self-compassion scale

CASE STUDY

When compassion is lacking

I completed my final acute-care placement on a busy medical oncology ward. One afternoon I took a client in a wheelchair and his wife down to the outpatients clinic to meet with the oncologist. I was tasked to accompany the client and to ask the oncologist to complete a signed consent form so the client's chemotherapy protocol could begin later that day. When I dropped the client off, I mentioned to the oncologist that the client was hard of hearing, so he would need to speak up and focus on the client directly. I excused myself and was told to come back to collect the client and his wife in 15 minutes. When I came back, the oncologist was still speaking with them, but he asked me to stay in the room. At this point, assuming they were wrapping up, I brought the consent form to the oncologist's attention, and he thanked me and continued speaking to the client, saying at a normal volume and while looking at his computer screen that he could not 'make' the client have the chemotherapy, that it was up to him to decide. The client said something that made it clear to me he was resistant to the treatment.

At this stage, the client's wife asked the oncologist, who was still keying notes into his computer, how long her husband would survive without the treatment. The oncologist looked up and said, in the same flat tone of voice, 'Oh, it's hard to say – maybe six to eight weeks'. Her husband did not hear that so the oncologist repeated it, this time louder. The client's wife then asked what the next step would be if her husband chose to have the treatment. Without looking at them, the oncologist said, 'It's difficult to tell – it depends on how the first treatment goes. It is possible we would have a second treatment, say, a month later. But it really depends on how he responds to the first one.' From the way the oncologist worded it, the implication was that it was unlikely he expected the client to respond favourably to the first treatment and have a second treatment. At this stage, both the client and his wife burst into tears. The oncologist said nothing.

Standing behind the client and his wife, I had been feeling uncomfortable about this exchange. When they both started crying, I leaned across to the oncologist's desk to grab a box of tissues (which he did not push towards me or them) and handed the client and his wife the box, then placed one hand on each of their shoulders. The oncologist continued keying in his notes. There was a long pause – maybe a minute – while the oncologist was on the computer and the client and his wife wept, before the oncologist finally said that he needed them to decide right then if they were going to consent to start treatment. He did not invite them to discuss it between themselves or give them time to consider it. He had the consent form in front of him. The husband agreed to start the treatment and the oncologist said, 'Great!' Then he said to me, 'Here's your form, take the file' as he signed it, before instructing me, 'Okay, you can all head back upstairs now.' I was quite shocked by the way he dismissed us all, but gathered the files and wheeled the client upstairs, with his wife walking alongside, crying the entire way.

QUESTION

As a student, what could you do next to exercise and demonstrate your compassion in this situation?

Kindness

We mention **kindness** here as it is a quality inextricably linked to caring, empathy and compassion, as discussed earlier in this chapter. For example, compassion is sometimes referred to as *intelligent kindness*, in that kindness shares the motivation to take action to address the needs or alleviate the suffering of others (Ballatt, Campling & Maloney 2020). At its heart, health care involves privileged and trusting relationships between healthcare professionals and the people they serve. We cannot do this (successfully) if we see people – particularly those with whom we have a professional caring relationship – as a 'generalised other' (Campbell 2017). To recognise and share the emotions of another, and to maintain the selfless motivation to take action in response to this, we need to see these others as *kin* – hence kinship and kindness (Ballatt et al. 2020; Campbell 2017). This brings to mind the importance of caring for others as we would like to be cared for ourselves.

Being in need or receipt of health care can leave individuals and families feeling frightened, anxious and vulnerable (Crock 2017). Caring for clients with dignity, sensitivity and kindness goes a long way towards mediating these feelings. Such gestures form lasting impressions on clients and their families, even when the prognosis or outcome is an unhappy one (Jones 2017). Accounts of such care often include comments such as, 'I'll never forget the nurse who took the trouble to … ' (Jones 2017, p. 66). According to Crock (2017), bullying, harassment, poor workplace culture, stress and burnout are also prevalent in our healthcare systems. It is well known that these workplace cultural issues 'impose high costs on health organisations through poorer staff performance, absenteeism, and sick leave. Poor staff behaviour is also directly linked to worse patient outcomes' (Crock 2017, p. 21). Our healthcare system is 'sick', and efforts to build a thoughtful, empathic and kind healthcare system are urgently needed.

Crock (2017) asserts that kindness has three functions. It makes the most of your team, who will respond to your kindness with their own kindness and feel inspired to help. Kindness fosters safety as people feel they can talk about and learn from their mistakes. Finally, kindness helps to improve client outcomes and satisfaction through quality person-centred care. Crock (2017, p. 21) refers to the work of Australian nurse ethicist Megan Jane Johnstone, who dismissed the claim that nurses are 'too busy to be kind', highlighting the restorative possibilities in health care, and that kindness needs to be 'instated as an essential adjunct to healthcare interventions'.

kindness an 'other-focused' quality or behaviour characterised by an ethical mindset, a friendly disposition, concern for others and the motivation to provide help and support

Video: 'The heart of nursing'

Prepare to be the best nurse you can be!

You might have looked at the title of this chapter and thought, 'Cheesy!' But it's important to consider the heart of nursing, what is at its very core, as you formulate your own perceptions of the profession and of yourself as a future nurse. This chapter began by looking at nursing from outside, examining what you might have thought about nursing before you started and what other people and systems think about nursing and nurses. Because your perceptions of nursing will evolve as your study and career progress, you must start thinking now about why you chose nursing, what kind of nurse you want to be, and how you want to act and be seen and known as a nurse.

We then asked you to consider your future professional identity and how you will integrate and reconcile your values, strengths and skills with the values and expectations of different nursing roles and settings, in order to provide the best client care. Perhaps you were motivated to become a nurse because you want to care for people, so we have discussed various caring theories that will underpin and influence your perception of nursing and your nursing practice and identity. It is imperative that nurses care for themselves too, and we have emphasised compassion (and *self-compassion*) practices that you can begin now to benefit you, your clients and your colleagues, and to help set you up for a long and rewarding nursing career.

SUMMARY

- A range of factors influence a person's and society's perspectives on nursing, including personal values, beliefs and experiences; the views of friends and family members; the ways in which a given society views women; other cultural and social norms; and the ways in which nurses are portrayed in popular culture, the media and social media. A nurse's own perspective on nursing is likely to change as their career progresses and their experience grows.
- The most common reason people want to become a nurse is to care for others, but other reasons might include the 'portability' of the profession (ability to travel) and opportunities to meet like-minded people. A person's decision-making regarding entering and staying in a particular profession will also include consideration of less-appealing factors such as relatively low pay, unsociable hours, emotionally charged work and the perception that nursing is a 'girl's job'. It is important that students are able to make sense of or reconcile these things through learning and socialisation in the profession, rather than acting exclusively on these predetermined perspectives. Nursing is a skilled, knowledge-based profession, and offers roles in clinical care, management, research and education. Nurses practice in a diversity of roles and settings (not just clinical care in hospitals), which can be a determining factor in a nurse's enjoyment of the profession.
- A nurse's professional identity develops through socialisation in the profession, and just as your individual perspective on nursing will change over time, your professional identity will be assembled and disassembled (change) as you progress through your undergraduate course, your graduate year and each time you change roles or jobs. It is important for student nurses to see themselves as nurses and to actively engage with the profession. Interaction with role models and mentors can be a valuable way to make sense of the experiences you have, to work through any challenges or dilemmas, and to reach conclusions about what it really means to be and act as a nurse.
- We contend that caring, compassion and kindness lie at the very heart of nursing. These concepts emphasise relational practice, genuine concern for others, the ability to perceive another person's reality and the motivation to take action to address the needs and alleviate the suffering of others. They also extend beyond care of your clients to care of yourself – a critical imperative in the complex and emotionally charged healthcare environment. This chapter has presented a range of theoretical perspectives, ideas and strategies for cultivating these qualities.

REVIEW QUESTIONS

1 What did Roach identify as the 6Cs of caring?
2 What is compassion and how can it be cultivated?
3 Why is self-compassion important for nurses?
4 What are some of the benefits or outcomes that come from kindness?
5 How is your professional identity formed?

Suggested responses

RESEARCH TOPIC

In what ways have media and social media created, affected and changed perceptions of what is at the heart of nursing? How might they influence the development of your own professional identity?

FURTHER READING

Andersson, E.K., Willman, A., Sjostrom-Strand, A. & Borglin, G. (2015). Registered nurses' descriptions of caring: A phenomenographic interview study. *BMC Nursing*, 14(16).

Gracia, M. (2016). So why did you become a nurse? Reflections from a second-year student. *British Journal of Nursing*, 25(13), 746

Post, S., Ng, L., Fischel, J., Bennett, M., Bily, L., Chandran, L., Joyce, J., Locicero, B., McGovern, K., McKeefrey, R., Rodriguez, J. & Roess, M. (2014). Routine, empathic and compassionate patient care: Definitions, development, obstacles, education and beneficiaries. *Journal of Evaluation in Clinical Practice*, 20(6), 872–80.

Tang, F.W.K., Ling, G.C.C., Lai, A.S.F., Chair, S.Y. & So, W.K.W. (2019). Four Es of caring in contemporary nursing: Exploring novice to experienced nurses. *Nursing and Health Sciences*, 1, 85–92.

Watson, C. (2018). *The language of kindness: A nurse's story*. New York: Tim Duggan Books.

REFERENCES

Andersson, E.K., Willman, A., Sjostrom-Strand, A. & Borglin, G. (2015). Registered nurses' descriptions of caring: A phenomenographic interview study. *BMC Nursing*, 14(16).

Ballatt, J., Campling, P. & Maloney, C. (2020). *Intelligent kindness: Rehabilitating the welfare state*, 2nd edn. Cambridge: Cambridge University Press.

Benner, P. (1984). *From novice to expert: Excellence and power in clinical nursing practice*. Menlo Park, CA: Addison Wesley.

Bennett, C.L., James, A.H. & Kelly, D. (2020). Beyond tropes: Towards a new image of nursing in the wake of CCVID-19. *Journal of Clinical Nursing*, 29(15/16), 2753–5.

Bluth, K. & Neff, K. D. (2018). New frontiers in understanding the benefits of self-compassion. *Self and Identity*, 17(6), 605–8.

Boykin, A. & Schoenhofer, S. (1993). *Nursing as caring: A model for transforming practice*. New York: National League for Nursing Press.

Bramley, L. & Matiti, M. (2014). How does it really feel to be in my shoes? Patients' experiences of compassion within nursing care and their perceptions of developing compassionate nurses. *Journal of Clinical Nursing*, 19–20, 2790–9.

Browne, C., Wall, P., Batt, S. & Bennett, R. (2018). Understanding perceptions of nursing professional identity in students entering an Australian undergraduate nursing degree. *Nurse Education in Practice*, 32, 90–6.

Campbell, D. (2017). Reflections on empathy. In M. Phillips (ed.), *Gathering of kindness anthology*. Melbourne: Hambone.

Campling P. (2015). Reforming the culture of healthcare: The case for intelligent kindness. *British Journal of Psychology Bulletin*, 39(1), 1–5.

Cowin, L.S. & Johnson, M. (2015). From student to graduate: Longitudinal changes in the qualities of nurses. *Journal of Advanced Nursing*, 71(12), 2911–22.

Crock, C. (2017). It's time for kindness. In M. Phillips (ed.), *Gathering of kindness anthology*. Melbourne: Hambone.

Davey, Z., Jackson, D. & Henshall, C. (2020). The value of nurse mentoring relationships: Lessons learnt from a work-based resilience enhancement programme for nurses working in the forensic setting. *International Journal of Mental Health Nursing*, 29(5), 992–1002.

Durgun Ozan, Y., Duman, M., Cicek, O. & Baksi, A. (2020). The effects of clinical education program based on Watson's theory of human caring on coping and anxiety levels of nursing students: A randomized control trial. *Perspectives in Psychiatric Care*, 3, 621–9.

Frogeli, E., Rudman, A. & Gustavsson, P. (2019). The relationship between task mastery, role clarity, social acceptance, and stress: An intensive longitudinal study with a sample of newly registered nurses. *International Journal of Nursing Studies*, 19, 60.

Gill, J. & Baker, C. (2019). The power of mass media and feminism in the evolution of nursing's image: A critical review of the literature and implications for nursing practice. *Journal of Medical Humanities*. Retrieved from https://doi.org/10.1007/s10912-019-09578-6.

Gracia, M. (2016). So why did you become a nurse? Reflections from a second-year student. *British Journal of Nursing*, 25(13), 746.

Haynes, S. (2020). How Florence Nightingale paved the way for the heroic work of nurses today. *Time,* 12 May. Retrieved from https://time.com/5835150/florence-nightingale-legacy-nurses/.

Health Navigator New Zealand (2021). Compassion (Website). Retrieved from https://www.healthnavigator.org.nz/clinicians/c/compassion.

Hevezi, J.A. (2016). Evaluation of a meditation intervention to reduce the effects of stressors associated with compassion fatigue among nurses. *Journal of Holistic Nursing*, 34(4), 343–50.

Hofmeyer, A., Toffoli, L., Vernon, R., Taylor, R., Klopper, H., Coetzee, S. & Fontaine, D. (2018). Teaching compassionate care to nursing students in a digital learning and teaching environment. *Collegian*, 25(3), 307–12.

Jeffrey, D. (2016). Empathy, sympathy and compassion in healthcare: Is there a problem? Is there a difference? Does it matter? *Journal of the Royal Society of Medicine*, 109(12), 446–52.

Joinson, C. (1992). Coping with compassion fatigue. *Nursing*, 22(4), 116–22.

Jones, R. (2017). A view from the other side. In M. Phillips (ed.), *Gathering of kindness anthology*. Melbourne: Hambone.

Kenny, G. (2016). Compassion for simulation. *Nurse Education in Practice*, 16(1), 160–3.

Leininger, M.M. (1991). *Culture care diversity and universality: A theory of nursing*. New York: National League of Nursing Press.

Levett-Jones, T., Palmer, L. & Wilson, A. (2019). Becoming part of a team. In J. Daly & E. Chang (eds), *Transitions in Nursing*, 5th edn. Sydney: Elsevier.

Lewis, M.J. (2014). Medicine in colonial Australia 1788–1900. *Medical Journal of Australia*, 201(1), S5–S10.

Lin, C., Yeh, J., Wu, M. & Lee, W. (2015). Religious orientation, endorser credibility, and the portrayal of female nurses by the media. *Journal of Religion and Health*, 54, 1699–711.

Lown, B., Dunne, H., Muncer, S. & Chadwick, R. (2017). How important is compassionate healthcare to you? A comparison of the perceptions of people in the United States and Ireland. *Journal of Research in Nursing*, 22(1–2), 60–9.

Mahon, M., Mee, L., Brett, D. & Dowling, M. (2017). Nurses' perceived stress and compassion following a mindfulness meditation and self-compassion training. *Journal of Research in Nursing*, 22(8), 572–83.

McClelland, L. & Vogus, T. (2014). Compassion practices and HCAHPS: Does rewarding and supporting workplace compassion influence patient perceptions? *Health Services Research*, 49(5), 1670–83.

McKenna, L., Brooks, I. & Vanderheide, R. (2017). Graduate entry nurses' initial perspectives on nursing: Content analysis of open-ended survey questions. *Nurse Education Today*, 49, 22–6.

National Health Service (NHS) (2016). *Compassion in practice: Evidencing the impact*. Retrieved from https://www.england.nhs.uk/wp-content/uploads/2016/05/cip-yr-3.pdf.

Post, S.G. (2011). Compassionate care enhancement: Benefits and outcomes. *The International Journal of Person Centered Medicine*, 1(4), 808–13.

Post, S., Ng, L., Fischel, J., Bennett, M., Bily, L., Chandran, L., Joyce, J., Locicero, B., McGovern, K., McKeefrey, R., Rodriguez, J. & Roess, M. (2014). Routine, empathic and compassionate patient care: Definitions, development, obstacles, education and beneficiaries. *Journal of Evaluation in Clinical Practice*, 20(6), 872–80.

Reinking, C. (2020). Nurses transforming systems of care: The bicentennial of Florence Nightingale's legacy. *Nursing Management*, 51(5), 32–7.

Roach, M.S. (1984). *Caring: The human mode of being Implications for nursing*. Toronto: Faculty of Nursing, University of Toronto.

——— (1992). *The human act of caring: A blueprint for the health professions*. Ottawa: Canadian Hospital Association Press.

——— (2002). *Caring, the human mode of being: A blueprint for the health professions*, 2nd edn. Ottawa: Canadian Hospital Association Press.

Rubbi, I., Cremonini, V., Artioli, G., Lenzini, A., Talenti, I., Caponnetto, V., La Cerra, C., Petrucci, C. & Lancia, L. (2017). The public perception of nurses: An Italian cross-sectional study. *Acta Biomedica*, 88(5S), 31–8.

Sinclair, S., McClement, S., Raffin-Bouchal, S., Hack, T., Hagen, N., McConnell, S. & Chochinov, H. (2016). Compassion in healthcare: Empirical model. *Journal of Pain Symptom Management*, 51(2), 193–203.

Sinclair, S., Raffin-Bouchal, S., Venturato, L., Mijovic-Kondejewski, J. & Smith-MacDonald, L. (2017). Compassion fatigue: A meta-narrative review of the healthcare literature. *International Journal of Nursing Studies*, 69, 9–24.

Soto-Rubio, A. & Sinclair, S. (2018). In defense of sympathy, in consideration of empathy, and in praise of compassion: A history of the present. *Journal of Pain and Symptom Management*, 55(5), 1428–34.

Sterchi, S., Brooks, S., Shilkaitis, M. & Ris, L. (2019). Reconnecting nurses to their passion and enhancing the patient and family experience. *Journal of Nursing Administration*, 49(9), 423–9.

Talley, C., Talley, H. & Collins-McNeil, J. (2016). The continuing quest for parity: HBCU nursing students' perspectives on nursing and nursing education. *Nurse Education Today*, 43, 23–7.

Tang, F.W.K., Ling, G.C.C., Lai, A.S.F., Chair, S.Y. & So, W.K.W. (2019). Four Es of caring in contemporary nursing: exploring novice to experienced nurses. *Nursing and Health Sciences*, 1, 85.

Tehranineshat, B., Rakhshan, M., Torabizadeh, C. & Fararouei, M. (2019). Nurses', patients', and family caregivers' perceptions of compassionate nursing care. *Nursing Ethics*, 26(6), 1707–20.

ten Hoeve, Y., Jansen, G. & Roodbol, P. (2013). The nursing profession: Public image, self-concept and professional identity – a discussion paper. *Journal of Advanced Nursing*, 70(2), 295–309.

Tierney, S., Bivins, R. & Seers, K. (2019). Compassion in nursing: Solution or stereotype? *Nursing Inquiry*, 26(1), e12271.

Timmons, S., Evans, C. & Nair, S. (2016). The development of the nursing profession in a globalized context: A qualitative case study on Kerala, India. *Social Science and Medicine*, 166, 41–8.

Traynor, M. & Butus, N. (2016). Professional identity in nursing: UK students' explanations for poor standards of care. *Social Science & Medicine*, 166, 186–94.

Ward, J., Cody, J., Schaal, M. & Hojat, M. (2012). The empathy enigma: An empirical study of decline in empathy among undergraduate nursing students. *Journal of Professional Nursing*, 28(1), 34–41.

Watson, J. (1979). *Nursing: The philosophy and science of caring*. Boston: Little, Brown and Co.

——— (1985). *Nursing: Human science and human care – a theory of nursing*. New York: National League of Nursing Press.

——— (1996) Watson's theory of transpersonal caring. In P. Hinton, P. Walker & B.M. Neuman (eds), *Blueprint for use of nursing models: Education, research, practice, and administration*. New York: National League for Nursing Press.

——— (2008). *Nursing: The philosophy and science of caring*. Boulder, CO: University of Colorado Press.

Wei, L., Zhou, S., Hu, S., Zhou, Z. & Chen, J. (2021). Influences of nursing students' career planning, internship experience, and other factors on professional identity. *Nurse Education Today*, 99. Retrieved from https://doi.org/10.1016/j.nedt.2021.104781.

Weng, H., Fox, A., Caldwell, J., Davidson, R., Stodola, D., Olson, M., Shackman, A. & Rogers, G. (2013). Compassion training alters altruism and neural responses to suffering. *Psychological Science*, 24(7), 1171–80.

Westwood, C. (2010). Nursing with compassion: What can you do? *Nursing Times*,
9 May. Retrieved from https://www.nursingtimes.net/nursing-with-compassion-
what-can-you-do/5014361.article.

Wiklund, G.L. & Wagner, L. (2013). The butterfly effect of caring: Clinical nursing
teachers' understanding of self-compassion as a source to compassionate care.
Scandinavian Journal of Caring Sciences, 27(1), 175–8.

Yu, H., Qiao, A. & Gui, L. (2021). Predictors of compassion fatigue, burnout, and
compassion satisfaction among emergency nurses: A cross-sectional survey.
International Emergency Nursing, 55. Retrieved from https://www.sciencedirect
.com/science/article/abs/pii/S1755599X20301336.

7

Philosophical underpinnings

Suzanne Bliss, Nick Arnott and Kerry Howells

LEARNING OBJECTIVES

At the completion of this chapter, you should be able to:

1 Outline the ways in which philosophy has relevance for nursing and why nursing needs a philosophical foundation.
2 Describe the philosophical underpinnings of nursing as a discipline and a profession.
3 Explain the main ideas behind Aristotle's conception of 'virtue', including the role of emotions in the acquisition of the virtues.
4 Appraise the virtue of gratitude and the role it can play in nursing education and practice.
5 Discuss the alignment of ends between the goal of nursing (excellence in the pursuit of *wellness*) and the goals of a 'good life' more broadly (flourishing as a human being).

Introduction

As a student nurse, you may be wondering what philosophy can offer nursing and why we believe nursing needs a philosophical foundation. One quick response would be to point out that a 'nursing philosophy' underpinning the curriculum is mandated by the accrediting body, the Australian Nursing and Midwifery Accreditation Council (ANMAC). But why does ANMAC require an underpinning philosophy? We believe it is because a rigorous philosophical position underpinning nursing theory and practice can provide a focus for the discipline in terms of practical reasoning and moral commitment.

While the word 'philosophy' may bring to mind ancient scholars and papyrus scrolls, it is relevant to everyone, including nurses. We discuss the reasons for this in the first part of the chapter. We also point out that nurses are required to be both knowledgeable and technically competent clinicians, and to have the emotional capacities and self-awareness that enable them to provide empathic, person-centred care (Stein-Parbury 2018). We refer to these as the 'knowledge' and 'caring' aspects of nursing. Any underpinning philosophy of nursing needs to recognise and accommodate these dual aspects.

The ancient philosopher Aristotle (1984) provided an ethical account of how we should live our lives in order to flourish to our full capacity. He did this by drawing on a conception of virtue. A virtue is a character trait, developed through intentional practice and habit, that is good for a person to have. In this chapter, we outline Aristotle's ideas and apply them to the 'knowledge' and 'caring' aspects of nursing practice. We introduce the concept of gratitude as an example of a virtuous character trait. Gratitude is now gaining currency in nursing theory, but it has long been recognised by philosophers as being a virtue or emotion that is a key element in fostering and maintaining harmonious social relations with others (Jackson 2016; Morgan, Gulliford & Kristjansson 2017).

Aristotle further recognised the importance of properly trained emotions for acquiring the virtues, thus his account is consistent with our emphasis on emotional intelligence and self-awareness. We show how excellent practice as a nurse aligns with doing well as a human being, based on Aristotle's account. The main point argued in this chapter is that Aristotle's conception of virtue can provide a philosophical 'basis for nursing that focuses on moral competence in a robust, coherent and systematic way, while at the same time accommodates the demand for discipline-specific knowledge and high levels of technical skill' (Bliss et al. 2017, p. 1). We contend that this underpinning philosophy allows the knowledge and caring aspects of nursing to be united.

What is nursing philosophy and why does nursing need a philosophical foundation?

REFLECTION 7.1

Why do you think 'philosophy' is important for nursing education and practice?

There are several ways in which philosophy has relevance for nursing. It is useful for its content matter, as a methodology and as a practice or way of life (Bruce, Rietze & Lim 2014). Let us briefly discuss each of these points in turn.

Philosophy as content matter

The content matter of **nursing philosophy** offers up ways of making sense of what nurses do and why they do it. When making practice-related decisions, nurses are frequently engaging with philosophical ideas (whether they are aware of it or not) as they work through questions about what nursing is, what good nursing practice amounts to and which kinds of knowledge are properly considered 'nursing knowledge' (Bruce, Rietze & Lim 2014). Nurse philosopher June Kikuchi (in Forss, Ceci & Drummond 2013, p. 105) vividly illustrated this point when she wrote about being 'shocked out of her complacency' as a postgraduate student when her instructor, Dr Helen Simmons, asked 'What is nursing?' Although she thought the answer would be straightforward, Kikuchi and her fellow students quickly realised it was not. They struggled to articulate exactly what nursing is, despite all being qualified nurses. The turning point came when Dr Simmons emphasised her reason for asking the question: 'It is only by defining nursing that we will know we are designing a nursing program and not, for example, a medical program' (Forss et al. 2013, p. 105). Simmons pointed out that we need philosophical inquiry to answer such a question. Kikuchi explained that understanding the nature of nursing requires more than simply being a nurse: it requires 'an understanding of such basic matters as the nature of reality, the human mind and free will' (Forss et al. 2013, p. 106), and this content (subject) matter is fundamental to philosophy as a discipline.

Philosophy as a methodology

Philosophy as a methodology is crucial in enabling nurses to analyse, critique and challenge situations that pose physical, psychological, emotional or moral risks to the client. This is because philosophy insists upon clarity of ideas, rigorous analysis of commonly used concepts and sound arguments to support a particular view. Philosophy as a methodology is 'critical thinking' *par excellence*: it teaches logical reasoning and alerts us to the presence of faulty reasoning or spurious claims. Philosophical methodology requires a person to be clear about their position and to provide substantial arguments to support it. Seedhouse (2000) pointed out that it is not good enough to recite platitudes or make vague, unspecified claims, as such claims could apply to most professions – they are not specific to nursing. Moreover, platitudes cannot provide guidance for individual cases, nor supply nurses with the personal resources to make appropriate judgements. Let us take the example of philosophy's concern with the analysis of concepts: if we apply this idea to nursing, we can see that the terms used to articulate a position must be defined clearly so that nurses understand just how to apply the ideas in practice. For example, the Nursing and Midwifery Board of Australia's (NMBA) Code of Conduct for Nurses (NMBA 2018) requires that nurses respect the dignity of people receiving care and treatment, yet there is no account of what dignity actually means or what respecting clients' dignity might actually involve. Nurses should, of course, respect the dignity of clients; however, without a clear definition of what dignity amounts to and how one might respect a client's dignity, there are likely to be challenges in applying this in practice. While the codes provide aspirational statements about how nurses should conduct themselves, they are necessarily vague and open to different interpretations, and can even be contradictory in some cases (Seedhouse 2000). Regrettably, this means that thoughtful nurses will often be unsure about whether they are complying with the codes appropriately, which can lead to moral distress or even burnout. Philosophy can assist with this by, for example, reflecting upon the situations or conditions under which a person is likely to lose their dignity (Seedhouse 2000). Applying these thinking processes (the methodology of philosophy) to such nursing concepts can assist nurses to recognise clearly (and quickly) when a client's dignity is being compromised.

Philosophy as a practice or 'way of life'

In more recent times, philosophy is often considered alongside ethics (and ethical practice), which refers to right and wrong, or good and bad conduct, in our dealings with other people, animals and the environment.

Philosophy as a way of life was an idea articulated and put into practice by the ancient Greeks. Aristotle, for example, believed that the aim of ethical inquiry was to discover how to *live well,* and focused on the personal qualities of the individual. This was then and remains quite a contrast to most contemporary accounts of **ethics**, which tend to put forward certain principles to assist us in making decisions when it is not at all clear what we should do. We find Aristotle's view particularly attractive as it emphasises 'the notion of *integrity,* where one's intellect and actions are aligned with one's character and motivations' (Bliss et al. 2017, p. 3). Incorporating philosophy as a *way of life* is especially relevant for nursing practice, for as nursing is a profession whose aims embody the essential preconditions for any good life, there is reason to expect that the requirements for achieving excellence as a nurse will be the same or similar to those for achieving excellence as a human being. Thus, nursing as a profession is particularly suited to incorporating philosophy as a way of life.

> **ethics** for Aristotle, ethics was the study of how we ought to live our lives

We believe that a clearly articulated philosophy of nursing practice, in which certain values are made explicit and appropriate behaviours are modelled by academics and clinical staff, can support nurses to cultivate the professional qualities, values and beliefs needed for excellence, while simultaneously representing nursing's purpose to other health professionals and the broader public (Mackintosh-Franklin 2016, p. 710). This is crucial if nursing is to be respected as a serious profession in its own right, rather than a 'watered-down' version of medicine. From a purely pragmatic perspective, the way nursing represents itself (as determined by its underpinning philosophy) will have certain political implications, such as whether it rightly has a place in the university (as a discrete academic discipline) and whether it is eligible for research funding (Risjord 2011, p. 490). These implications provide further support for our claim that philosophy has much to offer nursing.

Multiple-choice question

Two approaches to the question of how nursing should represent itself

As you may have gathered from some of the other chapters in this book, nursing can be considered both a discipline (a body of knowledge) and a profession (a field of practice for applying this knowledge). Being a *discipline* implies that nursing has its own body of knowledge that nonetheless overlaps with other disciplines, such as medicine. Nursing's disciplinary knowledge has a significant focus on knowledge that is evidence-based, in which 'fundamental physical and scientific/technical skills feature prominently' (Bliss et al. 2017, p. 1). The philosophical subdiscipline of **epistemology** (theory of knowledge) is particularly relevant to this aspect of nursing.

However, 'evidence-based knowledge' is not the only kind of knowledge that nurses need. As nursing is considered a 'caring profession', there is a long-held expectation that nurses will possess certain professional and moral qualities that are thought to embody non-evidential forms of knowledge (Carper 1978). This type of knowledge is often thought to be 'ineffable' – in other words, it can neither be put into words easily nor taught in a didactic way. It may develop over time but it also requires the nurse to form an intention to practise in certain ways, to reflect on their own practice and to seek constructive feedback from others. The philosophical subdiscipline of ethics is especially relevant to this aspect of nursing. As noted earlier, ethics considers questions of right and wrong, and what constitutes good and bad conduct in our dealings with others.

This relationship between disciplinary knowledge and ethical practice has stirred a debate in the literature about how nursing should represent itself to the broader public. Some scholars argue for prioritisation of a 'knowledge discourse' (Gordon & Nelson 2006; Paley 2002), while others promote a 'caring discourse', which aims to re-orient nurses to the 'heart of nursing' (see Chapter 6). This is construed as a caring relationship between the nurse and client that has humanistic values such as empathy and compassion at its core (Bliss et al. 2017). Although nurses should 'promote themselves as having rigorous, discipline-specific knowledge and high levels of technical skill', focusing predominantly on this aspect of nursing can lead to a devaluing of important character traits needed to provide holistic, person-centred care (Bliss et al. 2017, p. 3). 'Moreover, the insistence that practice must be evidence-based sets a 'standardising agenda' in relation to client care rather than promoting individually tailored care' (Bliss et al. 2017, p. 3; Thorne & Sawatzky 2014). If nursing is conceived exclusively (or primarily) in terms of having knowledge of illness and techniques for managing symptoms, there is a risk that the client may become simply 'the caesarean in room 203', rather than a new mother who needs to take as much care about how she raises herself up from the bed as she does when she holds her infant daughter. Prioritising the knowledge discourse 'has the effect of dehumanising the patient and devaluing their experiences – a clear breach of the ethos of patient-centred care' (Bliss et al. 2017, p. 3). In what follows, we show that an appropriate underpinning philosophy can accommodate both these aspects of nursing. A nursing philosophy that emphasises both the 'moral and intellectual *virtues* is a way of providing a moral foundation for the discipline by unifying the "knowledge" and "caring" discourses within nursing theory' (Bliss et al. 2017, p. 3, emphasis added). In the next section, we examine Aristotle's account of virtue, to flesh out these claims in further detail.

Aristotle's account of virtue

Virtue ethics is unique in that it focuses on the individual (the 'moral agent') and does not appeal to abstract principles (such as the four principles of bioethics) that claim to guide moral action. This makes virtue ethics particularly appealing as a

Short-answer questions

moral foundation for the healthcare professions, in which it is very difficult to devise general ethical rules that guide action (Bliss et al. 2017). After all, rules are necessarily general, but situations are very particular and sometimes differ from one another in subtle, although important, ways. We believe it takes wisdom to apply general rules to specific situations. But if wisdom is not to function simply as a pretext for doing whatever you want, no matter what the rules may be, it must be exercised with *integrity*. Aristotle's account certainly emphasises the importance of integrity, 'where one's intellect and actions are aligned with one's character and motivations' (Bliss et al. 2017, p. 3).

In his most famous treatise on ethics – the *Nicomachean Ethics* – Aristotle (1984) proposed that 'the good is what all men [sic] desire' (p. 1094a). The good, therefore, is the end (or goal) of all human activity – in other words, all our deliberate and purposeful actions have as their aim happiness or achieving a 'good life'. Of course, this does not mean that we enjoy everything we do – studying at university, for example, can be difficult and stressful at times, but we do it to attain something (an education) that will improve our chances of achieving a good life in the future.

Aristotle provided an account of the conditions that he believed would maximise the chances of human beings achieving a/the good life. The question he asked was, 'Under what conditions do human beings flourish or do well in life?' Aristotle thought that the character of **human flourishing** lay in our *shared common nature*, and he argued his case by means of his 'function argument'. He based this argument on the relationship 'between the *function* of a certain kind of thing, and *being a good thing of that kind*' (Bliss et al. 2017, p. 3). Aristotle purported that if the function of a particular object is to do something, then the function of a *good* object of that kind is to do that thing *well*. For example, if the function of a knife is to cut things, then the function of a good knife will be to cut things well (Bliss et al. 2017). Aristotle (1984) went even further, claiming 'that the criterion for something performing its function well is to perform it *in accordance with the virtue*' (p. 4). In this context, the term 'virtue' is simply a quality of a certain thing (or person) that allows it to perform its function. To use the knife example again, 'if the function of a knife is to cut things, then qualities like having a blade made from a metal that keeps a good edge will be a virtue [or signify *excellence*] of knives' (Bliss et al. 2017, p. 4).

So, this brings us to the question, 'What is the function of human beings?' Our answer to this question will provide clues to the kinds of virtues we need to *fulfil our function well*. As mentioned, Aristotle was looking for a 'common nature' that we all share. Of course, individuals are all different in various ways, but we have certain needs and capacities in common, such as the need for air to breathe, food and water. We share many of these needs and capacities with animals and even plants. For example, all living things need nourishment of some kind and have the capacity to extract nutrients from their food (or their environment, in the case of plants). Aristotle, however, wanted to identify the characteristic that makes human beings unique, and suggested that *rational thought* is the only capacity unique to humans. The function of the *good* human being, therefore, is to *live the life of rational activity well*. This requires us to cultivate virtues that enable us to fulfil this function. Aristotle (1984) claimed that human beings can live a good life if their lives are lived according to what he called 'the rational parts of the soul' (pp. 1102a5–30). He believed that if we are functioning correctly (by living the life of rational activity *well*), we will flourish as human beings.

human flourishing based on the Ancient Greek word *eudaimonia*, it literally means 'good spirit'. Aristotle's ethics is sometimes referred to as 'eudaimonic ethics'; contemporary translations emphasise human flourishing, happiness and wellbeing.

Multiple-choice questions

Nevertheless, Aristotle did acknowledge that we need a certain amount of luck to flourish. For example, we need luck to avoid being harmed by natural disasters, such as earthquakes, or to be living in a peaceful society in which there is a low risk of being harmed by others.

With this in mind, we consider Aristotle's account of rationality and explore his views on the virtues engendered by the different parts of the soul. We also highlight the necessity of properly trained emotions for developing Aristotle's virtues.

Theoretical and practical rationality

Aristotle suggested that human beings manifest rationality, both *theoretically* and *practically*. Theoretical reason aims to uncover truths about the world and has as its goal the systematic acquisition of knowledge. We utilise this aspect of our rationality in, for example, scientific inquiry or the diagnosis of illness. The qualities we need to reason theoretically align with what we call 'intellectual virtues' – character traits that help a person get to the truth, such as being thorough, studious or insightful. These traits are also known as 'epistemic virtues', which are different from 'moral virtues' or 'virtues of character'.

In contrast, practical reason allows us to resolve, through reflection, the question of what we should do in a particular situation. Practical reason is not so much concerned with knowledge as with *values*. The qualities we need to reason practically are the 'moral virtues', such as courage, compassion and justice. We now discuss Aristotle's account of both of these types of reasoning, in turn.

Theoretical reason

theoretical rationality one of the two main types of rational activity that is unique to humans; it (theoretical reason) aims to uncover truths about the world and has as its goal the systematic acquisition of knowledge

As mentioned, an intellectual virtue is a manifestation of our capacity for **theoretical rationality**. These character traits enable 'an individual to be in the best position to apprehend the truth, and this insight has led to the development of *virtue epistemology*' (Bliss et al. 2017, p. 4). Virtue epistemologists claim that acquiring knowledge requires certain intellectual qualities ('virtues') of the individual themselves, along with natural faculties of the mind (such as perception and memory) that are functioning correctly (Bliss et al. 2017). In order to be 'intellectually virtuous', a person must demonstrate consistency and reliability in their thinking and in the ways in which they form their beliefs. For example, they will be curious about the world and care about developing their knowledge base. Other intellectual virtues might include being thorough in their tasks and conscientious in their studies. As a nursing student, you are in no doubt familiar with the requirement for nurses to 'think critically', as emphasised in Standard 1 of the Registered Nurse Standards for Practice (NMBA 2016). To fulfil this standard appropriately, nurses need to make a conscious attempt to cultivate intellectual virtues such as those mentioned already.

Multiple-choice question

We can apply this conception of epistemic virtue to nursing's knowledge base, which requires robust intellectual engagement with ideas and, where there are empirical truths, to comprehend and apply this to practice. Nurses are expected to understand the biomedical model of disease and to appreciate the importance of evidence-based practice. A person cannot do this adequately unless they have certain cognitive and intellectual capacities, such as those mentioned. We can therefore extend the notion of virtue to the knowledge discourse within nursing by conceptualising epistemology as a *normative* discipline in much the same way that ethics is such a discipline. By 'normative', we mean that it gives rise to 'should' claims. Some 'should' claims (norms) are *ethical* in nature – for instance, we could say, 'He should have done more to ensure the client had all the knowledge he needed to make an informed decision.' Other 'should' claims are *epistemic* in nature – for instance, 'She should have been open-minded enough to consider the loss of electrolytes as a possible alternative to cardiac arrest.' Virtues such as open-mindedness give rise to norms of knowledge acquisition that are valuable 'because they enable the intellectually virtuous individual the best chance of apprehending the truth' (Bliss et al. 2017, p. 4).

Practical reason

The second way in which we manifest rationality is through our **practical rationality**. Aristotle believed that 'the moral virtues, such as courage, are virtues of practical reasoning applied to human action' (Bliss et al. 2017, p. 5). A practical reason that virtue is a state of character is that it is the average between two extremes, at which point one can make choices. For example, 'courage is the mean between foolhardiness (an excess of courage) and cowardice (a deficit of courage)' (Bliss et al. 2017, p. 4). If a person is truly courageous, then they will show courage whenever the situation requires it; however, 'a person is not considered courageous when taking the courageous course of action is the exception rather than the rule' (Bliss et al. 2017, p. 5). Nevertheless, acting courageously is not simply an automatic response for the courageous person; instead, the courageous person does not consider the cowardly action as a viable option (Bliss et al. 2017). The decision made by the courageous person will reflect what courage requires in a situation once relevant facts are considered. This means that, in some cases, avoiding a confrontation may be a more courageous response than standing up for oneself and fighting. Recognising when to 'fight' and when to walk away requires a degree of emotional intelligence (see Chapter 10), and we will look at the role of emotions in acquiring the virtues in the next section.

practical rationality the other type of rational activity that is unique to humans; it (practical reason) refers to our capacity to be rational in deciding how to act in the world – particularly in our dealings with other people

Video: 'Introducing virtue ethics'
Podcasts: Inspirational nurses

CASE STUDY

Does the family always want the best for their loved one?

You are a nursing student and have just started your first clinical placement at a suburban nursing home. One of your first tasks is to attend to the mouth care of some of the residents. Because they are elderly and infirm, many residents do not drink very much, and their mouths can become dry and sore. Many of the residents also wear dentures, and these sometimes cause problems such as denture-related stomatitis. This can result in mouth ulcers, oral thrush or other problems that are unpleasant and painful.

You are assigned to care for Mr R, who is a bedridden, 85-year-old man. Mr R has a number of medical problems, including some dementia or confusion and denture-related stomatitis. He has quite a large family and a number of grandchildren and great-grandchildren. Members of his extended family visit him regularly and he has several young great-grandchildren who are often present. Recently, Mr R's mouth has become very inflamed and sore, and the other nurses have instructed you not to replace his dentures after attending to his mouth care as they seem to be quite ill-fitting and are causing significant discomfort and irritation.

One afternoon, some family members arrive while Mr R is having a nap. His mouth is open and he is snoring softly. His granddaughter, Leah, notices this and asks you to replace the dentures. Her reason for this is that 'the children don't need to see him looking like that'. You explain to her that the dentures are causing a lot of discomfort and that Mr R really needs to do without them for a while. Nevertheless, she insists that the dentures be replaced, suggesting that 'if they're in for an hour or two that won't matter'. Mr R has now woken up and you ask if you can place the dentures. He turns his head away, but Leah insists they are put in his mouth. You place the dentures and see Mr R's face grimace in pain. Again, you tell Leah that it's not a good idea, but she just says, 'Don't worry, he'll be fine'.

QUESTIONS

1   What are the ethical complexities in this case (e.g. the competing ethical claims)? *Hint:* Try to think about what is at stake in this situation.

2   How would you have managed this situation if you were the student nurse? What virtues would be useful for dealing with a situation like this?

The role of emotion in acquiring the virtues

There are other types of moral considerations that also deserve attention in any discussion of virtuous attributes – considerations not only about what the virtuous person would do in certain situations, but also *how they would feel*. Many of Aristotle's virtues (and vices) relate to emotions. For example, a courageous person is a person who not only acts courageously when the situation requires it, 'but also fears just those things that are worth fearing' (Bliss et al. 2017, p. 5). For Aristotle, courage does not just involve overcoming fear, 'but also of experiencing fear *correctly* – that is, in relation to things that are worth fearing, to the right degree and under the right circumstances' (Bliss et al. 2017, p. 5). Aristotle further believed that we make judgements as part of our emotional experiences. This means that our emotions can either be reasonable or unreasonable responses to situations, as the judgements we make when appraising a given situation may be correct or incorrect. Take the emotion of anger. Anger is a painful form of *distress* that 'arises from the *belief* that you or those close to you have suffered a conspicuous harm, conjoined with a *desire* for revenge and even, in many cases, an anticipatory *pleasure* at the prospect of getting your own back' (Bliss et al. 2017, p. 5). As they say, 'revenge is sweet'! Let us imagine that my friend Bob is angry because a mutual acquaintance, Jane, snapped at him at work. If I happen to know that

Jane is about to undergo a major operation and that her husband has just lost his job, I can tell Bob that Jane is under a lot of pressure in her personal life, which may explain why she snapped at him. Giving Bob more information to change how he perceives the situation would be futile unless he were making a judgement as part of his emotional reaction.

Nevertheless, the judgements we make as part of our emotional experiences do not work in quite the same way as those we make when, for instance, we are considering the benefits and costs of a proposed course of action. The judgements we make as part of emotional experience rest upon certain presuppositions or biases that may not be part of our conscious experience. These types of biases may take many different forms, but one example is the sexist assumptions that many of us make (often without any intended malice). Imagine I have some spare tickets to a football match that I am unable to use. I offer them to Bob rather than Jane because I have unconsciously assumed that women do not enjoy watching football (and men do). My judgement that Bob would enjoy watching the match more than Jane might be completely unfounded, and although no malice was intended, my reasoning is based on a stereotype rather than the facts of the particular situation. While such implicit biases can be difficult to overcome, we can combat the cultural conditioning that makes us susceptible to them if we have the **self-awareness** that allows us to recognise (and do something about) our own shortcomings (Perry, Murphy & Dovidio 2015). The first way to 'reprogram' these judgements involved in strong emotions is simply to be aware that our judgement impacts how we feel – for example, angry.

As mentioned, this process of reprogramming requires a high degree of self-awareness, which is also crucial if we are to understand another person's experience (Carr & Cortina 2011). Developing self-awareness also requires constructive feedback from others who are supportive and empathic themselves. We refer to this process as the development of **emotional intelligence** (see also Chapter 10). Many factors determine how emotionally intelligent we are but a necessary condition for developing this capacity is that we have integrated our 'emotions into a coherent narrative of self-experience' – a continuous process that begins in infancy (Carr & Cortina 2011, p. 26). If an individual lacks emotional intelligence, their intersubjective abilities that allow them to validate and recognise the unique characteristics of others will be severely curtailed (Carr & Cortina 2011, p. 26; Nightingale et al. 2018). Thus, nurses who lack emotional intelligence and maturity are more likely to struggle to care for others empathically and compassionately.

We can improve our emotional intelligence by regularly interacting with people who are empathic and who provide understanding and recognition (Eisenberg, Spinrad & Eggum 2010). This demonstrates 'the importance of having people around us who are emotionally tuned in, a point Aristotle recognised millennia ago' (Bliss et al. 2017, p. 5). Because of this, we require reliable 'role models to support us in the process of educating our emotions', as we are unlikely to realise that we lack emotional intelligence unless we are around people who have appropriate emotional resources (Bliss et al. 2017, p. 5). Having these role models 'can help us to break bad habits of judgement and remove ourselves from the patterns of behaviour that reinforced them' (Bliss et al. 2017, p. 5). This is one reason why it is so important for nursing students to have positive role models, both at university and in the clinical setting (Felstead 2013).

self-awareness the conscious knowledge of one's own character, feelings, motives and behaviours

Multiple-choice question

emotional intelligence the ability to recognise, understand and respond appropriately to emotions in oneself and others

If emotions such as compassion are just as Aristotle suggested, then they may be an important element in justifying professional decisions and actions. Nurses should be able to 'feel and experience their emotions and act accordingly' (Bliss et al. 2017, p. 6) because the ability to feel one's (appropriate) emotions, such as compassion, empathy and distress, allows for empathic care. Having emotional intelligence affords us the ability to recognise the morally relevant features of the situations in which we find ourselves. For nurses, this ability is extremely important. This is because the ethical dimensions of a caring relationship will most commonly be in everyday interactions, where the nurse can humanise clients' experiences – something that most clients find very important (Griffiths et al. 2012). Care that is truly person-centred seems to require us to attend to ourselves first. This process involves 'an intention to consistently develop, hone and exercise certain character traits (virtues) over time' (Snow 2010; Bliss et al. 2017, p. 6). Let us now examine a virtue we believe is particularly important for nurses to cultivate: gratitude.

Gratitude in nursing

gratitude the appreciation of what is good, valuable and meaningful in one's life; a thankful appreciation for what an individual receives, whether tangible or intangible, often triggering a reciprocal, prosocial response

Multiple-choice question

Gratitude refers to an appreciation of what is good, valuable and meaningful in one's life. It affirms and 'amplifies the good in our lives: our awareness and interpretation of beneficial events' (Howells 2016), good memories and how we have been supported and affirmed by other people (Emmons 2010; Emmons & Smith 2020; Watkins & McCurrach 2016). Gratitude involves a thankful appreciation for the gifts and benefits we have received – big or small, tangible or intangible – accompanied by a force that encourages us to 'give back' or 'pay it forward' (upstream reciprocity) (Allen 2020; Cox 2018; Howells 2016). Gratitude has been described as 'relationship-strengthening' (Emmons 2010; Wong et al. 2020), in that it 'moves us into giving mode and [fosters] a greater sense of interconnectedness and empathy with those from whom we feel we have received' (Howells 2016, 2017).

Gratitude has been conceptualised as a moral virtue, an emotion, an attitude, a personality trait and a coping mechanism. Irrespective of any subtle differences in its defining features, we contend that gratitude aligns closely with many of the ideas discussed earlier in this chapter, and it is a concept worthy of further consideration in both nursing education and practice. In fact, in the context of 'virtues' discussed above, the Roman philosopher and statesman Cicero stated that 'gratitude is not only the greatest of virtues, but the parent of all others'. This suggests that gratitude is not just an episode, but a disposition or part of our character, and that when practised in conjunction with other virtues, gratitude can have a powerful and transformative influence in our own lives and on society as a whole (Howells 2017).

The existing body of gratitude research reveals three key areas in which gratitude could be cultivated in or for nursing:

- as a new 'disciplinary concept' to complement and reinforce core nursing concepts such as caring, compassion and person-centredness;
- as a 'therapeutic tool' to help enhance client engagement and satisfaction with care, and improve health outcomes, subjective wellbeing and quality of life; and

- as a 'self-care' resource to help moderate and protect nurses from emotional stress and burnout, thereby contributing to higher job satisfaction, organisational citizenship and retention in the profession.

Gratitude has long been a subject of great interest for classical scholars, philosophers, ethicists and theologians, but it has only been in recent decades that rigorous empirical inquiry into gratitude has emerged, particularly in relation to health and wellbeing (Arnott 2017; Emmons & McCullough 2003). While conceptual debates abound, there is a growing body of research that correlates the experience and expression of gratitude with enhanced physical health, subjective wellbeing, prosocial tendencies, stronger interpersonal relationships, optimism, resilience and overall positive functioning (Arnott 2017, Algoe, Fredrickson & Gable 2013; Arnott 2017; Emmons & Smith 2020; Howells 2017; Lavelock et al. 2016; Ma, Tunney & Ferguson 2017; Wong et al. 2020; Wood, Froh & Geraghty 2010).

Many of the identified qualities or benefits of gratitude appear to have a clear affiliation with the philosophy, values and therapeutic intent of nursing – particularly humanistic and relational characteristics such as caring, empathy, compassion and person-centredness (Arnott 2017; Dahlke & Stahlke Wall 2017; Fournier & Sheehan 2015; Howells 2017; Stein-Parbury 2018). Despite this correlation, gratitude has received limited attention in nursing research and practice. Most references to gratitude in nursing involve expressions of gratefulness directed *to* nurses *from* recipients of their care (clients and families) (Arnott 2017). This expression of gratitude – or what has been referred to as 'grateful to' gratitude (Lambert, Graham & Fincham 2009, p. 1194) – may well strengthen social bonds and relationships between clients and their care providers, enhance clients' satisfaction and their adherence to care regimens, and improve their perceived wellbeing and quality of life. However, little is known about the effects on the nurses receiving this gratitude, or the things that they themselves may feel grateful for or about, along with how this is expressed in the context of their nursing practice and the benefits that may come from this.

Our assertion is that the experience and expression of gratitude is equally, or at least interdependently, important for the caregiver or nurse (Arnott 2017; Hass 2020). Research has found that gratitude can help to moderate caregiver burdens (Bauer et al. 2013), act as a coping or protective mechanism in high-stress environments (Arnott 2017; Romanzini & Bock 2010), reduce the incidence of emotional exhaustion and burnout (Cheng, Tsui & Lam 2015; Converso et al. 2015), foster job satisfaction and organisational citizenship (Waters 2012), increase the motivation for prosociality or acting in kindness (Arnott 2017; Ma, Tunney & Ferguson 2017) and foster the adoption of a person-centred orientation to care (Fournier & Sheehan 2015).

While a detailed examination of gratitude is not our intention in this chapter, we want to introduce you to this emergent concept in nursing and encourage you to cultivate gratitude as part of your personal philosophy and identity as a nurse, and as a resource for your future learning and practice.

Short-answer question
Video + podcast: Gratitude

Cultivating an innermost attitude of gratitude

Gratitude may not be evident or come naturally to some people, but research has shown that it can be learned, cultivated and nurtured through intentional practice, introspection and reflection (Smith 2020; Wilson 2016). A quick internet search will reveal hundreds of gratitude practices and resources; here are a few you might like to try:

- *Count your blessings.* Set aside a few minutes each day or week to think about three to five 'blessings' that you have experienced (e.g. who or what you are grateful for; who or what has inspired you; things that have brought you happiness, comfort or peace). This practice can help you to acknowledge and affirm the 'good in your life'.
- *Keep a gratitude journal.* This is an extension of the above practice, but with an emphasis on recording your 'grateful recounting' in a journal. When you write in your journal is not important (e.g. before bed, when you wake up, in your lunch break) but it is important that you consistently take a few moments to consciously focus on your blessings. Some research suggests that benefits can flow from this practice after only a few days; however, we encourage you to commit to keeping a journal for at least a month (Chopra 2012; Emmons & McCullough 2003; Watkins, Uhder & Pichinevskiy 2015).
- *Write a gratitude letter.* Select someone who has had a profound effect on your life (a family member, friend, peer, teacher, client) and write them a thank-you letter in which you express gratitude for all the 'gifts' you have received from them. Some people benefit from simply writing the letter but, if possible, follow through by delivering the letter in person. Research has suggested that writing, delivering and receiving a gratitude letter can enhance the wellbeing of, and social bonds between, both the author and the recipient (Chopra 2012; Toepfer, Cichy & Peters 2011).
- *Be in a state of preparedness.* This activity has been developed in the context of education but is equally valid for your nursing practice. This practice specifically invites you to examine your outlook (regarding a class, a placement or a shift, for example) and to honestly evaluate whether you hold attitudes of gratitude or resentment. A state of preparedness does not automatically rid us of the negativity in our lives but it does encourage us to consciously choose a grateful perspective. The more we practise this state, the more gratitude can infuse our everyday encounters and help us to see beyond the negative without forcing it (Howells 2012, 2016).

NURSING PERSPECTIVE

Although my unit is getting the work done, staff engagement scores are not great, absenteeism is up and my own sense of job satisfaction is dwindling after five years in this role. How do we raise morale and make a much-needed attitude adjustment?

'Catching this deterioration before it impacts patient care is the key.' With perspectives from neuroscience and 'the emerging field of positive psychology, we're just beginning to understand the attitude of gratitude' and its influence on nursing.

The practice of gratitude is a key enabler of emotional intelligence and 'an essential skill set for leaders'. Gratitude has been called the 'secret sauce' to enhancing employee engagement. When we are expressing gratitude or reflecting on positives, our brains release dopamine and serotonin, which trigger positive emotions such as optimism and intrinsic motivation. The more we activate these 'gratitude circuits', the stronger the neural pathways become and the more likely we are to notice what is going right, rather than habitually being drawn to the negative.

A study on the psychological wellbeing of nurses found that gratitude 'is a consistent predictor of lower exhaustion and cynicism, fewer absences, higher job satisfaction, and more proactive behaviours'.

Other studies have shown that people who practise gratitude have less depression, better impulse control, greater optimism and higher self-esteem. They also have lower blood pressure, lower levels of cortisol and a stronger immune system … of all the character strengths, gratitude has been found to be the greatest predictor of wellbeing. Cultivating an attitude of gratitude can do a power of good for nursing practice and leadership, helping to strengthen engagement, relationships and the wellbeing of ourselves and others.

Source: Adapted from Cox (2018, p. 56).

Nursing as eudaimonic practice: The alignment of ends

If what we have said so far is correct, then the tension between the 'knowledge' and 'caring' discourses that we noted earlier is resolved: the moral and epistemic virtues are two sides of the same coin. If someone asked you 'Is the head (nursing knowledge) or the heart (empathic caring) the core of nursing?', we think you should reply, 'Both' – the two are not as different as people commonly suppose. This is because epistemic virtues like openness to alternatives or quick recollection of anatomical facts are qualities that allow us to exercise our rationality *successfully*. But we also do this by exemplifying moral virtues such as gratitude, compassion and justice. Each type of virtue informs the other. Feeling compassion for a client and acting accordingly may help them to feel more comfortable about disclosing sensitive information that is relevant to providing evidence-based care. Equally, understanding the physiology of the dying process, for instance, allows a nurse to exercise effective compassion for the client and their family.

We can think about it in the following way. Intellectual and moral virtues are qualities that make us good at the job of *being human*. So, what about the job of being a nurse? Could the qualities that would make you a good nurse be different from those that would make you a good person, or is being a good nurse one way of being a good person? If we apply Aristotle's ideas to these questions, we can see that nursing has as its end (goal) 'a *genuine social good*, without which human flourishing or "happiness" in its broadest sense would not be possible' (Bliss et al. 2017, p. 6). All of us are susceptible to illness and injury and may at some time need the assistance of nursing professionals. The healthcare professions 'are distinguished from other human pursuits, such as art, in that their technical artistry (for a nurse, this would include mastery of clinical reasoning, for example) must also serve a *moral* end' (Bliss et al. 2017, p. 6; Pellegrino 2007). Aristotle believed that it was not necessary for a great artist to also be a good human being; they 'would only need to possess the virtues that serve [their] artistic endeavours' (Bliss et al. 2017, p. 6). This is not the case for nurses, however. The goal of nursing is the welfare of a human being who is in need of a particular kind of help and has the specific good of those individuals at its centre, so the end or goal of nursing is *'the good of the patient'* (Bliss et al. 2017).

Aristotle (1984) suggested that the good of the client is *health*, and we think he was almost right about this – but not quite. It is generally understood that health 'is not an achievable end for many patients' (Bliss et al. 2017, p. 6). A more appropriate goal would be *wellness*, which captures the idea that health and illness are on a continuum rather than being a dichotomy. Wellness 'relates to the good of the whole person: biological, psychological, social, spiritual and personal' (Bliss et al. 2017, p. 6). There is something distinctive about nursing as a profession, in that nurses care for vulnerable individuals who are sometimes facing the prospect of serious life changes, or even death. The personal qualities of nurses are crucial for just this reason, for the very act of nursing practice takes place in a *moral* space. This is because nurses' work is striving to achieve this end (wellness) for the client. Nursing, at its core, is about assisting the client to achieve the 'good life' insofar as that is possible. Nurses very often need to take up the ethical pursuit of the 'good life' on behalf of their clients. They need to be able to anticipate and carry out certain tasks or actions, important for living *well*, which clients may not be able to perform for themselves. Nurses therefore have a uniquely and ethically demanding working life.

In short, because nursing as a profession promotes an end that is an essential precondition for any good life, there is a reason to hope that excellence in that profession (flourishing as a nurse) will coincide with flourishing as a human being. In other words, there is an **alignment of ends** between the goals of nursing and the goals of a 'good life' more broadly. Doing well as a nurse is one way of doing well as a human being, and nurses have a professional duty to themselves to preserve this coincidence. Clinical nurses, academics and students must work together to make sure that our working conditions – the concrete, specific settings in which we learn and exercise the nursing virtues – allow us to flourish as both nurses and human beings.

alignment of ends the proposition that the ends of nursing are the same as the ends of being a good (successful) human being, on Aristotle's account; being an excellent nurse is one way of being an excellent human

SUMMARY

- We identified two ways of thinking about nursing: the 'knowledge discourse', which focuses on 'discrete areas of evidence-based, discipline-specific knowledge' (Bliss et al. 2017, p. 6), and the 'caring discourse', in which the moral qualities needed for humanistic caring are at centre stage. While these two ways of understanding nursing are not mutually exclusive, there is a debate in the literature about how nursing should represent itself.
- Aristotle believed that acquiring virtues was a necessary condition for fulfilling our function as humans: to live the life of rational activity *well*. Aristotle distinguished two types of reason: theoretical and practical. Exercising these two forms of reason successfully requires the intellectual and character virtues, respectively. We develop these virtues through practice and habit, but emotions also have an important role. Aristotle's theories on emotions demonstrate a way for individuals to encourage the conditions within themselves that make holistic, person-centred care possible. We cannot acquire the capacity to care in this way without intentionally improving

our emotional intelligence and our ability to truly be there for another person (Bliss et al. 2017).

- An Aristotelian conception of virtue 'allows us to flesh out a theoretical basis for nursing that focuses on moral competence in a robust, coherent and systematic way, while at the same time accommodating the demand for discipline-specific knowledge and high levels of technical skill' (Bliss et al. 2017, p. 7). Thus, the apparent tension between the knowledge and caring discourses can be resolved. The notion of virtue can fruitfully be applied to nursing's theories in a way that accommodates both rigorous, evidence-based practice and the expectation that nurses should behave in a way that embodies humanistic caring values.

- The excellent exercise of practical and theoretical reasoning as it is manifested in the 'art of nursing' is one way a person can achieve Aristotle's account of happiness. The profession of nursing has a more intimate connection to happiness (and thereby *goodness)* than other professions or practices, whose ends are not so intimately connected with the essential preconditions of a 'good life'. Therefore, we can say that there is an alignment of ends between being an excellent nurse and flourishing as a human being.

- Gratitude is the appreciation of what is good, valuable and meaningful in one's life. Research has revealed many benefits and the value of gratitude for physical health, subjective wellbeing, interpersonal relationships, self-care and as a *state of preparedness* for education and practice, all of which highlight its relevance to nursing (and nurses). Gratitude can be cultivated through intentional practice, with various strategies being suggested in this chapter.

REVIEW QUESTIONS

Suggested responses

1 How can philosophy as a methodology assist practising nurses? Try to think of an example.
2 What are some of the risks of not having an underpinning philosophy of nursing?
3 What is 'practical reason' (sometimes referred to as 'phronesis') and how could it be applied to nursing practice?
4 Why does Aristotle think that emotions are an important part of cultivating the virtues?
5 Why are the 'ends of nursing' similar to, or the same as, the 'ends of being a human'?

RESEARCH TOPIC

Many people have thought (and still think) that emotions have no place in a professional context. Investigate the role and importance of the emotions, particularly relating to moral development and their role in providing person-centred care. Illustrate your findings with examples from nursing practice where emotions could have played a role in ensuring better-quality care.

FURTHER READING

Bliss, S., Baltzly, D., Bull, R., Dalton, L. & Jones, J. (2017). A role for virtue in unifying the 'knowledge' and 'caring' discourses in nursing theory. *Nursing Inquiry*, 24(4), doi:10.1111/nin.12191.

Day, L. (2007). Courage as a virtue necessary for good nursing practice. *American Journal of Critical Care*, 16, 613–16.

Fournier, A. & Sheehan, C. (2015). Growing gratitude in undergraduate nursing students: Applying findings from social and psychological domains to nursing education. *Nurse Education Today*, 35, 1139–41.

Greco, J. & Turri, J. (2016). Virtue epistemology. In E.N. Zalta (ed.), *The Stanford encyclopedia of philosophy*. Available from https://plato.stanford.edu/archives/win2016/entries/epistemology-virtue.

Kraut, R. (2017). Aristotle's ethics. In E.N. Zalta (ed.), *The Stanford encyclopedia of philosophy*. Available from https://plato.stanford.edu/archives/sum2017/entries/aristotle-ethics.

Kristjansson, K. (2013). An Aristotelian virtue of gratitude. *Topoi*, 34(2), 499–511.

Smith, J.A., Newman, K.M., Marsh, J. & Keltner, D. (eds). (2020). *The gratitude project: How the science of thankfulness can rewire our brains for resilience, optimism, and the greater good*. Oakland, CA: New Harbinger.

REFERENCES

Algoe, S.B., Fredrickson, B.L. & Gable, S.L. (2013). The social functions of the emotion of gratitude via expression. *Emotion*, 13(4), 605–9.

Allen, S. (2020). How gratitude relates to other emotions. In J.A. Smith, K.M. Newman, J. Marsh & D. Keltner (eds), *The gratitude project: How the science of thankfulness can rewire our brains for resilience, optimism, and the greater good*. Oakland, CA: New Harbinger, pp. 34–5.

Aristotle (1984). Nichomachean ethics. In J. Barnes (ed.), *The complete works of Aristotle: The revised Oxford translation (Vol. 2)*. Princeton, NJ: Princeton University Press.

Arnott, N. (2017). The grateful nurse: The possibilities and dilemmas of gratitude in nursing education and practice, paper presented to *11th Annual Graduate Research Conference – University of Tasmania*, Retrieved from http://ecite.utas.edu.au/121181.

Bauer, R., Sterzinger, L., Koepke, F. & Spiessl, H. (2013). Rewards of caregiving and coping strategies of caregivers of patients with mental illness. *Psychiatic Services*, 64(2), 185–8.

Bliss, S., Baltzly, D., Bull, R., Dalton, L. & Jones, J. (2017). A role for virtue in unifying the 'knowledge' and 'caring' discourses in nursing theory. *Nursing Inquiry*, 24(4).

Bruce, A., Rietze, L. & Lim, A. (2014). Understanding philosophy in a nurse's world: What, where and why? *Nursing and Health*, 2, 65–71.

Carper, B. (1978). Fundamental patterns of knowing in nursing. *Advances in Nursing Science*, 1(1), 13–23.

Carr, E. & Cortina, M. (2011). Heinz Kohut and John Bowlby: The men and their ideas. *Psychoanalytic Inquiry*, 31, 42–57.

Cheng, S.T., Tsui, P.K. & Lam, J.H. (2015). Improving mental health in health care practitioners: Randomized controlled trial of a gratitude intervention. *Journal of Consulting and Clinical Psychology*, 83(1), 177–86.

Chopra, D. (2012). 3 essential practices for gratitude. Retrieved from https://spirituality health.com/articles/2012/11/20/3-essential-practices-gratitude.

Converso, D., Loera, B., Viotti, S. & Martini, M. (2015). Do positive relations with patients play a protective role for healthcare employees? Effects of patients' gratitude and support on nurses' burnout. *Frontiers in Psychology*, 6, 470.

Cox, S. (2018). The power of gratitude. *Nursing Management*, 49(4), 56.

Dahlke, S. & Stahlke Wall, S. (2017). Does the emphasis on caring within nursing contribute to nurses' silence about practice issues? *Nursing Philosophy*, 18(3).

Eisenberg, N., Spinrad, T.L. & Eggum, N.D. (2010). Emotion-related self-regulation and its relation to children's maladjustment. *Annual Review of Clinical Psychology*, 6, 495–525.

Emmons, R. (2010). Why gratitude is good. *Greater Good Magazine*, 16 November. Retrieved from https://greatergood.berkeley.edu/article/item/why_gratitude_is_good.

Emmons, R.A. & McCullough, M.E. (2003). Counting blessings versus burdens: An experimental investigation of gratitude and subjective well-being in daily life. *Journal of Personality and Social Psychology*, 84(2), 377–89.

Emmons, R.A. & Smith, J.A. (2020). What gratitude is and why it matters. In J.A. Smith, K.M. Newman, J. Marsh, & D. Keltner (eds), *The gratitude project: How the science of thankfulness can rewire our brains for resilience, optimism, and the greater good*. Oakland, CA: New Harbinger, pp. 3–11.

Felstead, I. (2013). Role modelling and students' professional development. *British Journal of Nursing*, 22, 223–7.

Forss, A., Ceci, C. & Drummond, J.S (2013). *Philosophy of nursing: Five questions*. Copenhagen: Automatic Press.

Fournier, A. & Sheehan, C. (2015). Growing gratitude n undergraduate nursing students: Applying findings from social and psychological domains to nursing education. *Nurse Education Today*, 35, 1139–41.

Gordon, S. & Nelson, S. (2006). Moving beyond the virtue script in nursing: Creating a knowledge-based identity for nurses. In S. Nelson & S. Gordon (eds), *The complexities of care: Nursing reconsidered*. Ithaca, NY: ILR Press, pp. 13–29.

Griffiths, J., Speed, S., Horne, M. & Keeley, P. (2012). 'A caring professional attitude': What service users and carers seek from graduate nurses and the challenge for education. *Nurse Education Today*, 32, 121–7.

Hass, L. (2020). Why health professionals should cultivate gratitude. In J.H. Smit, K.M. Newman, J. Marsh & D. Keltner (eds), *The gratitude project: How the science of thankfulness can rewire our brains for resilience, optimism, and the greater good*. Oakland, CA: New Harbinger Publications Inc, pp. 158–63.

Howells, K. (2012). *Gratitude in education: A radical view*. Rotterdam: Sense.

——— (2016). A state of preparedness: Preparing our being with gratitude. Retrieved from http://www.kerryhowells.com/a-state-of-preparedness-preparing-our-being-with-gratitude.

——— (2017). Six pillars of gratitude. Retrieved from http://www.kerryhowells.com/six-pillars-of-gratitude.

Jackson, L. (2016). Why should I be grateful? The morality of gratitude in contexts marked by injustice. *Journal of Moral Education*, 45(3), 276–90.

Lambert, N.M., Graham, S.M. & Fincham, F.D. (2009). A prototype analysis of gratitude: Varieties of gratitude experiences. *Personality and Social Psychology Bulletin*, 35(9), 1193–207.

Lavelock, C.R., Griffin, B.J., Worthington, E.L., Benotsch, E.G., Lin, Y., Greer, C.L., Garthe, R. C., Coleman, J.A., Hughes, C.M., Davis, D.E. & Hook, J.N. (2016). A qualitative review and integrative model of gratitude and physical health. *Journal of Psychology and Theology*, 44, 55–86.

Ma, L.K., Tunney, R.J. & Ferguson, E. (2017). Does gratitude enhance prosociality? A meta-analytic review. *Psychological Bulletin*, 143(6), 601–35.

Mackintosh-Franklin, C. (2016). Nursing philosophy: A review of current pre-registration curricula in the UK. *Nurse Education Today*, 37, 71–4.

Morgan, B., Gulliford, L. & Kristjansson, K. (2017). A new approach to measuring moral virtues: The multi-component gratitude measure. *Personality and Individual Differences*, 107(1), 179–89.

Nightingale, S., Spiby, H., Sheen, K. & Slade, P. (2018). The impact of emotional intelligence in health care professionals on caring behaviour towards patients in clinical and long-term care settings: Findings from an integrative review. *International Journal of Nursing Studies*, 80, 106–17.

Nursing and Midwifery Board of Australia (NMBA) (2016). *Registered Nurse Standards for Practice*. Retrieved from https://www.nursingmidwiferyboard.gov.au/codes-guidelines-statements/professional-standards/registered-nurse-standards-for-practice.aspx.

——— (2018). *Code of Conduct for Nurses*. Retrieved from http://www.nursingmidwiferyboard.gov.au/Codes-Guidelines-Statements/Professional-standards.aspx.

Paley, J. (2002). Caring as a slave morality: Nietzschean themes in nursing ethics. *Journal of Advanced Nursing*, 40(1), 25–35.

Pellegrino, E. (2007). Professing medicine, virtue based ethics, and the retrieval of professionalism. In R.L. Walker & P.J. Ivanhoe (eds), *Working virtue: Virtue ethics and contemporary moral problems*. Oxford: Clarendon Press.

Perry, S.P., Murphy, M.C. & Dovidio, J.F. (2015). Modern prejudice: Subtle, but unconscious? The role of bias awareness in white's perceptions of personal and others' biases. *Journal of Experimental Psychology*, 61, 64–78.

Risjord, M. (2011). *Nursing knowledge: Science, practice, and philosophy*. Chichester: John Wiley & Sons.

Romanzini, E.M. & Bock, L.F. (2010). Conceptions and feelings of nurses working in emergency medical services about their professional practice and training. *Revista Latino-Americana de Enfermagem*, 18(2), 240–6.

Seedhouse, D. (2000). *Practical nursing philosophy: The universal ethical code*. Chichester: John Wiley & Sons.

Smith, J.A. (2020). How to cultivate gratitude in yourself. In J.H. Smit, K.M. Newman, J. Marsh & D. Keltner (eds), *The gratitude project: How the science of thankfulness can rewire our brains for resilience, optimism, and the greater good*. Oakland, CA: New Harbinger, pp. 158–63.

Snow, N.E. (2010). *Virtue as social intelligence: An empirically grounded theory*. New York: Routledge.

Stein-Parbury, J. (2018). *Patient and person: Interpersonal skills in nursing*, 6th edn. Sydney: Elsevier.

Thorne, S. & Sawatzky, R. (2014). Particularizing the general: Sustaining theoretical integrity in the context of an evidence-based practice agenda. *Advanced Nursing Science*, 37(1), 5–18.

Toepfer, S.M., Cichy, K. & Peters, P. (2011). Letters of gratitude: Further evidence for author benefits. *Journal of Happiness Studies*, 13(1), 187–201.

Waters, L. (2012). Predicting job satisfaction: Contributions of individual gratitude and institutionalized gratitude. *Psychology (Savannah, CA)*, 3(12), 1174–6.

Watkins, P. & McCurrach, D. (2016). Exploring how gratitude trains cognitive processes important to wellbeing. In D. Carr (ed.), *Perspectives on gratitude: An interdisciplinary approach* New York: Routledge.

Watkins, P.C., Uhder, J. & Pichinevskiy, S. (2015). Grateful recounting enhances subjective well-being: The importance of grateful processing. *The Journal of Positive Psychology*, 10(2), 91–8.

Wilson, J.T. (2016). Brightening the mind: The impact of practicing gratitude on focus and resilience in learning. *Journal of the Scholarship of Teaching and Learning*, 16(4), 1–13.

Wong, J., Brown, J., Armenta, C., Lyubomirsky, S., Allen, S., Gordon, A. & Newman, K.M. (2020). Why gratitude is good for us. In J.A. Smith, K.M. Newman, J. Marsh & D. Keltner (eds), *The gratitude project: How the science of thankfulness can rewire our brains for resilience, optimism, and the greater good*. Oakland, CA: New Harbinger, pp. 38–52.

Wood, A.M., Froh, J.J. & Geraghty, A.W. (2010). Gratitude and well-being: A review and theoretical integration. *Clinical Psychology Review*, 30 7), 890–905.

8

The history and evolving image of nursing

Mary Cruickshank, Penny Paliadelis, Swapnali Gazula and Margaret McAllister

LEARNING OBJECTIVES

At the completion of this chapter, you should be able to:

1 Explain the recent evolution of the nursing profession.
2 Reflect on the influences and meanings of positive and negative nursing images and stereotypes.
3 Discuss the importance of image in shaping how nurses are perceived and how nurses think about themselves.
4 Identify strategies to enhance understandings of the reality of nursing as a profession.

Introduction

The traditional stereotypical image of a nurse is closely linked to that of Florence Nightingale, the founder of modern nursing who established a training system to teach nurses how to be completely dedicated to the tasks of care, regardless of personal needs; to be dependent upon and deferential to authorities such as medical doctors and matron supervisors; and how to comport with modesty and femininity. Of course, contemporary nursing is no longer a profession exclusively female, nor does nursing work predominantly involve dependent actions. However, these outdated ideas remain strong in the minds of the public and are often repeated in popular culture.

The portrayal of nurses in the media has a powerful effect on perception by the public, clients and within themselves (Stanley et al. 2019). Sadly, their public image may not correspond with personal reality (Rauen et al. 2016), and this is the central argument in this chapter. Image is *a reflection* of an actual thing, not the thing itself. The image may be distorted or precise, contemporary and relevant, or embarrassingly outdated. What people take to be true about nursing and midwifery, because of what they read, see or hear in the media, may actually be more myth than reality, and myths can have a significant influence – both positive and negative.

Luckily for nursing, we have overwhelmingly been perceived as good – helpful, caring, ethical and practical. But occasionally nurses have been portrayed as evil and monstrous. This chapter explores the evolution of the nursing profession and considers the effects of image on contemporary nursing practice. It also invites you to reflect on whether these public perceptions have influenced you, your decision to be a nurse and your future actions. Reflecting on where we have come from and where we may be going is key to developing a nursing profession that meets the needs of future generations.

The evolution of the nursing profession

Modern nursing began in the 1850s with Florence Nightingale, who shot to fame (and ruffled some feathers) by becoming a nurse and caring for the sick and injured during the Crimean War. Nightingale was not a typical nurse of her day. She was born into a British upper-class family and, at 24 years of age, defied her parents by refusing to marry a suitable 'match'. Instead, she chose to study to become a nurse. She was a rebel and a trailblazer. In Australia, the early history of nurses caring for poor people is documented in a book titled *Poverty's Prison* by Ann O'Brien (1988), which shows how the Nightingale traditions were 'transported' to Australia.

Today, Nightingale's legacy continues to shape perceptions of the nursing profession as caring, selfless, devoted and honourable. These perceptions are both a blessing and a curse for professional nurses today, and into the future. They can limit understandings of the scope of the profession and the skills and knowledge required, by 'locking' nurses into 'just' being caring, compassionate and selfless – traits that are viewed as personal and feminine – thereby disregarding the diversity in present-day nursing (Hodges et al. 2017; Morrison-Beedy, Tzeng & Abriam-Yago 2017). This encourages the belief that some people are 'born' to be nurses and discounts the knowledge required to become a professional nurse in contemporary society. Some of the milestones in the evolution of nursing images and **stereotypes** over time and across geographic locations are summarised in the following section.

The evolution of nursing images and stereotypes

Prior to the image of nurses as composed and dutifully following orders, inspired by Nightingale, nurses were village healers, and before that they were male monks (Teodorescu & Preda 2018). From the Dark Ages through to the Middle Ages, the practice of nursing, as well as its image, underwent significant change. While not consistently or rigorously trained, nurses had a distinct role within society, to help people who were injured or ill. Nurses developed in-depth knowledge about the healing power of plants and herbs: chamomile and peppermint were frequently prescribed to calm physical pains; poultices were made to draw out infection; plants were used to initiate abortion in women who could not deal with a pregnancy. During the Dark Ages, when superstition and belief were rife, possession of nurses' secret knowledge was considered uncanny and untrustworthy, and some nurses and midwives were condemned as witches (Wright 2016, Ehrenreich & English 2010). The book and television series *Outlander* provide a fictionalised account of how nurses worked in the 1700s (Gabaldon 1991–2005; Moore 2014–).

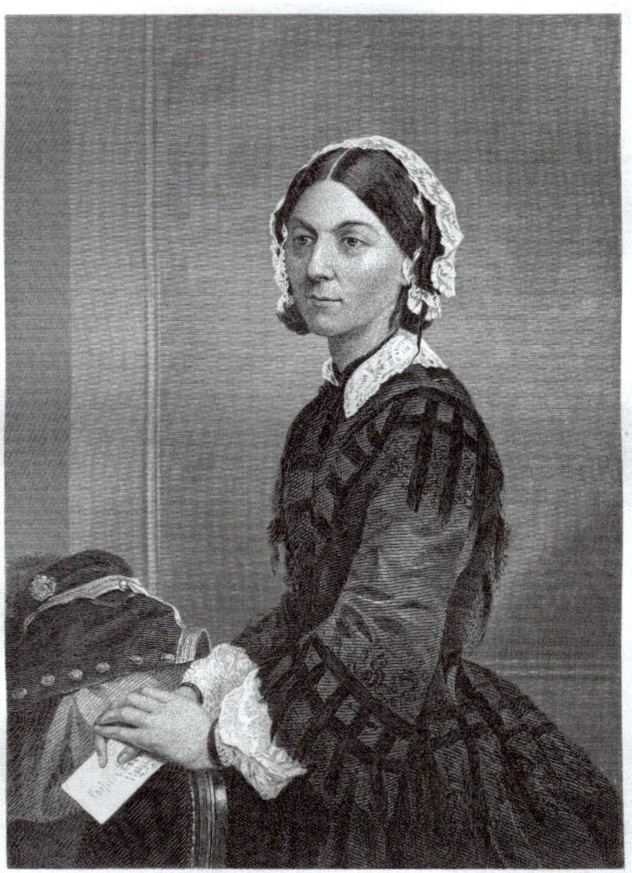

Figure 8.1   Florence Nightingale

In the Middle Ages, many nurses were male. Monks who tended wounded crusaders shared their wisdom with each other in documents that today resemble recipe books (Robles 2016). From this it is evident that nurses, even in earlier times, took their role in working with vulnerable people seriously. In the early Victorian era, prior to Nightingale's reforms, nursing's image hit an all-time low. During this time, there was no system-wide distribution of health care to ensure that those who were poor and needy had access to help. Nor was there any training for nurses. Standards were inconsistent and accountability was non-existent. Indeed, during this time nursing was so undervalued that most nurses were recruited from mental institutions ('madhouses'), workhouses and prisons.

In *The Life and Adventures of Martin Chuzzlewit,* a novel set in the mid-1800s by Charles Dickens (1999), the nurse Sairey Gamp embodies everything that was contemptuous and unflattering about nursing at this time. Sairey (or Sarah) was illiterate and untrained, selfish and unreliable, as well as frequently drunk and unsafe (Summers 1997). The image is shocking! Indeed, so influential was Dickens's harsh portrayal of nurses and the dreadful standards of care for those who were marginalised, poor and downtrodden in English and colonial societies at this time that healthcare reforms began to be instituted by governments and were spearheaded by the much-respected monarch, Queen Victoria.

So began what has come to be known as 'modern nursing'. During the Crimean War, Florence Nightingale – an educated woman who was looking forward to emancipation from her family and the excitement of living a public life – recruited women who were conservative, reasonably educated and willing to follow orders to help her form a nursing team to care for wounded soldiers on the Crimean Peninsula. These nurses completed training that emphasised special techniques Nightingale considered as embodying the art of nursing and taught through discipline and repetition. By maintaining routines and rituals, Nightingale believed that nursing could become consistent, and the care provided could be reliable. Nightingale argued that nursing required an image overhaul because it was providing a necessary service to society. Thus, all nurses needed to be sober, clean and literate. Rightly or wrongly, Nightingale linked nursing to being a 'good woman' (giving, devoted, selfless, sober and demure) with a 'calling' to care for the sick.

A dominant – and still prevailing – perception of what constitutes 'nursing work' has evolved out of what people believed was naturally 'women's work' – which in various times across history was or was not valued. It is easy to see why nursing constantly battles image problems and continues to encounter entrenched stereotypes – that the work is dirty, hidden or profane; that all nurses are the same and ought to be seen but not heard; that nurses will work for the love of it and thus do not need to be highly paid; and that nurses should endure a lower status when compared with some other health professionals (Ehrenreich & English 2010).

There are now many conflicting images of nurses in all forms of media, ranging from the view of nurses as motherly, virginal or heroic, to high-heeled sirens looking for romance, or grumpy and sadistic 'matrons'. Of course, the reality of nursing is not reflected in any of these shallow representations (Brideson et al. 2016; Gordon & Nelson 2005; Kelly, Fealy & Watson 2012; Summers 2015). Nursing is complex and diverse, and frequently involves independent actions in monitoring health and providing psychosocial support, diagnoses and treatments. Over centuries, nurses have come a long way from being subordinate to working alongside other healthcare team members (Dussault 2020). But it is alarming to note that, even in recent times, nursing has patronisingly been labelled as a 'clearly subordinate occupation dependent on knowledge produced by physicians in carrying out patient care' (Cockerham & Hinote 2015, p. 18).

That such an outdated idea continues to appear in contemporary discourse provides compelling evidence of the persistence of stereotypes – taken-for-granted ways of thinking that are allowed to recur and then maintained by failing to reflect on historical, gender and cultural biases about women and work. It is well known that, historically, 'women's work' was not easily spoken about because it was handed down from family member to family member, and often involved profane and taboo practices that were not to be discussed (Adam & Taylor 2014; Plessis 2016).

Like other images of women in popular culture, nurses are commonly represented as saintly and motherly. But, as we shall see, this is also a general stereotype – and so is the reverse idea: that nurses are bad, evil or monstrous.

Nursing is no longer so tightly bound to its religious, feminine or military roots, or to a sense of nursing being a 'calling'. The changes in uniform style reflect changing fashion trends, the expanding role and influence of women in the workforce (to emphasise practicality over decorum and gender differentiation) and the changing demands of the profession and workplace.

Representations of 'the good nurse'

The posters in Figure 8.2 show nursing in a positive light – the two world wars were a galvanising time for nurses, as they were seen in the world spotlight, and nursing became an esteemed and enviable career. At the time, such posters were very successful in mobilising a disengaged populace to buy war bonds, donate goods to the army and even to enlist as soldiers or train as nurses. Used in this way, nurses became the human face of war. Their nurturing skills were emphasised but also reduced to either a mothering or angelic image. The downside to this kind of representation is that the nursing image was appropriated by a propaganda machine to support the machine of war, and it set in train what would become commonplace and unchecked beliefs that nurses (a) were all female (when they were not) and (b) had an unlimited capacity for selflessness and gentility.

Tied to this notion of the 'good' nurse are values about behaviour that are culturally embedded and taken for granted. Many of these accepted beliefs about how nurses should behave need to be re-examined and replaced, because they have become outdated and are not conducive to a society that values equality over paternalism. For example, a century ago nurses were taught that they should be silent and impassive in the face of horrifying disease and suffering (Reverby 1987). Now, however, nurses are encouraged to speak out against injustice, to advocate for marginalised clients and to find their voice (Buresh & Gordon 2015; Lucatorto, Thomas & Siek 2016). McAllister and Brien (2020) challenged the concept of a 'good nurse', which locks nurses into an unrealistic and dehumanising portrayal and challenges a nuanced understanding

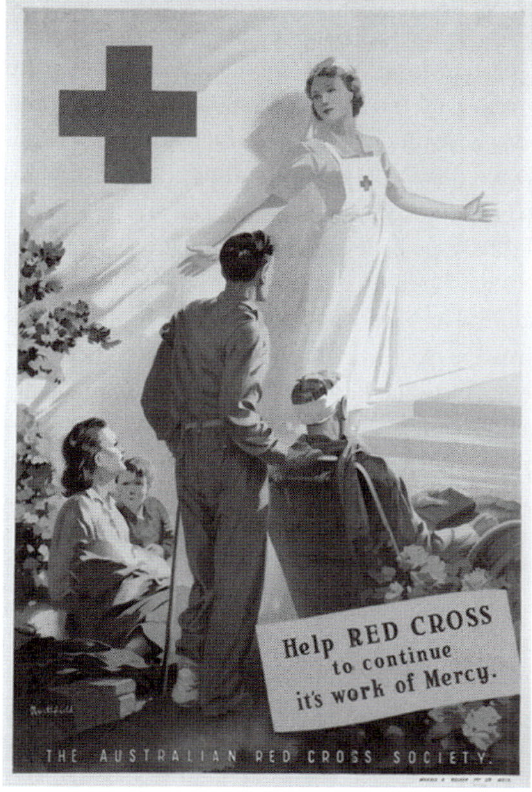

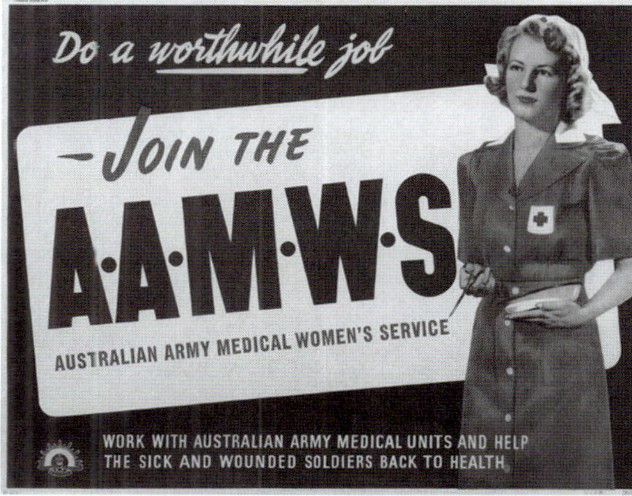

Figure 8.2   Australian war propaganda featuring nurses

Source: Australian War Memorial (ARTV00193; ARTV01081).

of a contemporary and realistic nursing image. The important role of nurses during the COVID-19 pandemic has highlighted that they are knowledgeable, brave and adaptable problem-solvers who have become the 'heroes' of stressed and overburdened healthcare systems in many countries (McAllister, Brien & Dean 2020; Thompson & Darbyshire 2020).

Despite this evolution in expectations, nurses are still often portrayed in popular culture in ways that reduce them to playing support roles to doctors, or even barely visible in the healthcare landscape. The medical television drama *House* is a clear example. As Summers (2015) comments, 'in hundreds of hours of programming seen by millions around the world, the physician characters just "happened" to spend half their time doing key tasks that nurses do in real life' (p. 52), such as taking a client's temperature and blood pressure or administering routine medications.

Closer to home, the Australian television series *Pulse* (Cruz-Martin 2017), in which the female nurse characters have non-speaking roles, seems to suggest that good nursing involves standing silently to one side, ready to be of assistance while the doctors provide all the care. Images of nurses that convey the ideal nurse as devoted and demure may be flattering on one level, but on another level they are patronising and simplistic, and may hinder the ability of nurses to have their work understood, valued and adequately resourced.

Multiple-choice questions
Short-answer questions

Representations of 'the bad nurse'

In contrast with the simplistic view of nurses as good, demure and selfless, are representations of 'bad' nurses – those who defy the social order and bring chaos and destruction, and about which nurses today have much to learn (Rezaei-Adaryani, Salsali & Mohammadi 2012). Nurses – like people – are not simply good or bad, and nor are they always able to deliver care that is consistent, compassionate, skilled and effective – no matter what the positive press would have us believe. There are many examples in recent times that provide evidence of this harsh reality. A shocking example is the Mid-Staffordshire scandal in the United Kingdom, where over 300 clients experienced needless suffering and even death due to widespread neglect from both nurses and medical staff (Francis 2010). A more recent example in Australia, based on a number of potentially preventable baby deaths in a Victorian regional hospital (King & Knight 2018), also highlights how health professionals (nurses, midwives and doctors) can become 'blinded' to a lack of robust safety and clinical governance processes, resulting in tragic outcomes.

Factual as well as fictional depictions of evil, corrupt or negligent nurses are important for all nurses to be aware of, because it is part of our history. And shared knowledge of the past advances our collective memory, which assists the nursing profession as a whole to identify what needs to be sustained or changed, and what lessons need to be learned so that nursing education and practice can be improved (Madsen et al. 2009). Fictional nurses, while they did not exist in reality, are still part of our history, because they are prominent in popular culture – a socialising agent that influences opinions and actions.

Nurse Ratched from *One Flew Over the Cuckoo's Nest* (Kesey 1962) is a memorable example. In the book and the film, set in the late 1950s, her character was the nurse in charge of an all-male forensic psychiatric unit. When this film was released, people were shocked at the treatment of clients in this ward, and it was the nurse character who had the biggest influence. Nurse Ratched came to represent all that was horrific about institutional care, and thus nursing was cast in a very bad light. While most people would say that Nurse Ratched was cold-hearted, there is an argument that she was being self-contained and rational in an environment that was chaotic and dangerous. Many people might also be critical of how detached and unfeeling Nurse Ratched was when confronted by the clients' distress. As Darbyshire (1995) argued, at least nursing's **power** was put into the spotlight within this fictional story, though it also reveals a deep-seated fear of women and, by association, nurses. It is interesting to note that in 2020 a 'spin-off' television series called *Ratched* was broadcast, which further demonstrates that this enduring and long-lived image of the uncaring nurse abounds.

Another well-known example of a bad nurse in popular culture is Annie Wilkes, the nurse played by Kathy Bates in the horror film *Misery* (Reiner 1990). Like Nurse Ratched, Wilkes is portrayed as skilled but damaged, and her ability to control, maim and destroy the male character has been read as a metaphor for all women – that if left unchecked, they will become monsters (Creed 1993).

As well as negative fictional representations of nurses, there are also many real cases of nurses committing terrible crimes and who have received notoriety in the media. In England, the case of Beverly Allitt (Katz 1993), a nurse who murdered children, is well known. In the United States, there was the case of Charles Cullen, a serial killer (Graeber 2014), and in Australia there have been cases of nurses deliberately

power a resource that can be used to influence and change for better or worse

committing acts of arson (Webb 2015). These real-life stories, like the extreme fictional narratives, may momentarily challenge the image of nurses as caring and trustworthy but they do not shift the stereotypes.

Perhaps this is because such stories are simply exceptions that prove the rule – or, in a cultural sense, stereotypes about nursing have become so deeply embedded in our social consciousness that they have become taken for granted, and thus will require significant challenging and re-education for them to be replaced. As Taguchi (2008) argues, this requires an **ethics of resistance** – one that the media, children and all students of nursing could benefit from developing.

Thinking about these negative images and reflecting on these cautionary tales may guide the profession to think about what not to do, how not to be and why nursing preparation requires extensive knowledge of ethics, legal and regulatory frameworks, and effective interpersonal communication (McAllister, Rogers & Brien 2015).

In this section, we have raised the notion that nurses who are powerful and unrestrained can also be used in the media to become symbols of danger. This view, like the notion that nurses are all saintly maternal figures, is simplistic. Unless audiences – particularly newcomers to nursing – appreciate that all these representations are fictitious, they may develop a rather unrealistic view of nursing.

ethics of resistance a learnt and collective response to overcoming unfair, oppressive practices

Video: *One Flew Over the Cuckoo's Nest*

The effects of nursing stereotypes

How do the stereotypical images of nursing affect nursing students' perspectives of the profession? ten Hoeve and colleagues (2017) surveyed nursing students over the first two-year period of their education to explore their changing attitudes towards nursing. They found that as students' awareness and understanding of what nursing really entails improved over time, so too did their perception of, and attitude towards, the profession. In Australia, a small number of prominent nurses have led the way in the evolution of nursing as a profession – for example, Vivian Bullwinkel (1915–2000), a nurse who served in Singapore during World War II, and Pat Slater (1918–90), who was instrumental in progressing nursing education from hospital-based apprenticeships to the university sector. In 2020, the public image of nurses in Australia was strengthened by regular press conferences by the Chief Nurse, Alison McMillan, talking about the important role of nurses in managing the pandemic and caring for their communities. These press conferences were picked up in the popular media and broadcast widely on the broadcast news. This type of media coverage contributes to an improved public understanding of the vital role of the professional nurse.

Unfortunately, numerous examples demonstrate that negative stereotypes of nurses continue to abound in the media (Pritchard 2013). For example, if you search the internet for 'naughty nurse' or 'battle-axe nurse', you will be inundated with images, blogs and commentaries that clearly indicate the prevalence of these sorts of stereotypes. 'Men-only' magazines regularly feature sexualised images of female nurses, and fancy dress shops have 'naughty nurse' costumes for hire. What do nurses make of such gendered and negative portrayals of their profession?

ten Hoeve and colleagues (2014) suggested that the stereotypical image of nurses constrains the profession's overall self-concept, which in turn increases the lack of visibility and poor status of nursing as a profession. These authors added that,

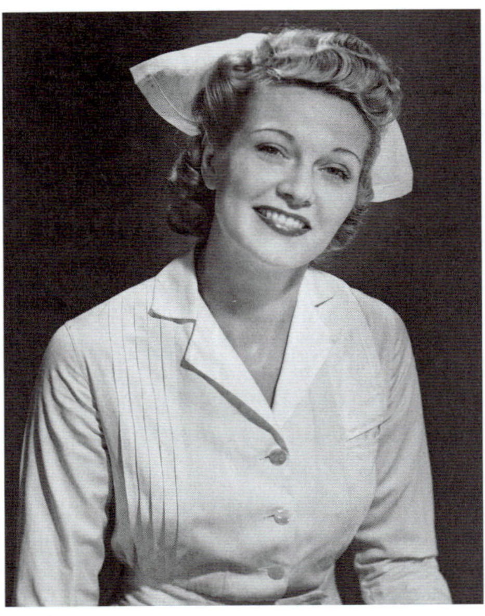

Figure 8.3   The traditional image of the nurse

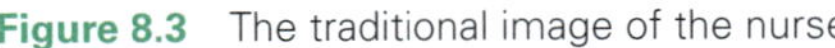

as the expectations for nursing research and education increase, these narrow stereotypical images are moving even further away from the reality of the profession. Therefore, it is incumbent on all nurses to challenge negative or demeaning perceptions of nursing and to correct public misconceptions.

It has been suggested that a negative self-image manifests as a tendency for nurses to remain silent about their profession. This is grounded in the belief that if nurses call attention to their own expertise, or the expertise of other nurses, then they are in some way 'showing off', or even tainting the caring and selfless image of the profession (Buresh & Gordon 2015). Diers (2004) argued that it is this professional reticence about what nurses actually do that 'makes it look easy to the untrained eye'. The layperson sees a nurse feeding a client, helping them to the toilet or washing them, and thinks that these are unpleasant but not difficult tasks. What is missing from this image is a public understanding of the knowledge, skills and *thinking* that underpin the 'doing' of these seemingly simple tasks.

Stereotypical ideas about nurses are also evident in the enduring positive perception that nurses are trustworthy, kind and caring (Brodie et al. 2004; Roy Morgan Research 2016). The fact that nurses are highly educated, skilled and professional is not evident in these popular perceptions of the profession and can actually devalue compelling evidence that well-educated, skillful nurses are essential in reducing mortality and negative health outcomes for the population (Aiken et al. 2014; McHugh et al. 2016; Vincent & Grimaldi 2016).

Shaping our own image

Although nurses constitute the greatest numbers of healthcare workers, their opinions are not often sought by the healthcare organisations that employ them, or by the media, when commentary is needed on topical health issues (Buresh & Gordon 2015; Mason 2020). When Buresh and Gordon studied media coverage of health issues, looking for nursing input, they found that nurses were virtually invisible on issues of healthcare planning, service delivery or policy. Sadly, nothing much had changed in nearly two decades, as Mason (2020) also found when reviewing nursing representation in the media. These authors have concluded that nurses' professional opinions are very rarely sought when health issues are discussed in the news, documentaries, current affairs reports or even women's magazines. This lack of nursing input into topical health debates may be one reason nursing is stuck with superficial and unrealistic stereotypes and is not seen as a high-profile professional career (unlike medicine, where it is easy to identify high-profile doctors).

Connecting with practice:
Nurse stereotypes
Short-answer questions
Video: Representation
in media

Unfortunately, nurses are still not viewed as skilled health professionals in the popular media, so the traditional enduring images of nurses as 'lesser' health professionals do not change. The Australian College of Nursing (ACN 2016) launched a white paper in which it lobbied for nurses to have a stronger voice in health and aged-care reform agendas, stating that, 'In Australia the nursing voice is not being heard and the profession is under-represented in strategic policy discussions and decisions' (p. 5). It is up to the nurses of today to actively seek opportunities to speak on a variety of health issues and showcase their expertise.

CASE STUDY

Media reporting on a community health issue

An article by Sean Parnell in the *Australian* newspaper (24 March 2017) discussed how important it is to be well informed about health matters. The article encouraged people to become better informed about a range of health concerns, to promote good health and prevent illness. The author suggested that overuse of antibiotics is a health concern that requires greater education and awareness. Several 'experts' from a range of universities, the World Health Organization (WHO) and the Australian and New Zealand College of Anaesthetists are quoted in the article, all urging for increased education to avoid overuse of antibiotics. However, no nursing experts are quoted and the role of nurses in consumer education is not mentioned.

QUESTIONS

1   This news story is about the appropriate use of antibiotics in the community. Do you think nurses do or should play a part in this issue? What roles do they play in educating clients about antibiotic usage?

2   Would a nurse's voice in this story have made a difference to what was said and perhaps what readers might do differently in relation to antibiotics?

3   Consider the notion that journalists need to develop an ethic of resistance towards nursing stereotypes. What could this journalist have done differently in his research and the resulting story?

REFLECTION 8.1

Find at least three recent articles on health topics published in popular magazines or newspapers.

- Were nurses asked to comment on these topics?
- What might this say about nursing's status and image, and where change is needed?
- What might a nurse's perspective add to the topics?

The looking-glass self

A socio-psychological concept, introduced by Charles Cooley (1902) a century ago, argued that representations of issues such as nursing – whether they are all good, all bad or inferior – are not inconsequential. They can shape a nurse's sense of self and, indeed, the profession's collective **identity**.

This idea is known as the **looking-glass self** (Cooley 1902). It means that during their development, a child will come to understand the self according to how they *think* others perceive them – that is, what they see in the mirror as others looking back at them. Coming to this self-assessment involves a combination of social interactions and self-talk. Whether we develop a sense of personal pride or shame is not only a psychological mechanism but also a complex interaction between the judgements of others about us, and whether we accept or refute those judgements. In addition, this concept suggests that a person's self-concept may change as society's perceptions of them and similar others change.

Applying this concept to nursing, it is possible that a student might start out thinking of themselves as capable and strong, but then they encounter others who reflect back to them different judgements – clients might think of the student as heroic but clinical colleagues may think of them as inexperienced and a burden. Depending on that student's psychological make-up and social effectiveness, the student might begin to see themselves as the client does, or as their clinical colleagues do. Thus, developing psychological as well as social strengths is an important asset in the development of a positive and strong public image.

Imagine yourself standing in front of three mirrors. In the first, you see your mother looking back at you. She thinks of you as warm-hearted, intelligent and generous. In the second, you see your spouse, partner or a friend looking at you. They think of you as funny, sexy and soft. In the third mirror, you see a stranger looking at you who has just been to see the movie *Misery* (or *One Flew Over the Cuckoo's Nest*), and has learned that you are studying to become a nurse. They think of you as smart and strong, but also scary.

identity who a person is, or the qualities of a person or group that make them different from others; positive identity can be a source of self-esteem

looking-glass self a social-psychological concept that describes the development, at a young age, of a sense of self that develops through social interactions – that is, we begin to see ourselves through the judgement of others

---

REFLECTION 8.2

Remembering Cooley's (1902) concept of the looking-glass self, which suggests that if we think others' evaluation of us is favourable then our self-concept is enhanced, identify the range of self-feelings that are generated within you when you apply the looking-glass self-concept to yourself.

Identifying strategies for enhancing understandings of the reality of nursing as a profession

Today, there are many roles and responsibilities for nurses, such as a client advocate, researcher, clinical nurse, educator and manager, across many specialised areas of nursing. However, as we have seen, the public's perception of nurses in today's healthcare environment often remains narrow and ill-informed. While members of the public are more knowledgeable today about their health care, the general population continues to be unaware of the evolving and complex roles and responsibilities of nurses.

The following strategies may be useful to consider in enhancing public understanding of the reality of nursing as a profession.

Nurses as advocates

Nurses need to become their own advocates and take every opportunity to correct public understandings of nursing by informing people of the influence of nurses on client outcomes and quality of life. According to Girvin, Jackson and Hutchinson (2016), when nurses discuss the effect they have on client outcomes and quality of life, they do so by presenting at nursing or health conferences or by publishing their work in nursing or health-related journals. As a result, nursing and other health professionals are informed – but not the general public. Nurses therefore need to promote a better public understanding of their role. This can be achieved by using informal sources such as taking every opportunity to talk about the changing role of nurses and the changing healthcare environment at local community forums and with their own families and friends.

Nurses as educators

Nurses also need to offer to speak to school children about their role and their influence, so children grow up having realistic perceptions of nursing as a career. This can also be done through children's literature, to accurately reflect contemporary nursing roles to receptive young minds (Carroll & Rosa 2016). Using social media to celebrate nursing achievements can also be a powerful tool to disseminate what nursing is really about to the general public (ten Hoeve, Jansen & Roodbol 2014).

Nurses as team players

It is important for nurses to work together as a profession. Nursing continues to be recognised as the most honest and trusted profession (Gallup 2020), and according to Girvin and colleagues (2016) we need to improve the health of the public by demonstrating our honest, responsible and ethical approach to our work. These authors challenge the nursing profession to implement a tactical plan to fully engage in wider debates about wellness, health and illness.

Nurses need to advocate for nurses. A lot has been written in the literature about the importance of nurses advocating for clients. However, in today's diverse and complex society, nurses also need to use advocacy skills to advocate for their profession (Mason 2020; Takase, Maude & Manias 2005). This may involve advocating from a nursing practice perspective – for example, advocating for change regarding workplace concerns and promoting positive workplace environments by becoming members of committees, boards and councils as well as quality improvement teams, thus advocating for both colleagues and clients.

Nurses need to advocate for each other from an educational perspective, or advocate for changes at the organisational level. According to Wood (2016), the healthcare environment presents many challenges and changes that offer opportunities for the nursing profession to lobby on its own behalf. Nurse advocates need to be politically 'savvy' to influence decision-makers and build collaborative relationships with major stakeholders, government, the media and the public.

Nurses as leaders

While it is important for nurses to lobby for each other, it is equally important for strong nursing leadership to guide the profession in an everchanging world. The Australian College of Nursing (2016) suggested that national policymakers consult with representatives of the nursing profession when making strategic healthcare policy decisions, to ensure that reforms are client focused and sustainable (Evans 2016). It was serendipitous that 2020 was commemorated as the International Year of the Nurse and Midwife, as it was the 200th anniversary of Florence Nightingale's birth.

Today, nurses are more visible than ever before, on the frontline of caring for people during the COVID-19 pandemic. Their role as community and team leaders has risen to prominence in the media, and the valuable work nurses do in society is increasingly appreciated.

Promoting excellence in nursing by conferring national awards enables the wider community to develop a more positive image of nursing (Finke et al. 2017).

Nurses as change agents

The scope of practice for nurses has changed in today's highly technological healthcare environment. The public needs to be made aware of the complex nature of nursing, which is by no means limited to following doctors' orders. The WHO (2016) acknowledged the global crisis caused by a critical shortage of skilled healthcare professionals. This means that the scope of nursing is constantly expanding to take a more active role in decision-making about client care, which leads to improvement in client satisfaction and reductions in mortality rates (Martínez-González et al. 2014). The advanced practice nursing role is gaining momentum worldwide, and there is huge scope for nurses to take a leading role in e-health (Williams 2016). Nurses are adept in the use of technology.

Nurses today need to communicate that they are highly educated, with the minimum requirement for entry to the profession being a bachelor's degree in most developed countries. In addition, continuing professional development is 'recognized as a necessary response to the complexity of patient's needs and the assurance of patient safety' (Girvin, Jackson & Sutherland 2016, p. 2). During their academic preparation to enter the profession, nursing students need to be taught client advocacy skills as well as self-advocacy skills that will equip them to become agents for change and leaders who can influence policymakers and governments. This will have a positive effect on the nursing profession and will also help to ensure that the public is better informed about the complex and changing role of nurses.

Nurses as researchers

Nurses play an important role in research, as our practice is built on an evidence-based foundation that is dynamic – as a profession, we are continuously generating questions and seeking answers. Research enables evidence-based practice and innovations in health care to provide safe, high-quality health care. Gray, Grove and Sutherland (2017) defined nursing research as 'a scientific process that validates and refines existing knowledge and generates new knowledge that directly and indirectly influences the delivery of evidence-based practice' (p. 15). This practice is not limited to healthcare settings; it includes education, management and other areas of nursing. Nurses play a vital role in actively participating as well as conducting research in healthcare settings (Young, Bakewell-Sachs & Sarna 2017). Nursing researchers are exploring complex areas including genome sequencing technologies, healthcare economics and client safety (Taylor et al. 2017).

In summary, nursing is a challenging and rewarding profession that is becoming increasingly diverse and complex. It is no longer possible to define nursing as merely a caring profession; in today's highly technological and demanding world, there is a need for nurses to be knowledgeable and skilled care agents as well as innovators, motivators and creative thinkers. The healthcare environment of today requires a generation of dynamic nurses who are agents of change and lobbyists who recognise the need to be heard by governments, policymakers and the broader community. While each nurse must take responsibility for communicating a contemporary image of the profession, it is imperative that everyone in the profession who is involved in education, practice, research, leadership and administration works together rather than in 'silos', to create greater visibility and increase the influence upon society.

Video: 'A tribute to nurses'

NURSING PERSPECTIVE

Voices of students are important to hear in this discussion of 'image', because it is students who might be most sensitive (and responsive) to their future profession's representation in the media. This story from a real-life nursing student in Australia reveals the influence of negative nursing stereotypes in the workplace.

During a critical-care placement I witnessed and felt the discomfort of bullying in the workplace by a visiting senior medical consultant. This doctor was a highly skilled and knowledgeable member of the critical care team, but bullied other (nursing) team members – particularly the nurse in charge. The other nursing staff also suffered critical remarks about our work practices: we were given the silent treatment if we asked questions and were subjected to eye-rolling when we spoke. This behaviour was a shock to me and undermined my confidence and self-esteem. The doctor seemed to delight in double-checking the nurses' work, belittling them in front of clients and families, and questioning why they were doing what they were doing. Sometimes this included criticism of their education and role. At the commencement of each shift, I saw that generally duties were divided up and the nursing staff talked and consulted together and with other medical staff to ensure that clients were cared for, yet I noticed that when this doctor was on the unit, the nurses stayed silent and looked downcast, in fear of being ridiculed. Luckily, this visiting doctor was only there for a few days of my placement and most of the other medical staff were supportive and helpful, but it helped me to realise how the role of nurses is still not out of the Dark Ages in the eyes of some doctors.

SUMMARY

- We explored the foundations of nursing and the legacy of Florence Nightingale by providing a brief history of the evolution of nursing in developed nations. In particular, it was noted that nursing had evolved from the traditional role of healer, through the Dark Ages, when nursing was seen to be a disreputable occupation, to an image that endures today.
- We presented and discussed examples of positive and negative stereotypes and the effects of these on the nursing profession today. Nursing images are commonly linked to goodness, dedication and subservience, and they have been used to 'promote' and glorify war. There are several examples of 'bad' nurses in some popular movies – including nurses who are uncaring and scary. There are also real-life examples of nurses who have engaged in heinous criminal activities. These extreme images do nothing to capture the reality of the modern nursing profession.
- We explored the ways in which nurses are seen and how they see themselves. The effects of traditional stereotypes were discussed, along with how this influences nursing students' view of the profession. The looking-glass self-activity reinforced the effect of that image on nurses' self-image.
- We suggested how nurses and nursing students could counter some of the negative influences of traditional stereotypes and improve the image of nursing. The strategies identified how nurses may be able to act as advocates, educators, team players, leaders, change agents and researchers to create a more realistic public perception of the nursing profession.

REVIEW QUESTIONS

Suggested responses

1 What image of nursing did you have before you commenced as a nursing student, and how was this image created?
2 How does the public image of nursing contribute to your personal and professional development?
3 How can the nursing profession change the common stereotypes of nurses?
4 How can nursing students contribute to the development of a nursing self-image that is more aligned with the reality of practice?
5 How do you intend to challenge stereotypes about nursing in your personal and professional life, in order to engage in an ethic of resistance?

RESEARCH TOPIC

Being a research-active professional means being a good consumer, or reader of research, and becoming a good conductor of research. This activity will prompt you to be more discerning about research in this area of nursing recruitment and retention.

Read the scoping literature review by Collard, Scammell and Tee (2020), which explored nurse retention and considered whether undergraduate nursing education adequately prepares new graduate nurses for the stresses and challenges they will face as novice nurses. Think about the four key themes that the authors identified as contributors to the retention of nurses in the workforce and reflect on how these might apply to your own experiences of nursing so far.

Collard, S.S., Scammell, J. & Tee, S. (2020). Closing the gap on nurse retention: A scoping review of implications for undergraduate education. *Nurse Education Today*, 84, 104253.

FURTHER READING

The journal articles below will provide food for thought as you consider the image, status and value of nursing. You might also like to have a look at the vast array of articles and resources available from the Greater Good Science Centre at the University of California, Berkeley (https://greatergood.berkeley.edu), which takes a perspective on some of the ideas in this chapter and suggests strategies to enhance your sense of purpose in life.

Bagnasco, A., Catania, G., Gallagher, A. & Morley, G. (2020). Media representations of nurses in the pandemic: Just doing our job? *Nursing Ethics*, 27(4), 901–5.

Bennett, C.L., James, A.H. & Kelly, D. (2020). Beyond tropes: Towards a new image of nursing in the wake of COVID-19. *Journal of Clinical Nursing*, 29(15–16), 2753–5.

Girvin, J., Jackson, D. & Hutchinson, M. (2016). Contemporary public perceptions of nursing: A systematic review and narrative synthesis of the international research evidence. *Journal of Nursing Management*, 24(8), 994–1006.

Kress, D., Godack, C.A., Berwanger, T.L. & Davidson, P. M. (2018). The new script of nursing: Using social media and advances in communication – to create a contemporary image of nursing. *Contemporary Nurse*, 54(4–5), 388–94.

McAllister, M., Brien, D. & Dean, S. (2020). The problem with the superhero narrative during COVID-19. *Contemporary Nurse*, 56(3), 199–203.

Perry, S.J., Richter, J.P. & Beauvais, B. (2018). The effects of nursing satisfaction and turnover cognitions on patient attitudes and outcomes: A three-level multisource study. *Health Services Research*, 53(6), 4943–69.

Stanley, D., Stanley, K. & Magee, D. (2019). Celluloid zombies: A research study of nurses in zombie-focused feature films. *Journal of Advanced Nursing*, 75(8), 1751–63.

Summers, S.J. & Broome, M.E. (2019). Improving representation of nurses in the media. *Nursing Outlook*, 67(1), 1–2.

REFERENCES

Adam, D. & Taylor, R. (2014). Compassionate care: Empowering students through nurse education. *Nurse Education Today*, 34(9), 1242–5.

Aiken, L.H., Sloane, D.M., Bruyneel, L., Van Den Heede, K., Griffiths, P., Busse, R. … Sermeus, W. (2014). Nurse staffing and education and hospital mortality in nine European countries: A retrospective observational study. *The Lancet*, 383(9931), 1824–30.

Australian College of Nursing (2016). *Nurses are essential in health and aged care reform*. A white paper by ACN 2016. Retrieved from https://www.acn.edu.au/wp-content/uploads/white-paper-nurses-essential-health-aged-care-reform.pdf.

Brideson, G., Willis, E., Mayner, L. & Chamberlain, D.J. (2016). Images of flight nursing in Australia: A study using institutional ethnography. *Nursing and Health Sciences*, 18(1), 38–43.

Brodie, D.A., Andrews, G.J., Andrews, J.P., Thomas, G.B., Wong, J. & Rixon, L. (2004). Perceptions of nursing: Confirmation, change and the student experience. *International Journal of Nursing Studies*, 41(7), 721–33.

Buresh, B. & Gordon, S. (2015). *From silence to voice: What nurses know and must communicate to the public*. Ithaca, NY: ILR Press.

Carroll, S.M. & Rosa, K.C. (2016). Role and image of nursing in children's literature: A qualitative media analysis. *Journal of Pediatric Nursing*, 31(2), 141–51.

Cockerham, W.C. & Hinote, B.P. (2015). PAs in a changing society: A sociologic perspective. *Journal of the American Academy of Physician Assistants*, 28(8), 18–20.

Cooley, C. (1902). *Human nature and the social order*. New York: Scribners.

Creed, B. (1993) *The monstrous feminine*. New York: Routledge.

Cruz-Martin, S. [Director] (2017). *Pulse* [TV series]. ABC TV.

Darbyshire, P. (1995). Reclaiming 'big nurse': A feminist critique of Ken Kesey's portrayal of Nurse Ratched in *One Flew Over the Cuckoo's Nest*. *Nursing Inquiry*, 2(4), 198–202.

Dickens, C. (1999). *The life and adventures of Martin Chuzzlewit*. Harmondsworth: Penguin.

Diers, D. (2004). *Speaking of nursing: Narratives of practice, research, policy, and the profession*. Sudbury, MA: Jones and Bartlett.

Dussault, G. (2020). From subordination to complementarity? *Revista latino-americana de enfermagem*, 28, 3355.

Ehrenreich, B. & English, D. (2010). *Witches, midwives and nurses: A history of women healers*, 2nd edn. New York: Feminist Press.

Evans, N. (2016). Nurses must get involved in implementing the cancer plan: National cancer director Cally Palmer outlines her vision. *Cancer Nursing Practice*, 15(6), 8–9.

Finke, M., Petto, P., Roberts-Turner, R. & Reggio, C. (2017). Nurse-led peer review committee promotes external recognition of nurses. Paper presented to the Creating Healthy Work Environments Conference 2017, Indiana. Retrieved from https://stti.confex.com/stti/chwe17/webprogram/Paper81904.html.

Francis, R. (2010). *Independent inquiry into care provided by Mid-Staffordshire NHS Foundation Trust, January 2005–9*. Richmond: Office of Public Sector Information.

Gabaldon, D. (1991–2014) *Outlander* [book series]. London: Random House.

Gallup (2020). Nurses continue to rate highest in honesty, ethics. Retrieved from https://news.gallup.com/poll/274673/nurses-continue-rate-highest-honesty-ethics.aspx.

Girvin, J., Jackson, D. & Hutchinson, M. (2016). Contemporary public perceptions of nursing: A systematic review and narrative synthesis of the international research evidence. *Journal of Nursing Management*, 24(8), 994–1006.

Gordon, S. & Nelson, S. (2005). An end to angels. *American Journal of Nursing*, 105(5), 62–9.

Graeber, C. (2014). *The good nurse: A true story of medicine, madness and murder*. New York: Atlantic Books

Gray, J., Grove, S. & Sutherland, S. (2017). *The practice of nursing research: Appraisal, synthesis and generation of evidence*, 8th edn. St Louis, MO: Elsevier/Saunders.

Hodges, E.A., Rowsey, P.J., Gray T.F., Kneipp, S.M., Giscombe, C.W., Foster, B.B., Alexander, V.R. & Kowlowitz, V. (2017). Bridging the gender divide: Facilitating the educational path for men in nursing. *Journal of Nursing Education*, 56(5), 295–9.

Katz, I. (1993). The verdicts: Beverley Allitt. *The Guardian*, 18 May.

Kelly, J., Fealy, G.M. & Watson, R. (2012). The image of you: Constructing nursing identities in YouTube. *Journal of Advanced Nursing*, 68(8), 1804–13.

Kesey, K. (1962). *One flew over the cuckoo's nest*. New York: Viking Press.

King, C. & Knight, B. (2018). Bacchus Marsh hospital staff remain 'badly damaged' by baby deaths as new obstetrics unit opens. *ABC News*, 27 June. Retrieved from https://www.abc.net.au/news/2018-06-27/morale-low-at-bacchus-marsh-melton-hospital-after-baby-deaths/9912470.

Lucatorto, M.A., Thomas, T.W. & Siek, T. (2016). Registered nurses as caregivers: Influencing the system as patient advocates. *Online Journal of Issues in Nursing*, 21(3), 2.

Madsen, W., McAllister, M. Godden, J., Greenhill, J. & Reed, R. (2009). Nursing's orphans: How the system of nursing education in Australia is undermining professional identity. *Contemporary Nurse*, 32(1), 9–18.

Martínez-González, N.A., Djalali, S., Tandjung, R., Huber-Geismann, F., Markun, S., Wensing, M. & Rosemann, T. (2014). Substitution of physicians by nurses in primary care: A systematic review and meta-analysis. *BMC Health Services Research*, 14, 214.

Mason, D. (2020). *Nurses representation in the media*. Retrieved from https://www.youtube.com/watch?v=6_5f2jfY7kM.

McAllister, M. & Brien, D. (2020) *Paradoxes in nurses' identity, culture and image: The shadow side of nursing*. London: Routledge.

McAllister, M., Brien, D. & Dean, S. (2020). The problem with the superhero narrative during COVID-19. *Contemporary Nurse*, 56(3), 199–203.

McAllister, M., Rogers, I.L. & Brien, D.L. (2015). Illuminating and inspiring: Using television historical drama to cultivate contemporary nursing values and critical thinking. *Contemporary Nurse*, 50(2), 1–12.

McHugh, M.D., Rochman, M.F., Sloane, D.M., Berg, R.A., Mancini, M.E., Nadkarni, V.M. … American Heart Association's Get With the Guidelines-Resuscitation Investigators (2016). Better nurse staffing and nurse work environments associated with increased survival of in-hospital cardiac arrest patients. *Medical Care*, 54(1), 74–80.

Moore, R.D [Series developer] (2014–). *Outlander* [Netflix television series]. Tall Ships Production.

Morrison-Beedy, D., Tzeng, H.-M. & Abriam-Yago, K. (2017). Building the pipeline of diverse nursing leaders: Reflections from the AACN Deans' mentoring program. *Journal of Professional Nursing*, 34(1), 9–11.

O'Brien, A. (1988). *Poverty's prison: The poor in New South Wales 1880–1918*. Melbourne: Melbourne University Press.

Parnell, S. (2017). Oversubscription of antibiotics helps superbugs spread. *The Australian*, 10 November.

Plessis, E. (2016). Caring presence in practice: Facilitating an appreciative discourse in nursing. *International Nursing Review*, 63(3), 377–80.

Pritchard, M.J. (2013). Comment on Stanley D. (2012), 'Celluloid devils: A research study of male nurses in feature films'. *Journal of Advanced Nursing*, 69(9), 2141–2.

Rauen, C., Jackson-Parkin, M., Jacobson, C., Marzlin, K.M. & Webner, C.L. (2016). Good witch or bad witch? *Critical Care Nurse*, 36(5), 66–9.

Reiner, R. [Director] (1990) *Misery*. United States.

Reverby, S. (1987). *Ordered to care: The dilemma of American nursing, 1850–1945*. Cambridge, MA: Cambridge University Press.

Rezaei-Adaryani, M., Salsali, M. & Mohammadi, E. (2012). Nursing image: An evolutionary concept analysis. *Contemporary Nurse*, 43(1), 81–9.

Robles, N. (2016). Saint John of God and the origins of nursing. *Hektoin International: A Journal of Medical Humanities*. Retrieved from http://hekint.org/saint-john-of-god-and-the-origins-of-nursing.

Roy Morgan Research (2016). Roy Morgan Image of Professions Survey 2016: Nurses still easily most highly regarded – followed by doctors, pharmacists and engineers. Retrieved from http://www.roymorgan.com/findings/6797-image-of-professions-2016–201605110031.

Stanley, D., Stanley, K. & Magee, D. (2019). Celluloid zombies: A research study of nurses in zombie-focused feature films. *Journal of Advanced Nursing*, 75(8), 1751–63.

Summers, A. (1997). Sairey Gamp: Generating fact from fiction. *Nursing Inquiry*, 4(1), 14–18.

Summers, S. (2015). *Saving lives: Why the media's portrayal of nursing puts us all at risk*, 2nd edn. New York: Oxford University Press.

Taguchi, L. (2008). An 'ethics of resistance' challenges taken-for-granted ideas in early childhood education. *International Journal of Educational Research*, 47(5), 270–82.

Takase, M., Maude, P. & Manias, E. (2005). Comparison between nurses' professional and their perceptions of their job. *The Australian Journal of Advanced Nursing*, 23, 28–33.

Taylor, J.Y., Wright, M.L., Hickey, K.T. & Housman, D.E. (2017). Genome sequencing technologies and nursing: What are the roles of nurses and nurse scientists? *Nursing Research*, 66(2), 198–205.

ten Hoeve, Y., Castelein, S., Jansen, G., Wiebren S. & Roodbol, P. (2017). Nursing students' changing orientation and attitudes towards nursing during education: A two year longitudinal study. *Nurse Education Today*, 48, 19–24.

ten Hoeve, Y., Jansen, G. & Roodbol, P. (2014). The nursing profession: Public image, self-concept and professional identity – a discussion paper. *Journal of Advanced Nursing*, 70(2), 295–309.

Teodorescu, S. & Preda, A. (2018). A brief history of nursing. *Practical Application of Science*, VI(18), 355–9.

Thompson, D.R. & Darbyshire, P. (2020). Nightingale's year of nursing: Rising to the challenges of the covid-19 era. *British Medical Journal*, 370, m2721.

Vincent, J.-L. & Grimaldi, D. (2016). Quick sequential organ failure assessment: Big databases vs. intelligent doctors. *Journal of Thoracic Disease*, 8(9), E996–8.

Webb, E. (2015). *Angels of death: Disturbing real-life cases of nurses and doctors who kill.* Melbourne: Five Mile Press.

Williams, S. (2016). Looking at advanced practice nursing roles: Expanded clinical roles are becoming more popular worldwide, but there are some differences in scope. *Nursing Management*, 23(6), 17.

Wood, P.J. (2016). Managing boundaries between professional and lay nursing following the influenza pandemic, 1918–1919: Insights for professional resilience today? *Journal of Clinical Nursing*, 26(5–6), 805–12.

World Health Organization (2016). *Global strategy on human resources for health workforce 2030*. Retrieved from http://apps.who.int/iris/bitstream/handle/10665/250368/9789241511131-eng.pdf;jsessionid=EF05A21B3150280CF29804E3ECD197BB?sequence=1.

Wright, M. (2016). Witchcraft and midwives: The fear behind the smoke. *The General: Brock University Undergraduate Journal of History*, 1, 48–54.

Young, H.M., Bakewell-Sachs, S. & Sarna, L. (2017). Nursing practice, research and education in the West: The best is yet to come. *Nursing Research*, 66(3), 262–70.

Thinking like a nurse

Joanne Porter and Alicia J. Perkins

With acknowledgement to Judith Lyons and Shireen Sewgolam for their
contributions to the first edition

LEARNING OBJECTIVES

At the completion of this chapter, you should be able to:

1 Describe the importance of critical thinking skills in the provision of safe and competent, person-centred nursing care, and discuss strategies to enhance critical thinking.
2 Develop an understanding of how clinical judgement applies to clinical practice.
3 Analyse the practice of clinical reasoning as an integral component of effective nursing practice and discuss ways to develop the necessary skills.
4 Demonstrate the concepts of reflective thinking and reflective practice, and their application to professional nursing education and practice.
5 Develop skills related to the development of a professional e-portfolio.

Introduction

Critical thinking, problem-solving, clinical reasoning, self-reflection and self-awareness are valued attributes of the contemporary nurse. These skills are essential for the provision of safe and competent, person-centred care to clients with ever-increasing acuity (care needs) and multiple, often complex comorbidities. This chapter focuses on critical thinking, clinical reasoning and reflective practice, and personal documentation using e-portfolios, along with strategies to assist beginning nurses in the development of these specific skills, which should be honed, practised and adapted to everyday clinical practice. The chapter also aims to assist the professional nurse to develop methods to demonstrate, document and evidence their personal and professional development through the use of e-portfolios.

NURSING PERSPECTIVE

To be a reflective practitioner, a nurse needs to develop a unique set of skills, which include the ability to self-regulate and self-monitor through reflecting on their actions, and being responsive to change. Reflective practice is not simply something that is done at the end of the shift; it should be incorporated into each planned action and, by doing so, nurses can aim to practice with capability and integrity. It is important to understand one's strengths and areas for improvement so that growth and learning can occur. Maintaining a career portfolio helps to track one's learning and development, while journaling helps to develop self-reflection.

From the first day you begin your nurse training, it is important to have an evidence-based practice approach to all that you do. When performing tasks, assessments or treatments, and in each interaction with a client, keep your professional consciousness (focus) sharp. Figure 9.1 shows how your professional consciousness works. The circle represents your professional consciousness (focus of attention) on the task or activity you are engaged in. The triangle, with its sharp points, represents your peripheral vision or awareness of the things that are outside of your immediate focus. Working like a radar,

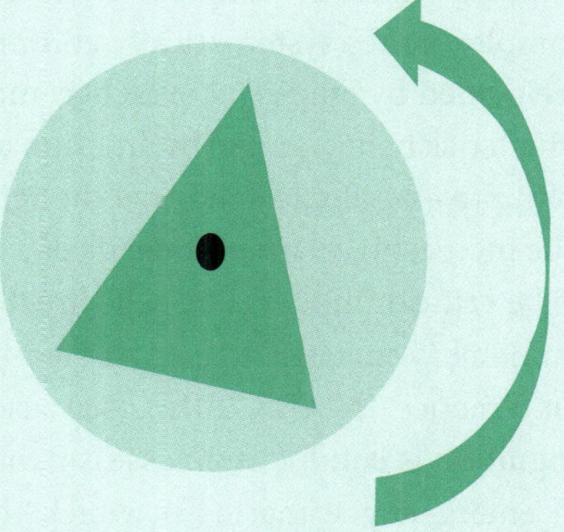

Figure 9.1 Professional consciousness diagram

the triangle moves slowly around the circle when you are performing a task, alerting you to (bringing into your consciousness) things that may need to be considered or addressed to perform the task safely and effectively. For example, suppose a nurse is dressing a wound and an item falls to the floor. The points of the triangle will alert the professional consciousness, reminding them not to pick up and use the item. The professional consciousness helps you learn and adapt in and to different situations, to better deal with the unexpected and not to cut corners. As your learning and experience grows, so too will your professional consciousness (the circle) but you need to keep your triangle points sharp throughout your career.

Critical thinking

Short-answer question

Critical thinking is widely thought to be a necessary element in the toolkit of a competent health professional. In the past, nurses were task-orientated clinicians who performed duties based on what doctors instructed them to do. Today, however, critical thinking has transformed professional nursing practice, and the ability of nurses to competently assess, identify anomalies, and formulate and initiate plans for client care is paramount. The notion of critical thinking and reflective practice in health care has become popular in recent times. So, what is critical thinking, and how can it be defined? Papathanasiou et al. (2014) defined critical thinking as 'the mental process of actively and skillfully perceive[ing], analys[ing], synthesis[ing] and evaluat[ing] collected information through observation, experience and communication that leads to a decision for action' (p. 283). Novice nurses and experienced nurses are continuously refining their critical thinking skills.

An alternative definition of critical thinking was developed by Papp and colleagues (2014), who posited that critical thinking is 'the ability to apply higher-order cognitive skills (conceptualization, analysis, evaluation) and the disposition to be deliberate about thinking (being open-minded or intellectually honest) that lead to action that is logical and appropriate' (p. 716). The National Council for Excellence in Critical Thinking defines critical thinking as 'The intellectually disciplined process of actively and skilfully conceptualising, applying, analysing, synthesising, and/or evaluating information gathered from, or generated by, observation, experience, reflection, reasoning, or communication, as a guide to belief and action' (Scriven & Paul 1987). Critical thinking transfers well into the healthcare setting, where it is essential to approach complex issues systematically and methodically, and to draw logical conclusions that are guided by empirical evidence and objectivity rather than sentiment and intuition, which risk being tainted by emotion and bias. However, no one is immune to periods of disruptive or illogical internal thoughts, particularly during highly stressful situations. The increasingly complex needs of working in the healthcare profession require nurses to be critical thinkers and self-directed learners (Rogal & Young 2009). In fact, critical thinking is specifically emphasised in Standard 1 of the Registered Nurse Standards for Practice (NMBA 2016) (see also Chapter 12). While this level of higher-order cognition is conducive in assessment and planning situations, translating this process to emergency scenarios in which the preservation of life is dependent upon rapid critical analysis and immediate responses requires practice.

Critical thinking attributes

Chan (2013) identified that the principles associated with critical thinking in nursing are constantly changing. Building on his earlier work, Ennis (2015) reviewed previous criteria and proposed the following updated set of 18 attributes as necessary for ideal critical thinkers to cultivate. These are the ability to:

1 Focus on a question.
2 Analyse arguments.
3 Ask and answer clarification questions.
4 Understand and use elementary graphs and maths.

5   Judge the credibility of a source.
6   Observe and judge observation reports.
7   Use existing knowledge.
8   Deduce and judge deductions.
9   Make and judge inductive inferences and arguments.
10   Make and judge value judgements.
11   Define terms and judge definitions.
12   Handle equivocation appropriately.
13   Attribute and judge unstated assumptions.
14   Think suppositionally.
15   Deal with fallacy labels.
16   Be aware of, and check, the quality of their own thinking.
17   Deal with things in an orderly manner.
18   Employ rhetorical strategies.

The principles associated with critical thinking (see Figure 9.2) provide nurses with a practical step-by-step guide to achieving a high level of critical thinking that is essential to ensuring that quality, safe care is delivered and that professional standards for practice are met. (See also Chapter 12, which examines these ideas in the context of professional standards, codes and regulations.)

Short-answer question

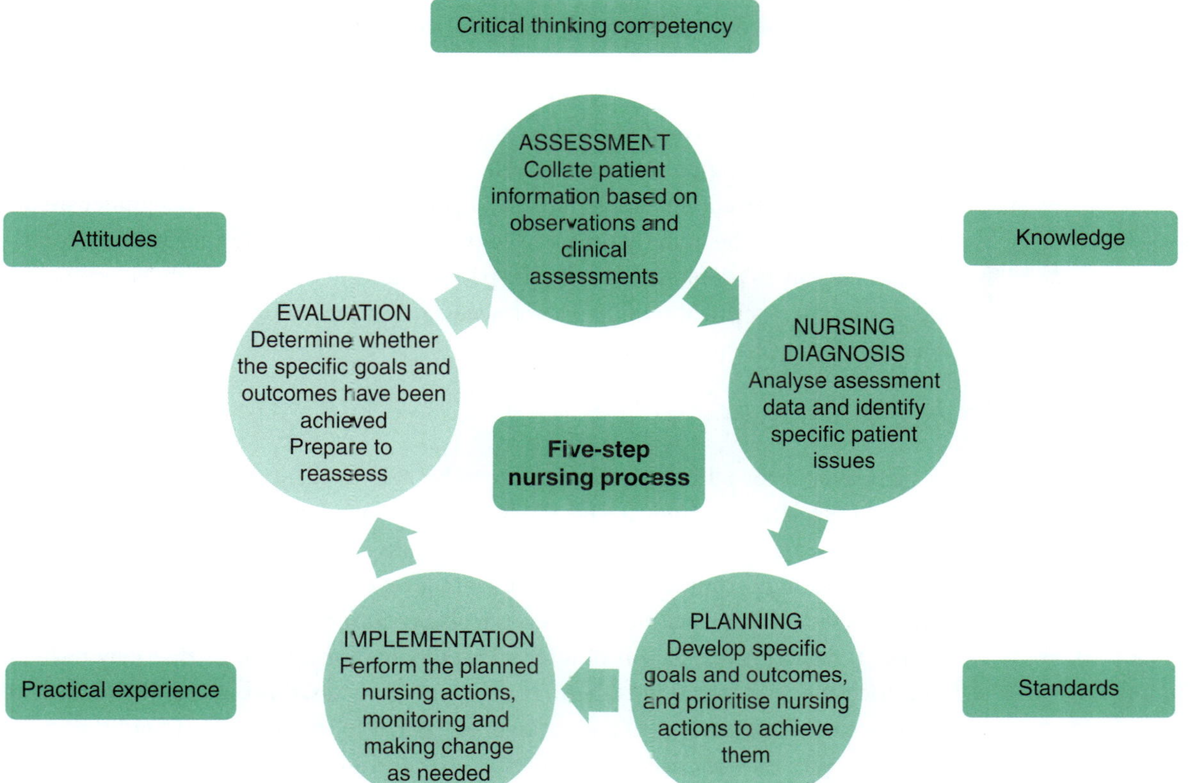

Figure 9.2   Five-step nursing process used as a decision-making approach to promote critical thinking in nursing

Source: Adapted from Kataoka-Yahiro and Saylor (1994).

Clinical judgement

clinical judgement the ability to apply higher-order cognitive skills and the disposition to deliberate about thinking critically

Clinical judgement is recognised as an essential skill for nursing but it is difficult to quantify. In order to establish excellent clinical judgement, the nurse must be able to apply higher-order cognitive skills and then have the disposition to be deliberate about thinking critically. With this intention, it is reasonable to assume that the nurse must possess a deep understanding of anatomy and physiology at a cellular level, and have clinical experience in caring for clients with complex diseases. But where does this leave the beginner nurse?

Scaffolding of clinical skills and knowledge has been successfully mapped and embedded into the tertiary nursing curriculum, and this is transferred into hospital postgraduate nursing programs, to enable the beginner nurse to develop the requisite skills to think critically and apply clinical judgement. The focus for the beginner should be on developing the underlying knowledge required to critically analyse a situation – not necessarily to problem-solve at a deep level but rather to identify that a problem is occurring. Here, critical thinking is not necessarily a case of understanding and fixing but identifying and escalating.

Short-answer question

A critical skill

A critical skill for all beginner nurses is to be able to identify anomalies and judge when to escalate care, and to have the underlying knowledge to justify their opinions and actions. Having the confidence to request a clinical review for a client perceived to be deteriorating certainly requires a sufficient level of clinical knowledge to be able to identify clinical abnormalities. However, it also requires a degree of logical reasoning, and at times an investigation of internal arguments for assertions that may have no empirical evidence to support them. For beginning nurses, this requires the courage to be able to construct a logical and rational argument for their concerns and the ability to convey it to relevant decision-makers, clearly and concisely. There are several client indicators that can lead a nurse to escalate care: ascertaining the client's level of pain or discomfort, carers' or family members' concern for the client and identifying a client as being 'not quite right' are all valid reasons to escalate care.

Elder (2007) saw critical thinking as a lifelong journey of self-directed, self-disciplined thinking. Based on this, critical thinking can only be achieved if nurses at all levels, from student through to expert (Benner 1982), are prepared to be accountable, and responsibly invest in their own professional, clinical and theoretical development through self-directed learning and through seeking opportunities for improvement in their individual clinical domains. Additionally, advances in treatment can result in rapidly changing clinical guidelines, which further reinforce the need for nurses to continually update their knowledge and skills, and to demonstrate continuing investment in their own professional development. Attaining continuing professional development, or CPD, points is a requirement of nursing registration; nurses are required each year to attend education and training sessions in order to reach the required number of CPD points to maintain clinical currency. By developing a deeper understanding of underlying principles, nurses can readily adapt to and embrace these changes.

Critical thinking is an important attribute of graduates across many disciplines and at most universities. Chan (2013) identified different perceptions of critical thinking among nurse educators, and suggested that this may create cognitive dissonance about whether the focus of nurse education should be to teach critical thinking or deliver course content, when in reality both are essential and should be seamlessly integrated into the education of nurses.

Brookfield (1987) postulated that to successfully transfer the skills of critical thinking at the tertiary level into the context of adult life, critical thinking should be seen as a practical and intentional activity, rather than just an academic construct.

The following strategies can be used effectively to develop critical thinking skills:

- Adopt a non-judgemental stance – demonstrate open-mindedness and acceptance of other cultures and other views.
- Seek the truth by actively investigating a problem or situation.
- Ask questions and admit to a lack of knowledge, then seek out additional information and evidence.
- Reflect on your own thinking process and the ways in which you reach conclusions.
- Indulge your intellectual curiosity – be a lifelong learner.
- View your clients with empathy and from a holistic perspective.
- Engage an experienced mentor and join a professional organisation such as the Australian College of Nursing (ACN).
- Advance your nursing education (Petrie 2020).

Be encouraged, motivated, inspired and empowered to seek the information required to develop your critical thinking skills. Assess your knowledge and employ a reflective dimension to promote your critical thinking abilities. By doing this, you will develop your learning capabilities and your clinical judgement.

CASE STUDY

Critical thinking skills in action

Ahmed, who is in the first six months of his graduate year, has started working the morning shift on a high-acuity surgical ward. He has been assigned his clients for the day and is working as part of a team with another registered nurse, Rebecca, in caring for eight clients. At lunchtime, when Rebecca is taking her break, Ahmed remains on the ward to care for their clients. Shortly after Rebecca leaves, Ahmed walks into the room of one of his clients to perform routine observations. Ahmed observes the client, Mrs Kempolous, who is at day three post-op following an open laparotomy, to be dyspnoeic and shivering. Ahmed performs a set of routine observations and notes that Mrs Kempolous's temperature is 38.1°C, her respiratory rate is 26 breaths per minute and her heart rate is 98 beats per minute. Mrs Kempolous's blood pressure is within the normal range and she is not complaining of pain or discomfort.

Ahmed remembers learning about systemic inflammatory response syndrome (SIRS) during his third-year pathophysiology course. He recalls that some of the criteria for SIRS were abnormal temperature and tachypnoea. Ahmed reassures Mrs Kempolous that he will be back shortly, and he approaches the team leader on the shift, Ligi.

Ligi tells Ahmed kindly that he is probably overreacting, as a temperature of 38.1°C and a respiratory rate of 26 are not very far outside normal parameters. Ahmed accepts Ligi's analysis of the situation and returns to Mrs Kempolous but he feels uncomfortable about her situation and is worried that she will deteriorate. Ahmed goes ahead and performs routine observations on his remaining seven clients.

Rebecca returns to the ward and Ahmed proceeds to go to lunch. While at lunch, Ahmed does an internet search for SIRS and is alarmed to find that Mrs Kempolous's observations fit not only the required two, but three, of the criteria for SIRS, and immediately feels annoyed with himself for not being more assertive when reporting Mrs Kempolous's condition to Ligi. Ahmed returns to the ward and reports his findings to Rebecca, who agrees with Ahmed's analysis of the situation and escalates care appropriately. Ahmed feels satisfied that Mrs Kempolous will now receive a medical review to initiate care and decrease her risk of developing SIRS but feels that if he had suitably escalated care with the team leader earlier, her risk of associated morbidity would be lessened.

QUESTIONS

1   What strategies could Ahmed, and Rebecca, employ now to facilitate the development of Ahmed's clinical judgement and critical thinking skills?

2   How should Ahmed manage similar situations in the future?

3   What activities could Ahmed engage in to improve his ability to be assertive and communicate his concerns to appropriately escalate clinical care in the future?

Video: Critical thinking tools
Short-answer question

Clinical reasoning

At the beginning of, and during, a nurse's career, proficiency in **clinical reasoning** is developed by the use of various cognitive processes (Kuiper & Pesut 2004). It is by engaging in dialogue that beginning nurses become more aware of how more experienced nurses use these thinking processes.

Learning clinical reasoning

The learning of clinical reasoning skills is to understand intuitive and analytical thinking processes, so that techniques are developed for storing knowledge that is clinically relevant. Clinical reasoning skills develop higher-level thinking in order to analyse and assess thinking, and therefore encourage reflection and change. The acquisition of these techniques is dependent on students' receptiveness to supervised practice with effective feedback. Clinical reasoning is the intended outcome of critical thinking (the intellectual work of the mind) that involves self-discipline in using particular skills (Kuiper & Pesut 2004). There is an enhanced expectation of these particular skills as it is evidenced in nurses who can credibly support their clinical decisions and judgements about client care (Grubbs 2017) Critical and reflective thinking combined are not only the key components of clinical reasoning but also a commitment to lifelong learning that determines professional growth and development.

When clinical reasoning is learnt, attitudes are developed that enable a nurse to recognise problems and search for credible evidence that supports understanding and decision-making in order to accurately sift through logically acquired evidence. Clinical reasoning is the ability to activate and apply appropriate emotional attitudes, such as feelings and emotions, when there is discomfort and dissonance in clinical practice. The ability to check in with one's emotions can assist the nurse in working towards informed decision-making in practice. Using vigilance, diligence and dedication, a nurse can learn about their own emotional reactions to a situation, define the emotions and thus understand the true cause of the problem. For example, nurses caring for clients who are under police custody need to understand their own feelings about social and criminal justice in order to care for clients, regardless of the circumstances surrounding their admission.

Nursing students need support and encouragement to test their thinking, validate their reasoning and reflect on credible evidence that underpins potential decisions and actions. The early recognition of barriers to effective clinical reasoning skills will set the precedent for confident and progressive practice.

Nurses with a humanistic philosophy of practice have been identified as having a high level of self-awareness and as being risk-takers due to the confidence they exude in their clinical reasoning and decision-making skills (Tanner 2006). Humanism involves an ethical structure that is based on the human values such as trust, honesty, courage, compassion and truthfulness. These values should be the basis of how all health care is organised (Kvesic, Galic & Vukojevic 2019). These are the nurses who exude power and influence in their practice areas. Clinical reasoning processes need to be meaningful to the clinical setting and context, so that nurses are able to tie

clinical reasoning the cognitive process that applies critical thinking to the current clinical situation, using available information to identify actions and make treatment decisions that will improve client outcomes

them to previous, current and future experiences, thereby ensuring that the process of reasoning remains available throughout the learning process. The learning itself is focused on self-regulatory strategies so that within a timeframe nurses may maximise the benefits of their diverse experiences and apply individual learning styles.

Practices that develop clinical reasoning skills

The following are examples of practices that help to develop clinical reasoning skills:

- Recognising the interaction between the cognitive needs (thinking) and metacognitive needs (reflection) of self-knowledge, environment and behavioural regulation
- Self-monitoring, to pay deliberate attention to the behaviour used to attain content and experience progress, and to motivate improvement in learning
- Seeking opportunities for self-evaluation and self-reinforcement, supported by evidence-based practice in a variety of situations
- Observing, recording and documenting role models' clinical reasoning behaviour in more critical and complex care
- Allocating time for yourself and taking opportunities for interprofessional and collegial debriefing as well as guided reflective journaling
- Identifying and including yourself in multiple opportunities to identify abnormal assessment findings and to prioritise assessments and interventions so that both clinical judgement and communication skills are practised
- Absorbing the role of both teacher and learner to foster creative strategies that improve psychomotor and communication skills. This is to ensure that you are not afraid to identify faulty thinking in yourself. The identification of the problem by self-realisation has the consequence of a relatively permanent change in behaviour and the acquisition of more defined clinical reasoning skills at a faster rate.

Practices that hinder clinical reasoning skills

Practices that hinder clinical reasoning skills include:

- Making decisions too fast, without considering the consequences
- Thinking and behaviour based on prior assumptions and preconceptions, in what is known as *ascertainment bias*
- Making judgements and decisions about clients and assigning the cause of medical conditions to the client rather than examining all situational factors
- Thinking that we know more than we do and acting on incomplete information. The actions then cannot be validated as they are based more on opinion than the collected evidence
- Applying premature closure, where a problem is identified and solved before it is fully verified.

The teaching and learning of clinical reasoning and its inherent skills result in a radical transformation in nursing practice and nursing education. Strategies for development of these inherent skills are essential to preparing the nurse for current and future practice.

Reflective practice

Nurses today practice in complex, dynamic healthcare environments, and need to be prepared to meet the evolving challenges of professional practice. The ability to reflect is regarded as an essential graduate capability for professional nursing practice that enables nurses to think and act professionally, which is an integral element of becoming a professional nurse.

The importance of reflection and **reflective practice** is acknowledged in nursing education and practice to develop and maintain competency of practice throughout your professional life (Taylor 2006). Nursing focuses on critical reflection for, in and on practice and experiences, to link theory to practice; to transfer what has been learnt to new situations and contexts; and to enable learning to be developed from prior experiences.

On your journey to becoming a nurse, you will be expected to think and write reflectively as part of your nursing studies, so as to develop higher-order, reflective thinking skills. You will be expected to record the creative process of your reflection and identify and evaluate the consequences and results that come from it. Your goal is to use tools and strategies to develop reflective writing and thinking skills in order to evaluate knowledge and improve practice.

reflective practice the intention to learn and develop as a result of reflecting upon current or prior experiences

What is reflection?

Taylor (2006) defined reflection as learning from experience to better understand yourself and to develop your practice. We reflect informally on everyday problems and situations. Reflection means throwing back from a surface or 'looking at the mirror image' of the situation. It involves engaging in attentive consideration to mull over recent events or to contemplate and deliberately think about what you are doing while you are doing it, or to consider, after the fact, why things went wrong. Reflection is a way of dealing with thoughts and feelings about difficult situations or days. This enables us to come to terms with our thoughts and feelings about the situation and to consider different ways of acting or responding to similar situations in the future. According to Higgins (2011), reflective practice ranges from 'questioning of presuppositions and assumptions, through to more explicit engagement in the process of critical and creative thinking in order to make connections between experience and learning in practice and practical action' (p. 583).

What does reflection involve?

Reflection can be descriptive or critical. Descriptive reflection is thinking about and describing what happened in each situation, while critical reflection engages in a process of analysis and evaluation to achieve a better understanding of a situation and to generate new learning and improved practice. Reflective thinking is a method of inquiry that involves a number of elements, including the abilities of engagement, pondering alternatives, drawing inferences and taking diverse perspectives; this is particularly important in situations that are complex and require a degree of situational awareness and understanding (Higgins 2011). According to Higgins (2011), the following elements are important aspects of reflective thinking:

- *Making sense of experience.* We know that not all experiences provide learning opportunities. However, through reflection we can analyse our experiences to make sense and find meaning in order to actively learn from the experience.
- *Standing back.* Sometimes it is difficult to reflect while we are caught up in the emotions and feelings of an event. Reflection on action provides the opportunity to 'think back' on the feelings and decisions made at the time and to explore new perspectives and solutions.
- *Repetition.* Reflection involves re-examining the situation – often several times – to clarify what happened from different perspectives.
- *Deeper honesty.* Reflection is being true to yourself and acknowledging feelings and thoughts that have influenced your actions, especially if you felt unsure or concerned about what others might think.
- *Weighing up.* Reflection involves taking into consideration all aspects – both positive and negative feelings and outcomes – of the experience and making balanced decisions.
- *Clarity.* Reflection provides clarity so that the situation can be improved if experienced again.
- *Understanding.* Reflection is about gaining insights, learning and understanding on a deeper level.
- *Making judgements.* Reflection involves drawing conclusions and changing behaviours to improve practice.

Schön (1987) differentiated between two types of reflection: reflection-in-action and reflection-on-action. He equated reflection-in-action with critical, spontaneous thought processes and acting while we are undertaking a task. It is a dynamic process in which 'thinking serves to reshape what we are doing while we are doing it' (p. 26). Reflection *on* action is exploring the event or situation in detail afterwards, to improve or learn from it. Further to this work, Gould, as cited in Redmond (2006), argued that there is a link between personal experience and organisational meanings and world views, and that both influence the learner's ability to undertake reflective practice.

Multiple-choice question

REFLECTION 9.1

- Select the most significant parts of an event or situation upon which you wish to reflect.
- Consider both the process and content for reflection.
- Look beneath the surface and employ critical reflection to explore and explain events, rather than just providing a description of the event.
- Reflect by revealing anxieties, errors and weaknesses, and strengths and successes. Using foresight, reflect into the future to do something differently, and reflect on the past to learn from it in hindsight and identify learning needs.

Short-answer question

Models of reflection

There are various models of reflection, based on philosophical approaches, to assist you to develop an understanding of critical reflection; however, the approach you use should help you achieve your learning outcomes. A list of different models is presented in Table 9.1. According to Martin and Fleming (2010), the approaches that encourage reflection should consider the individual needs of the student, be appropriate for the specific learning environment and help develop students' reflective skills. Approaches to critical thinking may include journaling, learning contracts, progress reports, reports and oral presentations that afford the student a the chance to hone their critical reflection abilities.

Table 9.1   Models of critical reflection

Model of critical reflection/framework	Description
Dewey's model of reflective learning	Using a pragmatic approach to review both past and present experiences, knowledge can be constructed. • Gibbs's model – cyclic approach • Stephenson's framework – set of cue questions
Habermas's model of critical reflection	Approach based on three areas of knowledge: technical, practical and emancipatory. • Taylor's framework – structured reflective model • Kim's framework – three phases of reflection
Kolb's model of reflexive learning	Integrates thinking and practice so that learning takes place when the lessons are learnt. • John's model – cue questions • Borton's framework – What? So what? Now what? • Rolf's framework – adds to Borton's framework by adding an element of reflexive learning

Source: Adapted from Rolfe, Freshwater and Jasper (2011).

What is reflective writing?

Reflective writing demonstrates your reflective thinking skills. It is more personal than other forms of academic writing but still requires a formal structure. This is when you would use one of the models or frameworks listed in Table 9.1 to help you reflect. The most common frameworks used in nursing are Gibbs's (1988) model, Kolb's (1984) reflective cycle and Taylor's (2010) framework. In the academic context, you may be required to use a formal structure to reflect. Your reflective thinking and writing can be organised using one of the models.

To proceed with reflective writing, take the following steps:

• First, identify the subject of reflection. This can be an event or a situation, something that happened that was positive or negative, a critical incident on placement, your results or grading that did not meet your expectations, or your progress.
• Second, examine closely what transpired during the event. Include your thoughts, feelings and reactions at the time. Include other people's reactions during the event. Conduct a detailed analysis of what happened, and the different assumptions and perspectives involved, and use evidence to explore and understand the event.
• Finally, think carefully about the lessons learnt. Include personal insights and how your understanding of the event developed. Identify key points that you would use should the situation arise again, both for personal and professional development.

Structuring your reflective writing

Personal reflective writing and journaling can be unstructured to help you explore ideas and experiences. However, in formal academic writing a well-structured piece of work is preferable, with descriptions, explorations, analysis and conclusions or judgements.

Useful phrases for reflective writing are:

- I felt …
- I thought …
- I realised …
- I was aware …
- I was comfortable/uncomfortable with …
- I learned …

Figures 9.3 and 9.4 show some useful examples.

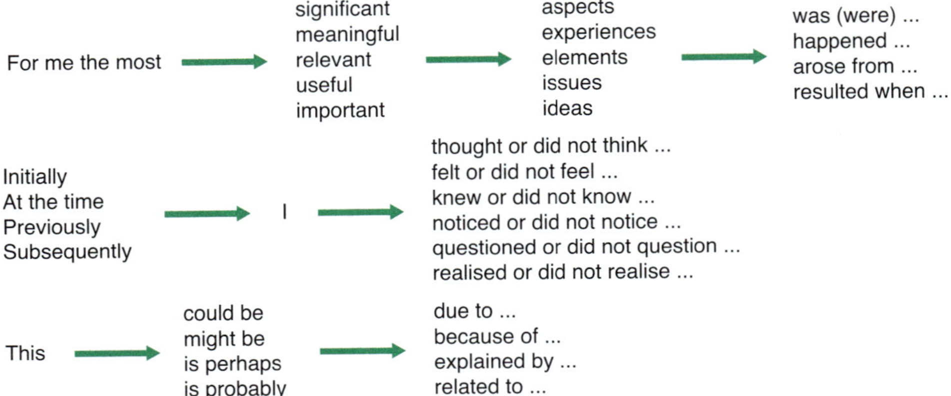

Figure 9.3 Useful analysis and interpretation phrases

Source: Adapted from Queen Margaret University (n.d.).

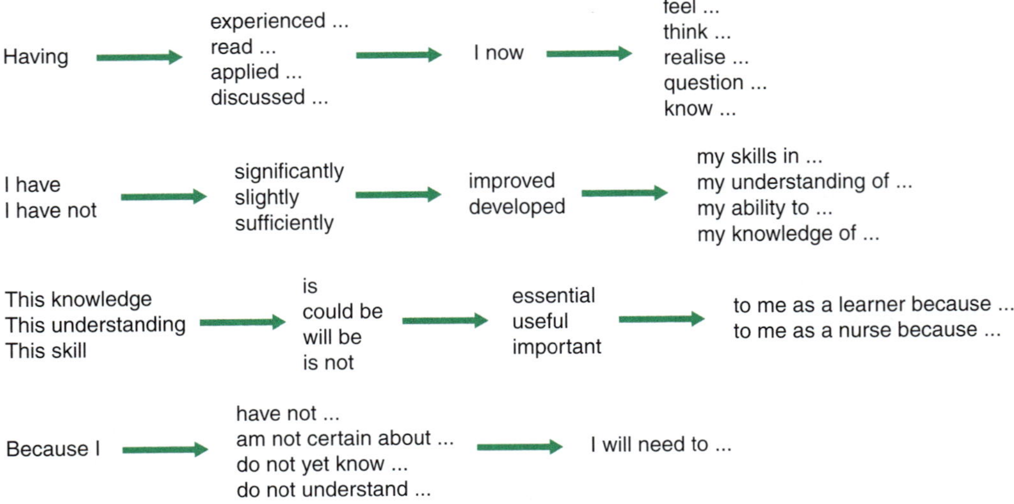

Figure 9.4 Useful outcomes and conclusion phrases

Source: Adapted from Queen Margaret University (n.d.).

Example 1: Borton's (1970) framework – a good starting point for reflective writing

- *What?* Describe a summary of what happened and when.
- *So what?* Explore how you feel about the situation, ask yourself why this is important to you, and what was concerning or useful.
- *What next?* Decide what you are going to do with the information. For example, you may seek out a mentor to ask for advice or a senior staff member to check on the best evidence-based approach that should be taken in such situations.

Example 2: Gibbs's (2001) reflective cycle

This example is the most commonly used model in nursing. Gibbs's (2001) reflective cycle (Figure 9.5) guides us through six stages of reflection (see Table 9.2).

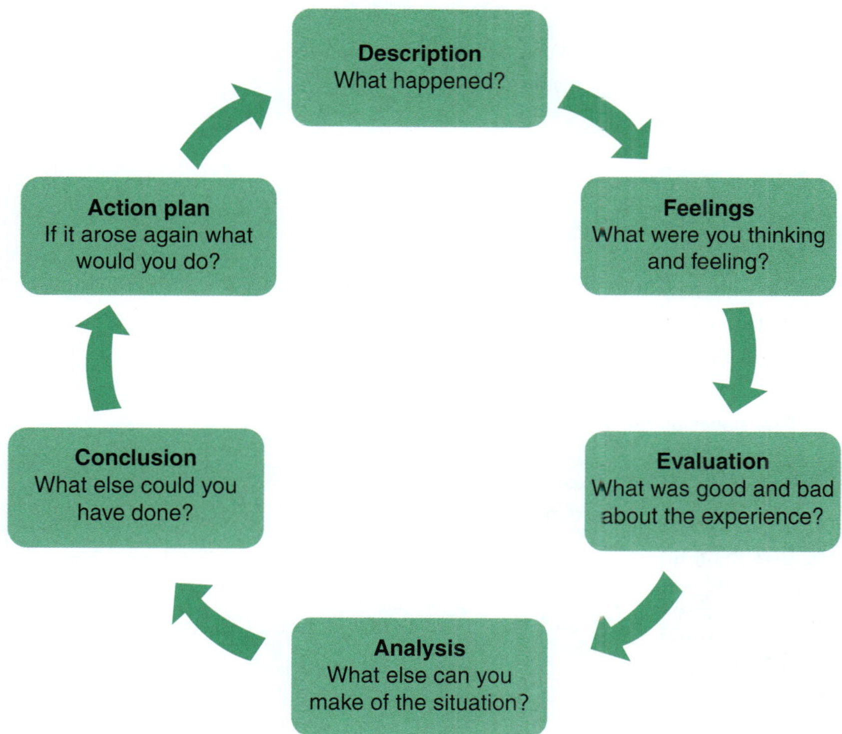

Figure 9.5   Gibbs's reflective cycle
Source: Adapted from Gibbs (2001).

Use informal writing to describe the event in detail, in the *past tense.* If you are reflecting on a specific model or theory, then is best to reflect in the *present* tense (e.g. 'Gibbs's model of reflection *identifies* … ').

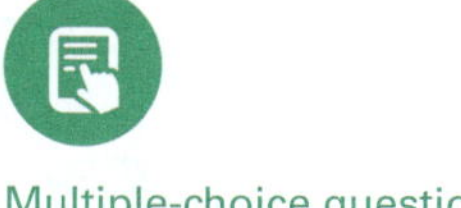

Multiple-choice question

Table 9.2   Structured reflection

Process	Reflective actions
1 Description – what happened?	What, where, when? Write down exactly what happened and when providing as much detail as you can.
2 Feelings – what were you thinking about?	Describe your feelings about the situation. How did that make you feel and why? How did your emotions affect your actions?
3 Evaluation – what was good or bad about the experience?	Think about all the elements that were useful, what was not useful and what did you learn from this experience?
4 Analysis – what sense can you make of the situation?	Compare theory and practice to help you to make sense of what happened.
5 Conclusion – what else could you have done?	Summarise what you have learned from this situation, what was done well and what areas need improvement.
6 What have you learnt for the future? What else could you have done?	What could you do differently next time and how could you prepare for this?

Source: Adapted from Gibbs (2001).

Video: Experiential learning
Short-answer question

Example 3: Kolb's (1984) reflection cycle

Kolb's (1984) reflection cycle is a four-stage process that includes incorporating experience, reflection, observation, conceptualisation, evaluation and creating a plan. Table 9.3 presents the stages of Kolb's cycle.

Table 9.3   The stages of Kolb's reflection cycle

Stage 1: Concrete experience	Life experiences provide opportunities for learning. Classroom, clinical placements, daily life experiences.
Stage 2: Reflective observation	Reflection involves thinking about what we have done and experienced. We can learn to be more deliberate about reviewing our experiences and recording them.
Stage 3: Abstract conceptualisation	In this stage we interpret our actions. Kolb termed this 'conceptualisation'. To conceptualise is to generate a hypothesis about the meaning of our experiences.
Stage 4: Active planning	In this stage we plan new actions, evaluate these actions or test hypotheses we have adopted. The new experiences will either support or challenge these. This will take us back to stage 1 of the cycle.

Source: Adapted from Kolb (1984).

Multiple-choice question

Example 4: Taylor's (2010) framework

Figure 9.6 and Table 9.4 present the key elements of the framework and the activities associated with developing reflective thinking skills.

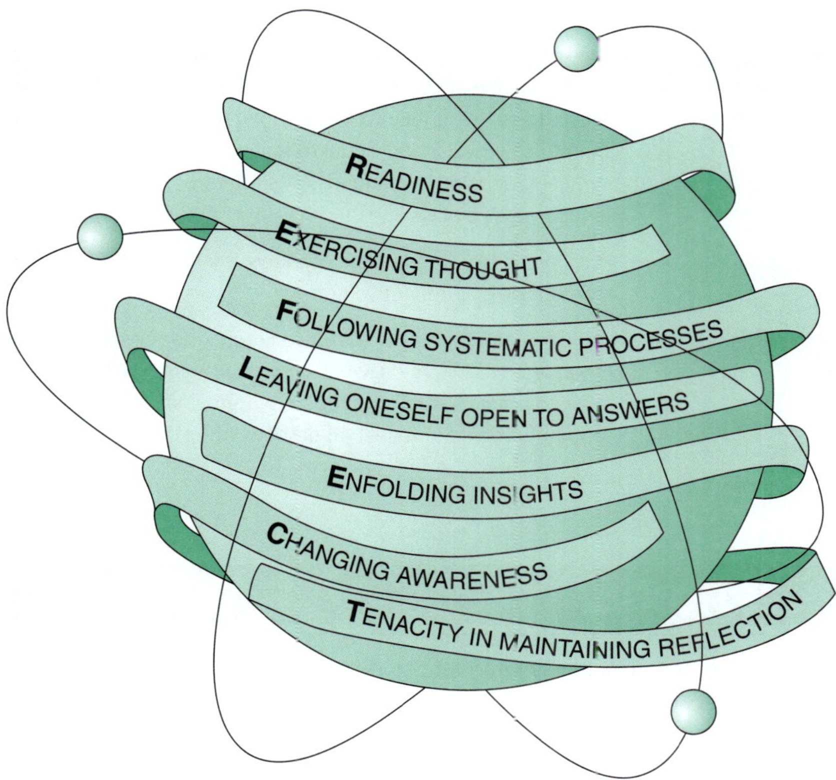

Figure 9.6 Taylor's framework

Source: Taylor (2006).

Table 9.4 Key elements of Taylor's framework

Process	Activities include reflection in nursing practice
Readiness	Being silent; centring; setting the intention; having reflective knowledge and skills; taking and making time; making the effort; being determined; having courage; knowing how to use humour
Exercising thought	Thinking about experiences Using inspiring and guiding strategies; being spontaneous; expressing freely Remaining open to ideas; choosing a time and place; being prepared personally; choosing suitable reflective methods
Following systematic processes	Processing activities Following systematic processes. For example: • *using technical reflection:* assessing, planning, implementing, evaluating • *using practical reflection:* experiencing, interpreting learning • *using emancipatory reflection:* constructing, deconstructing, confronting, reconstructing
Leaving oneself open to answers	Not jumping to early conclusions; being prepared for twists and turns; finding tentative multiple answers; living with uncertainty

Table 9.4   (cont.)

Process	Activities include reflection in nursing practice
Enfolding insights	Mixing new insights into present understandings; using a variety of group or individual reflective processes; enlisting critical friendships; letting insights rest a while; merging into deeper possibilities
Changing awareness	Making small, manageable changes; examining the emotional content of your reflective stories
Tenacity in maintaining reflection	Affirming yourself as a reflective practitioner; responding to the critiques; creating a daily habit; seeing things freshly; staying alert to practice; finding support systems; sharing reflection; getting involved in research; embodying reflective practice

Source: Taylor (2010).

REFLECTION 9.2

- Reflection *in* action is just as important as reflection *on* action.
- Critical reflection promotes deeper understanding and learning than descriptive reflection.
- The reflection process can be informal, or formally structured.
- Reflection allows us to reveal to ourselves the deep nature of our work, so that we can improve ourselves and our work procedures, interpersonal relationships and professional practices.

Professional portfolio

portfolio the term 'portfolio' comes from the Latin term *portate* – which means 'to carry' – and *foglio* – which means 'a sheet'

As employment opportunities become increasingly competitive, nurses need to consider a variety of ways in which to make an impression on prospective employers, and the traditional professional **portfolio** is no longer sufficient. An **e-portfolio**, incorporating additional information such as reflective journal entries, clinical reports and career aspirations, can enhance an application. e-Portfolios are relatively new in nursing, with many students and nurses opting to embrace the technology as a document-control strategy. An e-portfolio platform, with its filing system, makes for an easy storage system for electronic documents and certificates.

e-portfolio an electronic portfolio that is accessible anywhere the internet is available and on a range of devices, such as smartphones

Choosing an e-portfolio

The Australian Nursing and Midwifery Federation (ANMF) uses a platform called PebblePad (2017), which is an online storage system, as its recommended e-portfolio provider. Several universities have also adopted PebblePad as their e-portfolio platform. PebblePad can automatically store and hold certificates, CPD hours and learning activities in a single, easy online store. Journaling, blog and video-diary tools are also included in the platform. PebblePad is one example of a professional e-portfolio tool for nurses. There are hundreds of e-portfolio websites on the internet.

When choosing an e-portfolio, there are several important considerations:

- *The system needs to be accessible for life.* Many secondary and tertiary education providers have platforms you can use to create your e-portfolios; however, access may be linked to your enrolment. While some platforms may be mandated by your institution, if possible, choose a platform that will last the duration of your working life – one that will adapt to technological advances and will enable you to remain current in today's practice environment.
- *Choose a platform that has built-in IT support.* With so many platforms available, it is essential to choose one that has a help function and/or IT support – for example, online tutorials, examples and templates, prompts and the capacity to obtain email or phone advice.
- *Ensure you provide for advanced technologies.* We are becoming increasingly technologically advanced. Ensure the e-portfolio you choose has the capacity to create, store and run video, images and text. The e-portfolio should offer a mobile app to support recording on the go. In order to ensure your e-portfolio is accessible at all times, it needs to have the capacity to be opened, viewed and amended remotely.
- *The e-portfolio needs to be private and secure.* While it does need to be accessible remotely, and should be flexible and open, an e-portfolio also needs to remain under the control of the user. You can choose who can see what, and when. The site needs to have the option to create unique web addresses or hyperlinks, which can then only be accessed by those you choose to view your site.
- *Ensure you undertake reflective practice.* Nursing encourages reflective practice as a foundational skill; it is therefore essential that your e-portfolio site has the ability to prompt responses related to reflective entries, not simply allowing for an opportunity to write in a text box.

Creating an e-portfolio

When creating a professional portfolio, the following should be considered for inclusion:

- up-to-date resume or curriculum vitae
- cover letters
- statements addressing the key selection criteria
- list of referees and their contact details
- reference letters
- accomplishments
- examples of academic work
- conferences, workshops or seminars attended
- public speaking and presentations
- clinical reports and appraisals
- academic transcripts
- honours, awards and scholarships
- certificates.

This list is not exhaustive; you may think of other items that would enhance your professional portfolio. Using an inspirational quote that is reflective of your attitude towards the nursing profession is a great way to represent who you are.

Preparing the components of your portfolio

When preparing your professional portfolio, using the FOLIO acronym provides a step-by-step guide to assist with the process of development of the portfolio.

F – find what others have advised about format and content
O – online or paper-based
L – list what sections to include
I – insert information into each section
O – optimise your opportunities by reviewing regularly

Multiple-choice question
Video: Job application tips
Video: CPD
Connecting with practice:
Resume resources

The use of a photo in the portfolio is recommended but you will need to ensure that it is a professional photo and not a 'glamour' shot. Keep in mind that a simple layout allows the viewer to see all your essential documents and content. Use headings with a drop-down function; the viewer will open documents as needed.

SUMMARY

- This chapter has provided a contemporary definition and explanation of critical thinking and its application in twenty-first century nursing. Critical thinking involves higher-order cognition that requires knowledge of underlying processes in order to make appropriate clinical judgements and decisions. *Without a deeper knowledge, how can nurses be expected to think critically?* We also provided strategies for the beginner nurse to employ critical thinking at the beginner level by using careful and thorough client assessment, and by developing the confidence to know when to appropriately escalate care.
- Clinical judgement involves using all of your critical decision-making and analysis skills to come to a judgement about the best clinical action for the client.
- Clinical reasoning is the application of critical thinking and reflective practice to the current situation, to identify actions and make treatment decisions that will improve client outcomes. It is the ability to activate and apply appropriate emotional attitudes and thinking when there is discomfort and cognitive dissonance experienced in clinical decision-making. The chapter also outlined the practices that enhance and those that hinder clinical reasoning skills.
- The key ideas of reflection and reflective writing have been presented. The self-evaluation of one's actions, behaviours and lived experiences can result in development and enhancement of clinical knowledge, skills and professional practice.
- The chapter outlined how to go about preparing a professional portfolio, including strategies and examples of e-portfolios and the content required to successfully represent key skills and attributes.

REVIEW QUESTIONS

Suggested responses

1 List seven attributes necessary for ideal critical thinkers.
2 Which of the following practices would *not* assist in developing clinical reasoning skills?
    A – Seek opportunities for self-evaluation and self-reinforcement supported by evidence-based practice in a variety of situations.
    B – Observe, record and document role models' clinical reasoning behaviour in more critical and complex care.
    C – Make decisions too quickly without recognising the consequences.
    D – Allocate time to self and opportunities for interprofessional and collegial debriefing as well as guided reflective journaling.
3 True or false? Critical thinking and clinical reasoning go hand in hand in clinical practice and are considered to be the processes underpinning clinical analysis and decision-making.
4 What does the acronym FOLIO stand for?
5 What are the four stages of Kolb's reflective cycle?
6 True or false? Reflective writing is more personal than other forms of academic writing so there is no need to write a reflection using a formal structure.

RESEARCH TOPIC

Consider and undertake a literature review that addresses the following question: 'What are the most common obstructions to graduate registered nurses reporting concerns and escalating the care of clients in clinical settings?'

Read the following article to get you thinking about the issues related to commencing work as a registered nurse.

Meyer, G. & Shatto, B. (2018). Resilience and transition to practice in Direct entry nursing graduates. *Nurse Education in Practice*, 28, 276–9.

FURTHER READING

Brown, R.A. & Crookes, P.A. (2016). What are the 'necessary' skills for a newly graduating RN? Results of an Australian survey. *BMC Nursing*, 15(1), 23.
Caldwell, L. & Grobbel, C.C. (2013). The importance of reflective practice in nursing. *International Journal of Caring Sciences*, 6(3), 319–26.
Green, J., Wyllie, A. & Jackson, D. (2016). Electronic portfolios in nursing education: A review of the literature. *Nurse Education in Practice* 14(1), 4–8.
Hawkins, D., Elder, L. & Paul, R. (2010). *The thinker's guide to clinical reasoning*. Tomales, CA: Foundation for Critical Thinking.

REFERENCES

Benner, P. (1982). From novice to expert. *American Journal of Nursing*, 82(3), 402–7.
Borton, T. (1970). *Reach, touch and teach*. London: Hutchinson

Brookfield, S.D. (1987). *Developing critical thinkers: Challenging adults to explore alternative ways of thinking and acting.* San Francisco: Jossey-Bass.

Chan, Z.C.Y. (2013). A systematic review of critical thinking in nursing education. *Nurse Education Today*, 33, 236–40.

Elder, L. (2007). *The thinker's guide to analytic thinking.* Tomales, CA: Foundation for Critical Thinking. Retrieved from https://www.criticalthinking.org/data/pages/14/fd4e6f74cc717ed36a9faccc870b8a2e4fe0bd688b279.pdf.

Ennis, R. (2015). Critical thinking: A streamlined conception. In M. Davies & R. Barnett (eds), *The Palgrave handbook of critical thinking in higher education.* New York: Palgrave Macmillan, pp. 31–47.

Gibbs, G. (2001). *Learning by doing: A guide to teaching and learning methods.* Oxford: Further Education Unit, Oxford Polytechnic.

Grubbs, A.B. (2017). Boot camp: Enhancing clinical reasoning skills in MedVet to BSN students. *Kentucky Nurse*, 65(2), 18.

Higgins, D. (2011). Why reflect? Recognising the link between learning and reflection. *Reflective Practice*, 12(5), 583–4.

Kataoka-Yahiro, M. & Saylor, C. (1994). A critical thinking model for nursing judgment. *Journal of Nursing Education*, 33(8), 351–6.

Kolb, D. (1984). *Experiential learning: Experience as a source of learning and development.* Englewood Cliffs, NJ: Prentice-Hall.

Kuiper, R.A. & Pesut, D.J. (2004). Promoting cognitive and metacognitive reflective reasoning skills in nursing practice: Self-regulated learning theory. *Journal of Advanced Nursing*, 45, 381–91.

Kvesic, A., Galic, K. & Vukojevic, M. (2019). Humanism influencing the organisation of the health care system and the ethics of medical relations in the society of Bosnia-Herzegovina. *Philosophy, Ethics and Humanities in Medicine*, 14(12).

Martin, A. & Fleming, J. (2010). Cooperative education in outdoor education. *Australian Journal of Outdoor Education*, 14(1), 41–8.

Nursing and Midwifery Board of Australia (NMBA) (2016). *Registered Nurse Standards for Practice.* Retrieved from https://www.nursingmidwiferyboard.gov.au/Codes-Guidelines-Statements/Professional-standards/registered-nurse-standards-for-practice.aspx

Papathanasiou, I., Kleisiaris, C., Fradelos, E., Kakou, K. & Kourkouta., L. (2014). Critical thinking: The development of an essential skill in nursing students. *Acta Informatica Medica*, 22(4), 283–6.

Papp, K., Huang, M., Lauzon Clabo, L., Delva, D., Fischer, M., Konopasek, L., Schwartzstein, R. & Gusic, M. (2014). Milestones of critical thinking: A developmental model for medicine and nursing. *Academic Medicine*, 89(5), 715–20.

PebblePad (2017). Thinking about portfolio implementation? Here are 10 must-have requirements for your list [Blogpost]. Retrieved from https://www.pebblepad.co.uk/blogindex.aspx.

Petrie, B. (2020). The sentinel watch. American Sentinel University. Retrieved from https://www.americansentinel.edu/blog/2020/04/10/developing-critical-thinking-skills-in-nursing.

Queen Margaret University (n.d.). Critical thinking. Retrieved from http://archive.qmu.ac.uk/els/docs/critical%20thinking.pdf.

Redmond, B. (2006). *Reflection in action. Developing reflective practice in health and social services.* New York: Ashgate.

Rogal, S. & Young, J. (2009). Exploring critical thinking in critical care nursing education: A pilot study. *Journal of Continuing Education for Nursing*, 39(1), 28–33.

Rolfe, G., Freshwater, D. & Jasper, M. (2011). *Critical reflection in practice*, 2nd edn. New York: Palgrave Macmillan.

Schön, D.A. (1987). *Educating the reflective practitioner.* San Francisco: Jossey-Bass.

Scriven, M. & Paul, R. (1987). Critical thinking as defined by the national council for excellence in critical thinking. In *Proceedings from the National Council for Excellence in Critical Thinking*, 8th Annual International Conference on Critical Thinking and Education Reform.

Tanner, C. (2006). Thinking like a nurse: A research-based model of clinical judgement in nursing. *Journal of Nursing Education*, 45(6), 204–11.

Taylor, B.J. (2006). *Reflective practice: A guide for nurses and midwives.* New York: McGraw-Hill.

—— (2010). *Reflective practice for healthcare professionals: A practical guide*, 3rd edn. Maidenhead: Open University Press.

10 Understanding self and others

Nick Arnott, Penny Paliadelis and Mary Cruickshank

With acknowledgement to Danielle Williams for her contributions to the first edition

LEARNING OBJECTIVES

At the completion of this chapter, you should be able to:

1 Discuss self-awareness and its role in developing your professional identity and performance.
2 Examine diversity and culture as a means to understanding the unique world-views of others and in supporting professional relationships and care based on respect, empathy and compassion.
3 Explain the notions of social and emotional intelligence, and the role these play in understanding of self and others.
4 Explore the practice of mindfulness as a strategy to enhance your understanding of self and others, and to moderate the effects of stress.
5 Use critical reflection to help develop your social and emotional intelligence.

Introduction

As a society, we generally expect those working in professional roles to be 'professional', but this term is difficult to define. What does it actually mean to be professional? How can students develop their personal sense of self, and how might this interact with their professional identity and performance? This chapter explains self-awareness and the importance of understanding your own values, beliefs and motivations, which in turn will assist you to understand the diverse experiences and 'world-views' of others, and to develop and nurture the therapeutic and professional relationships that are essential in quality nursing practice.

The role of emotional and social intelligence in understanding ourselves and others is also explored in this chapter, as this concept is closely linked to self-awareness. Critical reflection and mindfulness are suggested as two of several possible strategies in fostering the development of self-awareness and self-care, which in turn may assist in caring for others with empathy, compassion and 'intelligent kindness'. In essence, enhancing your self-awareness, your self-care, and your understanding and compassion for others will help you to interact and communicate effectively, to reconcile differences or conflicts that may arise, and to cope with the emotional demands inherent in healthcare practice (Foster et al. 2015; Kelly, Runge & Spencer 2015).

Self-awareness

Self-awareness underpins personal success and growth, and lies at the root of happiness because it engenders a sense of purpose and meaning in our lives.

The benefits of attending to 'self' are many, including a heightened sense of wellbeing, an improved ability to self-evaluate and apply self-management, an increased capacity to learn, improved recognition of stressful situations and the development of adaptive coping skills (Silvia & Phillips 2013; van der Riet et al. 2015).

You have probably heard the saying 'be/stay true to yourself'. This may be great advice for both your personal and professional lives, but how can you 'stay true to yourself' (or even know that you want to) if you don't really know who you are?

Self-awareness (sometimes referred to as self-knowledge or introspection) is about knowing who you are and what makes you tick – the things that influence, motivate, inspire and challenge you. It is about understanding your own values and beliefs, your needs and preferences, your strengths and limitations, and your habits and behaviours. It involves recognising your thoughts and emotions and the ways in which you react to different situations or experiences, and understanding the internal resources you have for managing or regulating these things (Bradberry & Greaves 2009; Foster et al. 2017; Silvia & Phillips 2013).

self-awareness conscious knowledge of one's own character, feelings, motives and behaviours

When you are self-aware, you are far more likely to pursue the right opportunities, make good decisions, put your strengths to work and ensure your emotions do not hold you back through impulsive reactions or negative self-talk (Bradberry & Greaves 2009; Goleman, Boyatzis & McKee 2013). The more you pay attention to your values, emotions and the way you act, the better you will be at understanding why you do or say the things you do. The more you know about your habits, biases, reactions and behaviours, the easier it will be to regulate or improve them. Bradberry and Greaves (2009) profiled the characteristics of people from different walks of life. They found that highly self-aware people tended to be open and authentic, honest about their feelings and 'cool, calm and collected' in times of stress or crisis, whereas those low in self-awareness were more likely to project stress and urgency, be defensive, aggressive or demanding, and to fail to notice how they affected others.

Values, beliefs and attitudes

values the principles, standards or qualities that 'really matter' to an individual or group

beliefs the convictions or ideas that we believe to be true

attitudes the mental dispositions and behavioural tendencies a person may have and direct towards other people, groups, ideas or circumstances

As human beings, we all have our own **values**, **beliefs** and **attitudes** that contribute to our sense of who we are and how we view the world, and that influence the way we act or behave (McSherry et al. 2017). These are examined in this section (Drayton & Weston 2015; Moore 2017; New Zealand Government 2020):

- Values are those things that really matter to us: the principles, standards or qualities that an individual or group holds in high regard. Because they really matter, values greatly influence how we think, feel and behave, as well as the choices or decisions we make.
- Beliefs are the convictions or ideas that we believe to be true. Beliefs underpin our actions and behaviours, and they provide explanations for how we understand ourselves, our world and our experiences. Beliefs may be based upon certainties, probabilities, or matters of culture or faith. They may arise from different sources, including:
  - our own experiences or experiments;
  - the acceptance of cultural, familial and/or societal norms (e.g. religion); and
  - what other people say and do (e.g. education, mentoring, socialisation).
- Each person evaluates and seeks sound reasons or evidence for their beliefs in their own ways. Once a person accepts a belief as 'truth', it forms part of their belief system that they are willing to defend (although beliefs may change or cease, based on the person's experiences and evaluation of those experiences). Sometimes beliefs are described as values, based on the premise that certain beliefs may matter more, or be more important or valuable, to a person.
- Attitudes are a person's mental dispositions and behavioural tendencies, which they may direct towards other people, groups, ideas or circumstances. People primarily form their attitudes from underlying beliefs and values. Attitudes can sometimes reflect our values (things that really matter to us) but if they are not so important, they may be more like personal opinions.

Our work as health professionals involves establishing and maintaining meaningful and empowering relationships with clients and colleagues, who may sometimes have very different values and beliefs from our own. Sometimes, our own attitudes can cause us to overlook other people's values and beliefs, lead us to behave or respond in a certain way towards a person or group (stereotyping), or can cloud our judgement in meeting people's needs (basing decisions on what *we* think someone should do, rather than their own choices and preferences). As such, being aware of – reflecting upon and critically evaluating – our values, beliefs and attitudes is particularly important for professional development and improvement.

self-management understanding your emotions, needs and behaviours, and using this understanding in beneficial ways

self-improvement improvement of one's knowledge, character and abilities by one's own effort or actions

Self-awareness is a key requisite for **self-management** and **self-improvement**. Being mindful of your weaknesses enables you to set goals and implement strategies to better manage these limitations. Paying attention to your strengths can also contribute to self-improvement by developing ways in which you can more readily harness and deploy these positive resources in times of stress, emotional turmoil or conflict. Bulmer Smith and colleagues found that, 'As frontline healthcare workers, nurses form and maintain relationships within emotionally charged environments' (2009, p. 1625), and provide complex care for people who are emotionally vulnerable due to physical or mental illness (Foster et al. 2015). Every situation or experience will evoke an emotional reaction, derived from your own value base or belief system – your personal world-view. There may arise a dilemma, in that in many interactions and experiences these emotions manifest subconsciously, making self-management and self-improvement much more difficult. So, while the 'what' and 'why' of self-awareness can easily be defined, the actual ability to *be* self-aware, and to bring this awareness to your interpersonal interactions, requires dedicated focus and practice.

There are many ways to cultivate greater self-awareness, including:

- meditation or mindfulness training
- goal-setting – working out where you want to go in life and how you will get there
- keeping a journal
- regularly reflecting on and evaluating your ideas, behaviours and performance
- learning to give and receive honest and constructive feedback
- asking trusted colleagues, friends or family members to provide honest appraisals of how they perceive you and your particular strengths and weaknesses
- taking psychometric tests.

Connecting with practice: Personality tests

Awareness of others

Developing self-awareness requires us to be mindful of **diversity** – that is, understanding the unique experiences and world-views of others. Understanding the values, beliefs, needs and emotions of others is the key to achieving **empathy**, which is especially critical for healthcare professionals, whose work often involves complex and sensitive emotional encounters (Bulmer Smith et al. 2009; Foster et al. 2015). Empathy is the ability to perceive and share in another person's reality, or to feel *with* another person (Stein-Parbury 2017). Empathy requires us to 'tune in' to what someone else might be thinking or feeling about a particular situation, even if it differs from our own perception of that situation. It does not involve a judgement about the validity of someone's feelings; it is simply an attempt to understand those feelings, regardless of whether we feel the same way (Faguy 2012).

diversity involves recognising each person as unique and respecting individual differences

empathy the ability to perceive and share in another person's reality

Diversity and culture

Diversity recognises that each individual is unique and has different traits, characteristics and world-views that may distinguish them from others in society (Australian HR Institute 2020). At its core, diversity is simply a reflection of these individual differences; however, in most professional domains – especially those such as nursing, which are centred on human relationships (Bulmer Smith et al. 2009) – diversity is mostly viewed as a positive orientation underpinned by respect and acceptance of these differences. Diversity is often considered in relation to age, gender, socio-economic status, race, ethnicity, religious beliefs, physical abilities,

Video: Diversity in
Australia

culture refers to the customs and beliefs, art, way of life and social organisation of a particular country or group (Oxford Dictionary 2020)

sexual orientation, political beliefs, personal interests and passions (Australian HR Institute 2020). While these 'macro' factors undoubtedly influence people's thoughts, feelings, decisions and actions, as nurses we need to be careful that our understanding of others is not clouded by preconceived notions or stereotypes about such things – for example, that women are physically weaker than men, or that men are unable to express emotions.

Culture is another concept or term that is sometimes used interchangeably with diversity. While there are obvious similarities, there are also some differences. These are particularly evident when culture is defined and considered through the narrow lens of 'ethnicity'. As such, we explore culture here as an element of diversity.

Culture refers to the ideas, customs and social behaviours of a particular people or society. It includes human values, beliefs, customs, ethics, gender roles, languages and traditions, as well as the material objects and practices that are common to a group or society. Culture is reflected in how people express their ideas, creativity, history and heritage. In the Universal Declaration on Cultural Diversity, the United Nations Educational, Scientific and Cultural Organisation (UNESCO 2001) states that 'culture should be regarded as the set of distinctive spiritual, material, intellectual and emotional features of society or a social group, and that it encompasses, in addition to art and literature, lifestyles, ways of living together, value systems, traditions and beliefs'.

In striving to be culturally aware, health professionals need to understand that cultural differences exist, and to be sensitive towards and respectful of those differences when interacting with people and groups whose beliefs, customs and world-views are be different from our own. This may sound reasonable in principle; however, when we identify comfortably with our own culture (especially if this is a dominant or mainstream culture), our awareness and openness to the cultural nuances, norms and needs of other people and groups can be overlooked. We all have the *potential* to connect with one another but developing our *capability* for culturally informed practice requires that we expand our awareness, knowledge and skills through learning, reflection and story telling, in order to improve and enhance these connections in new and diverse contexts (Australian Government 2015).

This requires professional curiosity and a willingness to objectively examine and discuss the values, beliefs, traditions and perspectives of both our own and other cultures, and to evaluate situations and make decisions that are free from judgement, assumptions or stereotypes. This empathetic and inclusive approach helps to promote 'cultural safety', a concept drawn from Māori nurses in New Zealand, describing 'an environment that is spiritually, socially and emotionally safe, as well as physically safe for people; where there is no assault, challenge or denial of their identity, of who they are and what they need. It is about shared respect, shared meaning, shared knowledge and experience, of learning together with dignity and truly listening' (author unknown but commonly attributed jointly to Williams 1999, pp. 213–14 and Bin-Sallik 2003, pp. 21–8). Cultural safety is underpinned by respectful and trusting relationships with our clients, their families and significant others. It involves listening to their stories, valuing their lived experiences and world-views, and building meaningful connections that support and promotes their cultural knowledge, identity and sense of belonging (Kickett 2020).

People and organisations valuing diversity and inclusion demonstrate practices and behaviours that recognise the uniqueness of each individual and that are open to exploring these unique experiences and world-views of 'others' (Australian HR

Institute 2020). To empathise with (feel *with*) someone, nurses must move beyond their personal perspectives and experiences, and must pay careful attention to cues from the other person – what they say, their tone of voice, facial expressions, body language and behaviours – to fully comprehend that person's unique experience and reality (Faguy 2012; McSherry et al. 2017). Embracing diversity starts with managing our own attitudes, emotions and behaviours, which stem from our awareness of self and others. Recognising and celebrating individual differences and the strengths and advantages that diversity can bring to our lives and our practice are key to building positive, safe and inclusive environments that foster personal and professional growth.

Contemporary healthcare also demands a person-centred approach (see also Chapter 11), in which healthcare professionals 'develop the ability to form therapeutic interpersonal relationships that elicit the true wishes of clients and their families and recognise and respond to their needs and emotional concerns' (Kornhaber et al. 2016, p. 538). It is widely acknowledged that understanding and accepting diversity is implicit in person-centred practice, which involves:

- treating each person as an individual;
- respecting a person's culture, values, rights and preferences;
- empowering choice and self-determination;
- protecting a person's dignity; and
- forming collaborative and respectful partnerships between health professionals, their clients or patients and others significant to them, built on mutual respect, trust and understanding (McCormack & McCance 2016; NMBA 2016).

Our self-awareness is key to understanding others. Greater self-awareness creates a clearer lens through which to see other people as distinct individuals, and to understand their particular perspectives, emotions and behaviours, without judgement. For example, a less self-aware nurse may view their client entirely from the perspective of how they or another client may have felt or reacted in a similar situation. If they do not 'tune in' to what this person is really thinking or feeling about their situation, the nurse may well misinterpret or misunderstand important signs or cues, or perhaps be too preoccupied or distracted by other things to even notice at all. Their responsiveness to this client may be compromised by a tendency to subjectively evaluate or judge this person's experience as good or bad, right or wrong, important or trivial, rather than trying to understand the person's own unique reality – the meaning they make from this health event or experience (Stein-Parbury 2017).

Self-awareness does not automatically make you more aware of others but it can promote more mindful attention to those around you. This can help to identify your likely feelings and reactions to various situations, enable you to recognise the triggers for these emotional responses, and give you the ability to use these insights to inform improvements required to be more responsive to the unique, subjective world of those with whom you are interacting (Adams & Iseler 2014; Stein-Parbury 2017). Likewise, exploring the emotions, needs and views of others may help to recognise, affirm, accept or change certain aspects of your own 'self', thereby making you more 'present', authentic and **compassionate** in your interpersonal relationships with others. In developing our self-awareness, however, Goleman (2011) warns us to be careful of crossing the line from introspection to self-absorption:

compassionate able to *feel* another person's pain, struggles or suffering; compassion is similar to empathy but is accompanied by the motivation to 'take action' to alleviate these feelings

Video: Inside others' hearts

Self-absorption in all its forms kills empathy, and particularly compassion. When we focus on ourselves, our world contracts as our problems and preoccupations loom large. But when we focus on others, our world expands. Our own problems drift to the periphery of the mind and so seem smaller, and we increase our capacity for connection – or compassionate action (p. 54).

Developing effective 'people skills'

Developing your awareness of self and others contributes to improvements in your interpersonal skills, or 'people skills'. This is important in all walks of life, but it is especially critical for nurses, whose work is largely about 'relational practice', in which the nurse needs to demonstrate an authentic interest in the client's experiences and to 'use skills such as active listening, observation and inquiry to advocate for and promote independent and self-actualised care' (Robertson-Malt, Norton-Westwood & Pearson 2017, p. 94). Stein-Parbury (2018) asserts that 'the more nurses are aware of themselves, the more likely it is that their interpersonal skills will be used in an authentic and natural way' (p. 61). Newman (2016) suggests that being more attentive to ourselves and our relationships can help us to translate our values into action and to live and act more authentically.

So far, this chapter has emphasised 'people skills' in the context of therapeutic relationships with clients or patients, their families and significant others. While this is obviously a core focus in nursing, nurses (including students) also need to establish and maintain professional relationships with a range of other people, including colleagues from the same or other disciplines, healthcare administrators, academics, members of professional bodies and the general public. Embracing diversity by valuing the different backgrounds, perspectives and experiences of others provides a foundation for supportive, respectful and collaborative relationships and communication (Stein-Parbury 2017).

Working with diverse groups of people who are often going through difficult, stressful or traumatic experiences can take a significant emotional toll on health professionals. Building genuine, authentic and compassionate relationships, having respect for each other in the workplace and providing meaningful recognition of others' work can contribute to quality outcomes for clients and can also help to mediate compassion fatigue, reinvigorate the passion for caring and enhance job satisfaction and engagement for ourselves and our colleagues (Moore 2017, Kelly, Runge & Spencer 2015). Effective 'people skills' help us to demonstrate integrity in our relationships and to promote the confidence and abilities needed to successfully navigate complex personal and professional situations, and to initiate self-care strategies in times of stress or emotional overload. These respectful relationships and compassion for ourselves and others can also reduce the likelihood of conflict in the workplace, and can help in the resolution of any conflict that may arise.

We have all experienced times when our responses to others have been less than positive or constructive, where we have said or done something that has inflamed a situation, or we have acted on strong feelings without thinking through the consequences (Faguy 2012). By developing our self-awareness and situational awareness, we build on the ability to monitor and regulate our actions and reactions, in order to more readily draw upon our strengths and to identify and take action to address any limitations. As nurses, awareness of self and others will improve communication, enhance relationships and promote self-care – all of which are essential for success as a health professional.

Evaluating and improving your self-awareness and self-management skills

The opposite of self-awareness is self-deception, and we can all fall prey to this at times. We may sometimes fool ourselves or hold unrealistic views about our own strengths and weaknesses, and the ways in which our thoughts, feelings, actions and behaviours affect others. Being an effective, lifelong learner requires critical reflection on our experiences, to think about what has worked well, what has not, what we have learned from positive and negative outcomes, and how to embed these insights into our future actions and practices (Deutschendorf 2018; Steiner 2014).

One practical way to build your self-awareness and practise self-management is to keep a journal or professional portfolio (see Chapter 9), in which you regularly record your thoughts, feelings, actions and interactions (Harrison & Fopma-Loy 2010; Tjan 2015). Deutschendorf (2018) recommended setting aside a few minutes every day to reflect on such things, thereby creating a substantive record from which specific insights, patterns, triggers and behaviours can be identified and analysed. You may choose to keep this journal private so that you can be totally honest with yourself but remember that 'critical reflection' requires a willingness to open your perspectives to scrutiny and feedback from (trusted) others, so try to think about what you might like to share, when and with whom.

REFLECTION 10.1

Each time you write in your journal, consider these questions:

- What was the situation or experience?
- With whom did you interact?
- What is your relationship to that person?
- What emotions did you feel and how strong were they?
- Were you able to control your emotions and behaviours?
- Was the experience generally positive or negative, and why?

Once you have kept this journal for a time, it is useful to reflect more deeply on your entries by asking yourself:

- Do particular people or situations make you react in a certain way?
- Do some situations cause you to have strong feelings and reactions?
- Are you able to identify your feelings, triggers, reactions and behaviours accurately?
- Are you able to regulate or manage your feelings and emotions effectively to achieve positive outcomes?
- What do you need to improve on, and how might you do it?

As noted earlier, self-awareness is intrinsically linked to self-improvement. Keeping a journal can provide a consistent and disciplined method for reflecting on your strengths and weaknesses, the things you do well and not so well, and any knowledge or skills requiring improvement (Harrison & Fopma-Loy 2010). Remember, though, that improvement is not achieved by simply identifying the need for it. Successful reflective practice also requires you to 'close this loop' by developing and implementing proactive and realistic plans for achieving your desired improvements.

Short-answer questions

CASE STUDY

Self-awareness in practice

While on a clinical placement at a community palliative care service, a final-year nursing student witnessed an incident that they *perceived* to be an example of poor professional practice and miscommunication. The incident involved a 52-year-old registered nurse and a 45-year-old client who had been receiving community palliative care since having been recently diagnosed with an aggressive cancer that had metastasised to his bones.

Since diagnosis, the client had rapidly declined within only a matter of weeks, from being a fit, healthy and active man to becoming almost entirely bed-bound. Despite this decline, he believed he could beat the cancer using alternative therapies. He had already refused the next round of chemotherapy, based on the medical advice that it was unlikely to succeed, and had sourced information about meditation and diet that he believed would rid his entire body of the aggressive cancer. It is important to note that this man was well educated and had devoted many hours of research to exploring alternative treatment options. He felt he was making an informed and well-considered decision in refusing chemotherapy and opting for the alternative treatment. He spoke about his decision with great motivation and displayed a strong sense of hope at the prospect of embarking on this new treatment regimen.

The registered nurse and student listened carefully to the client. The registered nurse then gently told him that the treatment he was about to embark upon was unlikely to work and was not based on scientific evidence, and that it was very likely he would die within weeks. The client was clearly disturbed by these comments and the student felt that it had been disrespectful, mean and unprofessional for the registered nurse to dash the client's hopes in this way.

After the visit, the registered nurse spent an hour debriefing with the student. She clarified that her relationship with the client was based on an agreement to be absolutely honest with each other, which they had discussed when the client was first diagnosed. The experienced palliative care nurse also explained that terminally ill clients often 'grasp at straws' – even when, within themselves, they probably know that their situation is hopeless. By being honest, the registered nurse felt she was actually assisting the client to face the unpleasant truth about his situation and to better prepare for his continuing and rapid decline. This would enable the client to focus on getting his affairs in order and to spend precious time with his family and friends, rather than being distracted by a futile search for miracles.

The registered nurse added that this was a difficult part of the role, but that direct and honest communication supported clients to move past self-deception and denial, and to hopefully achieve greater self-awareness and acceptance in their final phase of life.

QUESTIONS

This scenario is not presented as the *right* or *only* way of approaching a situation such as this. It is offered as a 'reflective prompt' to help stimulate the development of your own self-awareness and self-improvement.

1   How do you think the nursing student could use this experience to enhance their self-awareness?

2   What were your feelings about this scenario, and how do you think you might react or behave in a similar situation?

3   Based on your reflection, what changes or improvements would you like to bring to your own future practice, and how might this be achieved?

Social and emotional intelligence

What does it mean to be 'intelligent'? We often think of the narrow and rather old-fashioned definition of intelligence as being knowledgeable, clever or learned, but in more recent times 'social and emotional intelligence' has emerged as an important component of intelligence overall, and is seen as vital to the development of well-rounded, or 'balanced', individuals (Goleman, Boyatzis & McKee 2013; Mayer, Caruso & Salovey 2016; Snowden et al. 2015).

Philosophers including the novelist Dostoevsky (1962) have long debated whether to follow one's 'head' or one's 'heart'. Many healthcare scholars have landed on the side of 'rational thought', arguing that critical thinking, knowledge and technical expertise are the core competencies required for enacting clinical decisions that positively influence client outcomes (Cherry 2018; Faguy 2012). While this is true in part (see Chapter 7), there is now growing recognition that in a profession that articulates 'caring' as a core concept, nurses are professionally obligated to develop their **emotional intelligence** and to integrate both cognition *and* emotions. This integration can help to enhance relationships, improve the quality of clinical decision-making and assist in managing or coping with emotionally laden situations and complex communication challenges encountered in practice (Bulmer Smith et al. 2009; Raghubir 2018; Stein-Parbury 2018). Mayer, Salovey and Caruso (2008) argued that a truly healthy and successful individual cannot rely on thought or emotion alone but must functionally integrate these major psychological processes. In his seminal work on emotional intelligence, Goleman (1998) set out to illustrate this point by evaluating the cognitive and emotional competencies of both star and average performers in 40 companies. He found that the 'stars' were 27 per cent more likely to score high in cognitive ability than 'average' performers and 53 per cent more likely to score high on emotional competency, thereby concluding that emotional competencies were twice as important in contributing to excellence than pure intellect and technical expertise.

Although there is no common definition of emotional intelligence, it is generally accepted that it involves the ability to perceive and understand one's own and others' emotions and to use this information to guide thinking and behaviour (Craig 2020; Mayer et al. 2016). Emotional intelligence involves four interrelated components: *perceiving* emotions in ourselves and others; *understanding* the messages conveyed by these emotions; using this emotional input to *facilitate* thinking; and *managing* emotions by promoting actions and behaviours that benefit ourselves and our relationships (Goleman et al. 2013; Mayer et al. 2016; Shanta & Gargiulo 2014).

emotional intelligence the ability to recognise, understand and respond appropriately to emotions in oneself and others

Video: Emotional intelligence

Emotional intelligence is often considered to be a range of core emotional abilities or competencies. Five such competencies, based on an amalgam of work by leading emotional intelligence scholars Daniel Goleman, Peter Salovey and John Mayer, are outlined in this section (Cherry 2018; Faguy 2012, p. 241):

- *self-awareness* – understanding one's own emotions and abilities
- *self-regulation* – managing one's emotions well
- *motivation* – using one's preferences to stay focused on goals and to cope with setbacks
- *empathy* – being sensitive to and aware of others' feelings
- *social skills* – using sensitivity to emotions to interact effectively with others (e.g. to lead, motivate or resolve disagreements).

As emphasised throughout this chapter, awareness of self and others is integral to emotional intelligence. Likewise, the importance of social skills and our earlier exploration of diversity and empathy have prompted us to extend this focus to **social intelligence**, which emphasises the ability to understand and manage our own and others' emotions in order to act wisely in our personal, therapeutic and professional relationships (Craig 2020; Goleman 2011).

social intelligence sensitivity to emotions and the ability to use this emotional information to enhance relationships with others

The concepts of social and emotional intelligence were first used in the 1920s with reference to the skills needed to decipher one's own and others' emotions and to act in a socially acceptable manner (Arghode 2013). Today, a nurse with social and emotional capability is able to interact effectively by being aware and mindful of others' feelings and reactions, and adjusting their own thinking and behaviour to time, space, context and situation (Silvia & Phillips 2013). They practise emotional intelligence by being self-aware and applying self-regulation and management, which is central to quality decision-making and the maintenance of genuine, authentic and compassionate relationships (Bulmer Smith et al. 2009; Raghubir 2018; Stein-Parbury 2018). They can effectively integrate their cognitive and emotional abilities to support critical thinking, problem-solving and conflict resolution (Foster et al. 2015; Mayer et al. 2016). In addition, they are able to use this social and emotional intelligence to help moderate the effects of emotionally charged situations and chaotic environments, and protect against their own stress and burnout (Kelly, Runge & Spencer 2015; Kinman & Leggetter 2016; Ruiz-Aranda, Extremera & Pineda-Galan 2014).

In the context of social and emotional intelligence, the term 'social skills' refers to a wide range of relationship and interpersonal abilities. These include rapport-building, communication, leadership, cooperation, negotiation, conflict resolution, change management, team-building and collaboration. These abilities, or skills, enable us to demonstrate respect and empathy for the feelings of others, and to regulate our own emotions and behaviours in order to better adapt to diverse social situations and to find effective solutions to any differences or conflicts that may arise. Bear in mind that our motivations and intentions are critical to success in these encounters, as demonstrating genuine interest or empathy for another person's reality will rarely be achieved through impulsive, 'fake' or scripted responses. Appearing interested, saying the right things or laughing at the right times can all be legitimate interpersonal strategies, but if the motivation is selfish, based on preconceived ideas, or on sympathy (feeling *sorry for*) rather than empathy, these interactions or relationships may come across as inauthentic, judgemental or disrespectful (Emmerling & Boyatzis 2012).

There is a link between emotional intelligence and the concept of 'emotional labour', which involves concealing your true or natural emotions and displaying those that are considered professionally desirable or in keeping with the expectations of service provision (Stein-Parbury 2018). While this 'surface-acting' – the overt expression of emotions you are not actually feeling – may sometimes be a necessary part of emotional self-regulation, it has been criticised in nursing literature for being inauthentic, for disrupting the building of trust in the therapeutic nurse–client relationship and for its link to emotional exhaustion, burnout and poor job satisfaction (Kinman & Leggetter 2016; Stein-Parbury 2018). With all this taken into consideration, it is clear that self-awareness, self-management and self-improvement are vital in the development of social and emotional intelligence, and in building effective relationships with others.

Short-answer questions
Connecting with practice:
Emotional intelligence quiz
Multiple-choice questions

NURSING PERSPECTIVE

One day, as a student nurse, Cathy had been allocated responsibility for a client who had been referred to as 'a difficult lady' in handover. She tells the story.

I went to see her first, deciding to get her out of the way so I could enjoy the rest of my day. 'Good morning, Anna,' I said. 'GOOD?' she snapped back. 'Try your useless platitudes on someone else.' She sat in bed glaring at me as I delivered a steaming bowl of water for her wash. She dipped a finger into it. 'Too hot,' she announced. I took a deep breath and said, 'Sure, Anna. I'll just get you another one.' I wrestled the bowl back to the pan room and adjusted the contents. On my return, she rolled her eyes in frustration. 'You really are incompetent' she said. 'Too cold!' Feeling like Goldilocks, I brought back the bowl a third time, and this time it really was just right. Anna then berated me for expecting her to use an 'old' face washer, the one she had probably used on her bottom yesterday. 'I require two. And different colours so that they can't be mixed up.' By the time I had finished all my fussing, the water had gone cold again. I was near boiling point and on the verge of letting this malicious old lady know about it when I noticed tears cascading down her cheeks. Anna whispered, 'Thank you, nurse. You're the only person here who has been nice to me, and I am so very frightened.'

Source: Wilson and Wilson (2011).

How to enhance social and emotional intelligence

According to Bradberry and Greaves (2009), emotional intelligence is the single biggest predictor of high performance in the workplace. The good news is that social and emotional intelligence can be developed, but not so much through theoretical content, homework, written tests or formal exams; rather, it takes hands-on learning and problem-solving, self-evaluation and critical reflection (Arghode 2013; Deutschendorf 2018; Shanta & Gargiulo 2014). Keeping a reflective journal or professional portfolio, as suggested earlier in this chapter (see also Chapter 9), can be a valuable learning tool, particularly during clinical placements when you encounter real people and enter into relationships requiring a depth of emotional involvement and sensitivity (Foster et al. 2017; Stein-Parbury 2018). Bear in mind that stress, tiredness and emotional fatigue can impair your social and emotional abilities. In other words, if you are tired, cranky or overwhelmed, you may not be at your best when interacting with others (Littlejohn 2012). Cultivating awareness of self and others through strategies such as reflection and mindfulness can help you to recognise when your reactions or behaviours are less than ideal, and can assist in developing self-care strategies to manage or moderate the effects of stress. Some good news is that research has shown that emotional and social intelligence develops in most people over time (Foster et al. 2017; Littlejohn 2012), so stick at it!

REFLECTION 10.2

Reflect on the following questions and then record your responses in your reflective journal or professional portfolio. An experience from clinical practice would be ideal for this exercise, but if you have not yet completed any clinical placements, any other professional or personal experience would be fine.

- Briefly describe a situation in which your personal values, beliefs, emotions or feelings controlled what you said or how you behaved.
- Explain the outcome of that situation.
- What outcome would you have preferred?
- How could you achieve this preferred outcome if a similar situation arose in the future?

Mindfulness

mindfulness purposefully and non-judgementally giving awareness and attention to the present moment or experience

One way of enhancing self-awareness and building social and emotional intelligence is to practise **mindfulness** (Ponte & Koppel 2015). You have probably heard the merits of 'multi-tasking'; in contrast, mindfulness is about purposefully paying attention to the 'here and now' and being fully present in your immediate experiences, without judgement (Krasner et al. 2009). It involves being *present* and *focused* on the particular feelings, thoughts, actions and interactions you are experiencing in that moment, and giving your undivided 'attention to your intentions'. Mindfulness 'is based on the premise that while both pleasant and unpleasant experiences arise in daily life, the habit of judging or resisting those experiences heightens their impact' (Hassed et al. 2009, p. 389). Thus 'acceptance' also sits alongside focus and attention as core elements of mindfulness practice.

With its roots in Eastern meditation practices, mindfulness training is now being used in schools, healthcare organisations and industry to provide people with the tools to be more focused on their everyday practice, to recognise and respond to their own needs, to improve their decision-making and to manage and cope with the emotional demands and stress they may experience (Bedson 2016; Hulatt 2015). Evidence suggests that mindfulness practice may help to develop self-awareness, facilitate the development of empathy and compassion, enhance relationships and communication with others, improve mood and productivity, build personal resilience and coping skills, foster self-compassion and mental wellbeing (see Chapter 6), and improve physiological functions such as boosting immune responses, reducing high blood pressure and increasing tolerance to pain (Bedson 2016; Hassed et al. 2009; Keng, Smoski & Robins 2011; van der Riet et al. 2015).

CASE STUDY

Research highlights

Hassed and colleagues (2009) used surveys and interviews to measure the effects of a program of mindfulness, stress management and lifestyle on the psychological wellbeing and quality of life of first-year undergraduate students at an Australian university. The study found that participants in the program experienced significantly improved physical and psychological wellbeing, and enhanced the students' quality of life, despite the fact that the post-program evaluation was undertaken immediately prior to mid-year exams, when there is often an expected decline in mental health.

Schwind and colleagues (2017) studied the influence that instructor-guided mindfulness practice, conducted at the beginning and end of class, had on undergraduate nursing and community service students' feelings of stress, anxiety and overall sense of wellbeing. Participants in the study self-reported a greater sense of relaxation and wellbeing, decreased anxiety and stress, and an increased capacity to focus on academic tasks. Instructors observed that brief mindfulness practice at the beginning of class helped students to feel more grounded, focused and engaged in course content and class activities.

Krasner and colleagues (2009) conducted a study to determine whether an intensive, mindfulness-based communication and self-awareness program was associated with improvement in primary care physicians' wellbeing, psychological distress, burnout and capacity to relate to clients. The study demonstrated that participation in the program contributed to improved personal wellbeing, decreased emotional exhaustion and burnout, improved mood, and positive changes in empathy and psychosocial beliefs, which are both indicators of a person-centred orientation to care.

Mindfulness practice

There are now numerous websites, apps, books, training programs and self-directed activities available to assist people to develop mindfulness skills. Many formal and informal mindfulness practices can assist in developing self-awareness, reducing stress and building social and emotional intelligence – for example, guided mindfulness meditation (in person or online), mindfulness movements (e.g. walking, yoga, tai chi) and body-scan (a process for developing greater sensory awareness). Mindfulness can be practised in everyday situations, such as while brushing your teeth, taking a shower or going for a walk. A recent trend has involved the use of colouring books to encourage mindfulness, based on the idea that colouring intricate patterns helps people to focus on the 'here and now' and to give complete attention to their immediate thoughts, actions and intentions.

Simple mindfulness activity: Mindful breathing

You can do this simple mindfulness exercise standing or sitting, anytime and anywhere. Why not try it now?

- You need to focus on your breathing for one minute. Do this by being aware of breathing in through your nose and out through your mouth.
- Be aware of the feeling of the air entering your nose, travelling into your lungs and then out through your mouth. Focus on this and let go of any other thoughts.
- Focus on your senses. What does it feel like to breathe slowly and effortlessly? How does the rest of your body feel? Are your shoulders relaxed? What are you hearing, smelling, seeing in this moment?
- If your mind wanders to other things, gently bring it back to focus on your breathing and how that feels.
- Extend this exercise beyond breathing by focusing your undivided attention on other things you are doing or thinking.

Connecting with practice: Smiling Mind

SUMMARY

- Self-awareness is about knowing who you are and what makes you tick – the things that influence, motivate, inspire and challenge you. It involves recognising your values, beliefs, thoughts and emotions, and the way you react to different situations or experiences. It also helps you to identify and understand the internal resources you have for managing or regulating these things in both personal and professional contexts.
- Greater self-awareness creates a clearer lens through which to see other people as distinct individuals, and to better understand their particular perspectives, emotions and behaviours, without judgement. This awareness of self and others is a key requisite for self-management, self-improvement and self-care, and for the development of a person-centred orientation that recognises and respects diversity, and enables culturally safe care based on empathy, compassion and empowerment.
- Social and emotional intelligence involves the ability to perceive and understand our own and others' emotions, to use this information to guide thinking and behaviour, and to act wisely in our personal, therapeutic and professional relationships. These concepts are closely aligned with self-awareness, self-management and self-improvement, and support our ability to think and act like nurses, to care for ourselves, and to feel and express empathy and compassion for others.
- Mindfulness is about intentionally paying attention to the here and now. It involves being aware, awake and fully engaged in the current moment, and bringing an attitude of curiosity and acceptance to each experience, rather than habitual patterns of judgement and criticism. Research has shown that mindfulness practice can enhance wellbeing; improve self-awareness, empathy and compassion; and help to build

personal resilience and coping skills. A range of resources is now readily available to assist people to develop and apply mindfulness skills for improved learning, practice and self-care.

- Throughout this book, we have encouraged you to reflect critically on your experiences – to think about what has worked well and not so well, what you have learned from positive and negative outcomes, and how to embed these insights into your future actions and practice. This chapter has emphasised critical reflection as a valuable strategy for developing your social and emotional intelligence, and has suggested the use of a personal journal (or professional portfolio, as a record or description of your experiences and as a prompt for deeper reflection on the issues, patterns or triggers revealed and the ways in which such insights can inform improvements to your future practice.

REVIEW QUESTIONS

Suggested responses

1 How does awareness of self and others contribute to your personal and professional development?
2 What differentiates sympathy, empathy and compassion?
3 What might the five core emotional intelligence abilities or competencies referred to in this chapter actually look like or involve in your own practice? How might you achieve or enact these things?
4 What are some of the benefits for people who regularly practise mindfulness or related relaxation techniques?
5 How can reflective practice and keeping a journal or professional portfolio support lifelong learning, practice development or improvement, and our own self-care?

RESEARCH TOPIC

Evidence from research has shown that almost one in five nurses leave their position (or the profession altogether) in their early years of practice (e.g. Kovner et al. 2014; Kinman & Leggetter 2016). Investigate the importance and benefits of 'emotional self-care' in nursing practice and identify some achievable self-care strategies that you could add to your own professional 'toolkit'.

FURTHER READING

Bulmer Smith, K., Profetto-McGrath, J. & Cummings, G. (2009). Emotional intelligence and nursing: An integrative literature review. *International Journal of Nursing Studies*, 46(12), 1624–36.

Craig, H. (2020). The theories of emotional intelligence explained. Positive Psychology Program. Available from https://positivepsychologyprogram.com/emotional-intelligence-theories.

Stein-Parbury, J. (2017). Interpersonal communication skills. In J. Bloomfield et al. (eds) *Clinical nursing skills: An Australian perspective*. Melbourne: Cambridge University Press.

——— (2018). Nurse as a therapeutic agent. In *Patient and person: Interpersonal skills in nursing*. Sydney: Elsevier.

Check out the vast array of relevant articles and resources from the Greater Good Science Centre at the University of California, Berkeley. Available from https://greatergood.berkeley.edu.

REFERENCES

Adams, K.L. & Iseler, J.I. (2014). The relationship of bedside nurses' emotional intelligence with quality of care. *Journal of Nursing Care Quality*, 29(2), 174–81.

Arghode, V. (2013). Emotional and social intelligence competence: Implications for instruction. *International Journal of Pedagogies and Learning*, 8(2), 66–77.

Australian Government (2015). *Aboriginal and Torres Strait Islander Cultural Capability Framework*. Retrieved from https://www.apsc.gov.au/sites/default/files/aboriginal-and-torres-strait-islander-cultural-capability-framework.pdf.

Australian HR Institute (2020). *Diversity and Inclusion*. Retrieved from https://www.ahri.com.au/resources/ahriassist/diversity-and-inclusion.

Bedson, P. (2016). The heart of mindfulness: Developing courage and self-compassion. *The Hive*, 16, 10–11.

Bin-Sallik, M. (2003). Cultural safety: Let's name it! *The Australian Journal of Indigenous Education*, 32, 21–8.

Bradberry, T. & Greaves, J. (2009). *Emotional intelligence 2.0*. San Diego, CA: TalentSmart.

Bulmer Smith, K., Profetto-McGrath, J. & Cummings, G. (2009). Emotional intelligence and nursing: An integrative literature review. *International Journal of Nursing Studies*, 46(12), 1624–36.

Cherry, K. (2018). 5 Components of emotional intelligence. *Very Well Mind*. Retrieved from https://www.verywellmind.com/components-of-emotional-intelligence-2795438.

Craig, H. (2020). The theories of emotional intelligence explained. Positive Psychology Program. Retrieved from https://positivepsychologyprogram.com/emotional-intelligence-theories.

Deutschendorf, H. (2018). *The other kind of smart: Simple ways to boost your emotional intelligence for greater personal effectiveness and success*. Nashville: Harper Collins Focus.

Dostoevsky, F. (1962). *The letters of Fyordor Michailovitch Dostoevsky*. New York: Horizon Press.

Drayton, N. & Weston, K.M. (2015). Exploring values in nursing: Generating new perspectives on clinical practice. *Australian Journal of Advanced Nursing*, 33(1), 14–22.

Emmerling, R.J. & Boyatzis, R.E. (2012). Emotional and social intelligence competencies: Cross-cultural implications. *Cross Cultural Management: An International Journal*, 19(1), 4–18.

Faguy, K. (2012). Emotional intelligence in health care. *Radiologic Technology*, 83(3), 237–53.

Foster, K., Fethney, J., McKenzie, H., Fisher, M., Harkness, E. & Kozlowski, D. (2017). Emotional Intelligence increases over time: A longitudinal study of Australian pre-registration nursing students. *Nurse Education Today*, 55, 65–70.

Foster, K., McCloughen, A., Delgado, C., Kefalas, C. & Harkness, E. (2015). Emotional intelligence in pre-registration nursing programmes: An integrative review. *Nurse Education Today*, 35(3), 510–17.

Goleman, D. (1998). *Working with emotional intelligence*. New York: Bantam Books.

——— (2011). *Social intelligence: The new science of human relationships*. New York: Random House.

Goleman, D., Boyatzis, R.E. & McKee, A. (2013). *Primal leadership: Unleashing the power of emotional intelligence*. Cambridge, MA: Harvard Business Press.

Harrison, P.A. & Fopma-Loy, J.L. (2010). Reflective journal prompts: A vehicle for stimulating emotional competence in nursing. *Journal of Nursing Education*, 49(11), 644–52.

Hassed, C., de Lisle, S., Sullivan, G. & Pier, C. (2009). Enhancing the health of medical students: Outcomes of an integrated mindfulness and lifestyle program. *Advances in Health Sciences Education*, 14(3), 387–98.

Hulatt, I. (2015). Mindfulness for practice nursing: Fad, fantasy or the future? *Practice Nursing*, 26(8), 408.

Kelly, L., Runge, J. & Spencer, C. (2015). Predictors of compassion fatigue and compassion satisfaction in acute care nurses. *Journal of Nursing Scholarship*, 47(6), 522–8.

Keng, S., Smoski, M.J. & Robins, C.J. (2011). Effects of mindfulness on psychological health: A review of empirical studies. *Clinical Psychology Review*, 31(6), 1041–56.

Kickett, G. (2020). What is cultural safety? (Blog post, 3 August). Australian Childhood Foundation, Centre for Excellence in Therapeutic Care. Retrieved from https://cetc.org.au/blog/what-is-cultural-safety/

Kinman, G. & Leggetter, S. (2016). Emotional labour and wellbeing: What protects nurses? *Healthcare*, 4(4), 39.

Kornhaber, R., Walsh, K., Duff, J. & Walker, K. (2016). Enhancing adult therapeutic interpersonal relationships in the acute health care setting: An integrative review. *Journal of Multidisciplinary Healthcare*, 9, 537–46.

Kovner, C., Brewer, C., Fatehi, F. & Jun, J. (2014). What does nurse turnover rate mean and what is the rate? *Policy, Politics, and Nursing Practice*, 15(3–4), 64–71.

Krasner, M.S., Epstein, R.M., Beckman, H., Suchman, A.L., Chapman, B., Mooney, C.J. & Quill, T.E. (2009). Association of an educational program in mindful communication with burnout, empathy, and attitudes among primary care physicians. *JAMA*, 302(12), 1284–93.

Littlejohn, P. (2012). The missing link: Using emotional intelligence to reduce workplace stress and workplace violence in our nursing and other health care professions. *Journal of Professional Nursing*, 28(6), 360–8.

Mayer, J.D., Caruso, D.R. & Salovey, P. (2016). The ability model of EI: Principles and updates. *Emotion Review*, 8, 290–300.

Mayer, J.D., Salovey, P. & Caruso, D.R. (2008). Emotional intelligence: New ability or eclectic traits? *American Psychologist*, 63(6), 503–17.

McCormack, B. & McCance, T. (2016). *Person-centred practice in nursing and healthcare*. Oxford: Wiley-Blackwell.

McSherry, W., Bloomfield, S., Thompson, R., Nixon, V.A, Birch, C., Griffiths, N., Fisher, S. & Boughey, A.J. (2017). A cross-sectional analysis of the factors that shape adult nursing students' values, attitudes and perceptions of compassionate care. *Journal of Research in Nursing*, 22(1–2), 25–39.

Moore, S. (2017). Influence of personal values on nursing home staff's attitudes to care. *Nursing Times*, 113(8), 37–40.

New Zealand Government (2020). *Personal beliefs, values, attitudes and behaviour*. Ministry of Business, Innovation & Employment, Immigration Advisers Authority. Retrieved from https://www.iaa.govt.nz/for-advisers/adviser-tools/ethics-toolkit/personal-beliefs-values-attitudes-and-behaviour.

Newman, K.M. (2016). Can mindfulness help you to be more authentic? (Blog post, 31 October). Greater Good Science Centre. Retrieved from https://greatergood.berkeley.edu/article/item/can_mindfulness_help_you_be_more_authentic.

Nursing and Midwifery Board of Australia (NMBA) (2016). *Registered Nurse Standards for Practice*. Retrieved from http://www.nursingmidwiferyboard.gov.au/Codes-Guidelines-Statements/Professional-standards/registered-nurse-standards-for-practice.aspx.

Oxford Dictionary (2020). Culture. Retrieved from https://www.oxfordlearnersdictionaries.com/definition/english/culture_1.

Ponte, P.R. & Koppel, P. (2015). Cultivating mindfulness to enhance nursing practice. *American Journal of Nursing*, 115(6), 48–55.

Raghubir, A.E. (2018). Emotional Intelligence in professional nursing practice: A concept review using Rodgers's evolutionary analysis approach. *International Journal of Nursing Sciences*, 5(2), 126–30.

Robertson-Malt, S., Norton-Westwood, D. & Pearson, A. (2017). Patient assessment. In J. Bloomfield et al. (eds), *Clinical nursing skills: An Australian perspective*. Melbourne: Cambridge University Press.

Ruiz-Aranda, D., Extremera, N. & Pineda-Galan, C. (2014). Emotional intelligence, life satisfaction and subjective happiness in female student health professionals: The mediating effect of perceived stress. *Journal of Psychiatric and Mental Health Nursing*, 21(2), 106–13.

Schwind, J.K., McKay, E., Beanlands, H., Schindel Martin, L., Martin, J. & Binder, M. (2017). Mindfulness practice as a teaching-learning strategy in higher education: A qualitative exploratory pilot study. *Nurse Education Today*, 50, 92–6.

Shanta, L. & Gargiulo, L. (2014). A study of the influence of nursing education on the development of emotional intelligence. *Journal of Professional Nursing*, 30(6), 511–30.

Silvia, P.J. & Phillips, A.G. (2013). Self-awareness without awareness? Implicit self-focused attention and behavioral self-regulation. *Self and Identity*, 12(2), 114–27.

Snowden, A., Stenhouse, R., Young, J., Carver, H., Carver, F. & Brown, N. (2015). The relationship between emotional intelligence, previous caring experience and mindfulness in student nurses and midwives: A cross-sectional analysis. *Nurse Education Today*, 35(1), 152–8.

Stein-Parbury, J. (2017). Interpersonal communication skills. In J. Bloomfield et al. (eds), *Clinical nursing skills: An Australian perspective*. Melbourne: Cambridge University Press.

—— (2018). *Patient and person: Interpersonal skills in nursing*, 6th edn. Sydney: Elsevier.

Steiner, P. (2014). The impact of the self-awareness process on learning and leading (Blog post, 19 August), New England Board of Higher Education. Retrieved from http://www.nebhe.org/thejournal/the-impact-of-the-self-awareness-process-on-learning-and-leading.

Tjan, A.K. (2015). 5 ways to become more self-aware (Blog post, 11 February). Retrieved from https://hbr.org/2015/02/5-ways-to-become-more-self-aware.

UNESCO (2001). *Universal Declaration on Cultural Diversity*. Retrieved from http://portal.unesco.org/en/ev.php-URL_ID=13179&URL_DO=DO_TOPIC&URL_SECTION=201.html.

van der Riet, P., Rossiter, R., Kirby, D., Dluzewska, T. & Harmon, C. (2015). Piloting a stress management and mindfulness program for undergraduate nursing students: Student feedback and lessons learned. *Nurse Education Today*, 35(1), 44–9.

Williams, R. (1999). Cultural safety – what does it mean for our work practice? *Australian and New Zealand Journal of Public Health*, 23(2), 213–14.

Wilson, A. & Wilson, M. (2011). What I wish I knew about nursing. Retrieved from http://whatiwishiknew.com/nursing/.

11 Foundations of nursing practice

Rhian Cramer, Nicole Coombs, Judith Lyons and Jeong-ah Kim

LEARNING OBJECTIVES

At the completion of this chapter, you should be able to:

1. Discuss the concepts of quality and safety in nursing practice in relation to evidence-based practice and person-centred care.
2. Demonstrate an understanding of the key concepts underpinning evidence-based practice in nursing.
3. Recognise the importance of person-centred practice to contemporary nursing.
4. Develop a foundation of effective therapeutic and interpersonal communication capabilities as a basis for professional nursing practice.

Introduction

Becoming a nurse is more than just being able to demonstrate clinical skills or understand disease processes. It is about critical thinking – understanding *why* we do what we do and *how* to do it in ways that optimise quality and safety. Achieving the best outcomes for clients is always paramount. This chapter explores the foundational principles of contemporary nursing practice: evidence-based practice, person-centred care, and therapeutic and professional communication; all contribute to a safe practice environment. It also introduces the growing role of technology in health care and looks at how numerous factors come together to influence health outcomes for the individual client.

Quality and safety in nursing practice

The World Health Organization (WHO 2017, p. 1) defined client safety as a 'fundamental principle of health care'. As a nurse, your top priority is the **safety** of those in your care and the provision of high-quality nursing care. Nurses are at the core of **quality** health care, as they are usually the primary caregivers and spend the most time working directly with clients in healthcare settings. This makes nurses the best-placed health professionals to significantly influence the quality of care provided in healthcare settings.

safety protection from, or unlikely to cause, danger, risk or injury

quality a standard of excellence, compared or measured against a similar product, service or experience

Technology has enabled advancements in medical treatments available to consumers of health care but it has also placed safety and quality at the forefront of health care, in terms of protecting clients and staff alike. Workplace health and safety (WHS) procedures recommend and describe the safest way to complete our work as nurses, often incorporating these technologies. The guiding principle is always to protect yourself first, no matter what else is happening for clients. If we do not ensure our own safety, we cannot be useful to anyone. Easily identifiable examples are removing traditional manual-handling techniques, and using mechanical beds and lifting machines to mobilise and position clients. Safety needles have also been designed to prevent needle-stick injuries to healthcare practitioners.

Eliminating human error is an important focus of contemporary health care, as errors can be harmful and costly to clients as well as the health service overall. Safety has become the main focus of contemporary health technology development and underpins the implementation of new innovations. Medication errors, for example, have been significantly reduced by the introduction of automated medication dispensers (Kang, Jin, Jin & Lee 2018). After a medication is prescribed by the medical practitioner, the nurse can only access and administer the medication once the automated dispensary has recognised all the required client identifiers and checked that the order is correct against the accepted safety standards (Risor, Lisby & Sorensen 2017), thereby significantly reducing medication errors.

While the prevention of adverse outcomes remains important, the reality of the nurse's role in providing safe and quality care is far greater and is growing in complexity as the health system evolves and changes. The evidence clearly shows that the major factor in improvement is understanding and accounting for the complexity of healthcare organisations and systems, care processes and client needs. The foundation of quality and safety improvement initiatives needs to be centred on systemic factors, not on individual factors (Sherwood & Barnsteiner 2017). Individual practitioners still play an important role but we must be creative and innovative in our approach.

While healthcare settings are constantly evolving to best suit the needs of the community, and technology is getting 'smarter', the underlying principles and concepts in our nursing practice remain the same. Being able to accept and adapt to change is a key factor in ensuring our practice is current, efficient and equitable for all who need it. No matter what technologies or resources are available in your health setting, the way to achieve the best possible outcomes for your clients is to adhere to the principles of *evidence-based practice* and *person-centred care*, using the best possible research evidence and resources available, and the client's values, preferences and individual circumstances to inform your comprehensive, quality nursing care plans.

Advances in nursing practice and technology are intended to improve healthcare and client outcomes, but we cannot ignore the legal and ethical considerations they raise. Client privacy and the confidentiality of health information are of particular interest and can be controversial, as there is potential for access by multiple health practitioners in diverse roles and settings (Kluge 2017; Moss et al. 2017). A common fear that concerns clients and health practitioners alike is unauthorised access to electronic medical records and private data, whether through human error or cyber-attack. Another concern is that digital systems can fail, resulting in loss of access or restricton of vital health information when it is needed most. New technologies in health care are likely to continue to increase and evolve rapidly, so it is vital that nurses understand their role, their legal and ethical responsibilities and how to safely adapt their practice and professional conduct to the changing healthcare environment.

Evidence-based practice

Evidence-based practice (EBP) involves making clinical decisions based on consideration of the most reliable evidence and current quality research; the nurse's clinical experience; the context of the healthcare setting; and the client's experience and preferences (Kim, Mallory & Valerio 2020). EBP must also consider the context of the healthcare setting and the policies and procedures of the organisation or healthcare provider. While it sounds simple, EBP can be a difficult balancing act, having to juggle influencing factors on all sides. The principles of EBP are very strongly related to person-centred practice (Ellis 2019), and the two often work in unison to consider the client's reality and healthcare preferences in light of the body of evidence available. Figure 11.1 illustrates the complexity of these influencing factors on the nurse's clinical decision-making.

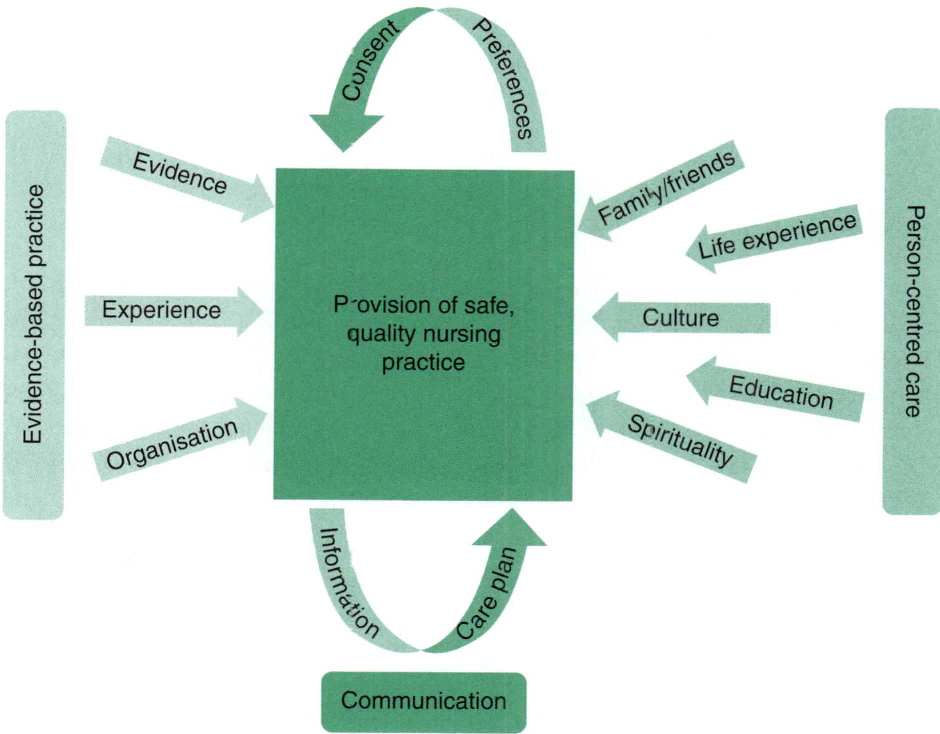

Figure 11.1 Evidence-based practice

REFLECTION 11.1

Every person, regardless of who they are, has their own unique view of the world. They have beliefs and values shaped by their experiences that help form an individual identity and help to interpret the world around them. While it is an unavoidable part of the human experience, as nurses these values and beliefs we hold may interfere with the way we communicate and engage with the people in our care. This may include unconscious or subconscious biases, or personal views on matters that relate to health care.

Reflection is an incredibly valuable tool in your development as a nurse; it is a good way to figure out where your unconscious or subconscious biases or values may be in conflict with that of your clients. By reflecting in a very deliberate and systematic way, you can identify any personal biases or potential challenges to open communication and collaborative care. Once identified, you can examine these in a conscious way and figure out how to separate your personal opinions or values from that of your professional nursing responsibilities.

Consider your thoughts and feelings on the following scenarios. What can you do to ensure your personal values do not affect the nursing care you provide to the following clients?

- A man declines a life-saving blood transfusion as this treatment is not acceptable for their spiritual wellbeing, since it goes against their religious teachings and beliefs.

> - A pregnant woman drinks alcohol throughout her pregnancy, despite the potential effects on the health of her baby.
> - Parents elect not to vaccinate their children.
> - A teenage boy is transferred from a correctional facility for care after an assault.

In the past, nurses were educated in an apprenticeship-style training program, provided within the hospital setting (Department of Health 2013). They were taught both knowledge and skills by the senior nurses on the wards, and they learned how the hospital operated by experiencing it first-hand. This style of education is no longer considered useful or appropriate, as it resulted in nursing practices being taught that were not always safe and effective; rather it reflects the adage of 'that's the way it has always been done'. An example of this is the practice of attending to all hygiene activities like assisting with showers first thing in the morning. There is no evidence that this is preferable for every client or that it makes a difference to client wellbeing, and it is certainly not consistent with person-centred care, but despite this the practice is still common in many healthcare settings today.

Contemporary nursing education takes place in partnership between universities and healthcare providers. The students are educated at university on the most up-to-date skills and develop a solid foundation of knowledge before entering clinical placements, where they consolidate and apply their knowledge and develop their skills in a diverse range of healthcare settings. Students are taught to underpin every nursing decision and action with the principles of evidence-based and person-centred practice, to ensure optimal health outcomes for their clients (Australian Nursing and Midwifery Accreditation Council 2019).

Types of research evidence

The first rule of evidence is that not all sources are created equal. There are dozens of ways we can find out information on a given topic, and each has its place in the puzzle of EBP. Your role is to ask yourself 'What do I need to know?' and 'Why?' It seems simple, but it is important to ascertain the answers to these two questions, to guide you to the right source for your purpose.

Textbooks are fantastic in helping to establish foundation-level understanding of a subject. They can give definitions and explanations on key components – for example, the anatomy and physiology of a health condition. However, they are not always suitable in informing the nurse (or student) about current population data or research outcomes, as they are a snapshot of the time when they were produced.

With immediate access to the internet, more and more clients are getting information, or even self-diagnosing and treating their medical conditions, using online search engines such as Google and Bing. As not everything on the internet is truthful or regulated, misinformation is common, and this can have a significant effect on a person's health or understanding of their condition. We discuss the internet as a source of information because we need to know what clients are accessing online and to be able to guide them to more reputable and reliable sources.

Websites can be a very useful tool if we use them to engage clients in their own health care. There is a simple rule when considering a website: look at the end of the main web address. Websites ending in .gov (government website), .org (not-for-profit organisation) or .edu (educational institution) are almost always preferable to a .com (commercial or personal website). Ask yourself: 'Why is this being published? What's in it for the publisher/s?' (Ellis 2019). If the answer may be financial gain, it is often best to seek an alternative source of information to confirm or dispute the recommendations of a person or organisation with purely financial motivations.

Most evidence from nursing and health research is published in articles and reports, which can be accessed from libraries, specialist search engines and databases. They are usually the most up-to-date sources, with new articles being published daily, and provide data on the safety and efficacy of care and treatment options as well as giving us insights into the experience of health conditions, treatment and care options. Research can seem a little daunting at first. There is so much jargon and unfamiliar terminology that it can be quite intimidating. But it does not have to be: there are a few basic principles to help you wade through the literature and find relevant, applicable and reliable evidence to use in your assessments and to guide your practice decisions. More importantly, these same basic steps will help to ensure you remain informed and able to maintain high standards of EBP throughout your career, not just as a student.

In general, you want to find the most recent evidence available, which has looked at the largest population of participants in the most rigorous way possible. Figure 11.2 shows the hierarchy of evidence (the pyramid on the left) compared to the population or number of participants involved (the inverted pyramid on the right). This is applicable to both qualitative and quantitative research, though broadly speaking, quantitative research projects will generally have far larger numbers of participants than qualitative research projects.

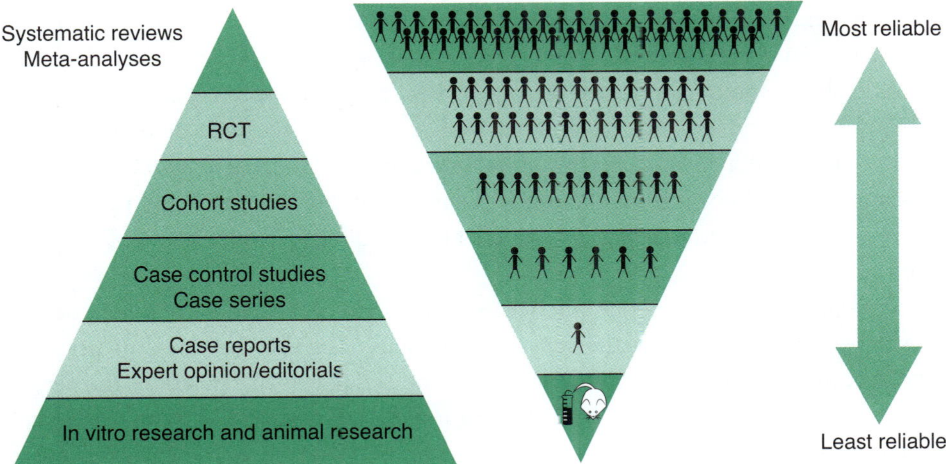

Figure 11.2   Levels of evidence

With all sources of information, it is good to consider how recent the information is and whether it is still relevant to contemporary practice (Ellis 2019). Healthcare research is published daily and information can become out of date quickly (Kim, Mallory & Valerio 2020). Be sure to maintain your skills in seeking out reliable, contemporary evidence to inform your practice, beyond your studies and into your career in nursing. Evidence-based practice underpins many of the Registered Nurses Standards for Practice (Nursing and Midwifery Board of Australia 2016), which you need to meet in order to achieve and maintain your registration as a nurse in Australia. The best way to develop these skills is to attend a session with your university librarian, who has expertise to help you find the most recent evidence available (SCONUL Working Group on Information Literacy 2011). They can teach you how to best define and refine your topic into key words; navigate the databases most relevant to the discipline; and access EBP repositories, reliable websites and other resources.

Multiple-choice questions
Short-answer questions
Connecting with practice:
NMBA Standards

Person-centred practice

What does person-centred practice (PCP) mean? Although the term sounds logical, putting the person at the centre of our nursing care is not necessarily a natural trait for many nurses. In addition, our health system sometimes fails to accommodate for it. There is no 'one size fits all' approach to client care. Practice must be unique for every individual client, must protect the client's dignity, rights and preferences, and must ensure therapeutic relationships are based on trust and mutual understanding (Australian College of Nursing 2019).

Remember that a client is not just a client: they are first and foremost a person. They have different backgrounds, family, culture, values, beliefs, education and social circumstances that make them all unique. Nurses care for people when they experience some kind of self-care deficit – be it physical or emotional. It may only be for a few hours or days, or it could be for the remainder of the person's life. When accepting the role of carer, nurses are entering *their* world. It is important to be mindful that the majority of clients previously existed as functioning individuals without nurses, who were able to function in society, look after themselves and possibly others, make decisions and communicate their needs and wants. Why, then, is this less important when a person becomes ill?

PCP places the *person* at the centre of healthcare provision. Care is provided holistically and individually, enabling choices in the care received or required, and facilitating maintenance of personal responsibilities, if capable (McCormack & McCance 2017). Recognising and appreciating the importance of enabling self-care where possible and advocating for our clients are fulfilling components of a nurse's role.

Changing perceptions of our practice from 'What do I need to do?' to 'What does the person want or need?' places the *person* as the focus of care, rather than the practices involving medical interventions, treatments, time and place. This positions the person at the centre of the process of care (see Figure 11.3). Using a PCP framework, such as that developed by McCormack and McCance (2017), ensures the client is kept at the centre of the care being provided. This includes ensuring adequate prerequisites for PCP (professional competence, values and commitment), having an environment that enables PCP care (appropriate staff mix, shared decision-making, innovation), person-centred processes (working with client values, client engagement) and PCP outcomes (satisfaction with care, involvement, therapeutic culture).

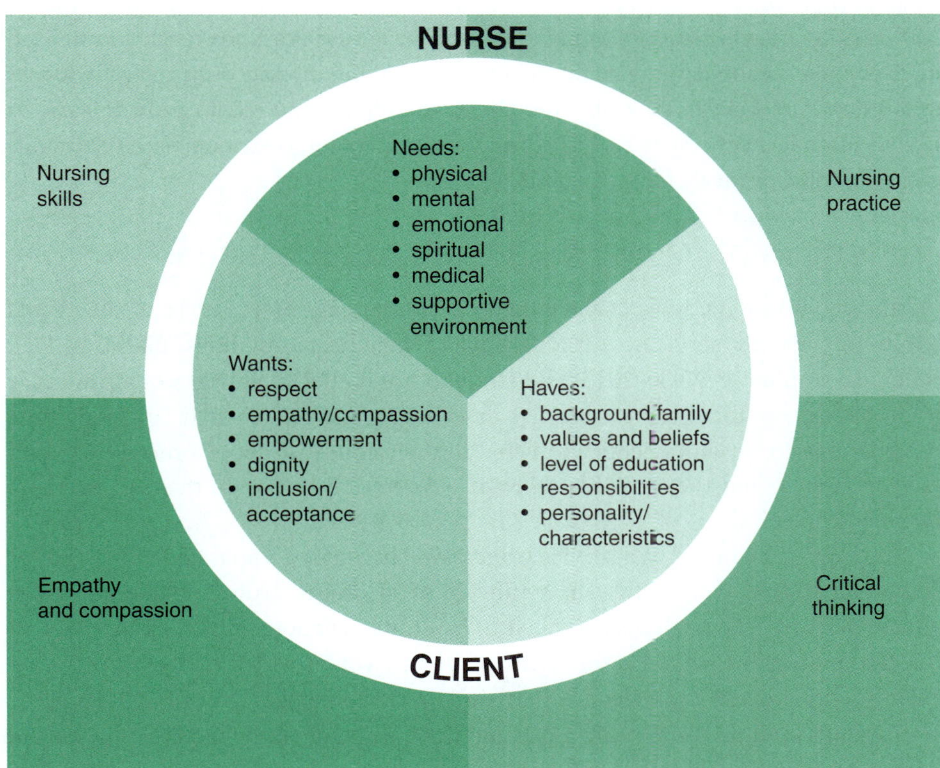

Figure 11.3   Person-centred practice

Benefits of person-centred practice

PCP does not mean surrendering responsibility or forsaking the knowledge, experience and expertise of the healthcare staff. Instead, PCP offers clients opportunities and accountability for their health choices. By providing appropriate information and facilitating discussions of care options, it enables clients to make informed decisions and to invite the nurse into their world.

Feeling respected and valued as a capable individual is very empowering for clients. Engaging with their care will ensure accountability for their own health, and clients may be more accepting of the care and health education provided. This collaborative approach enables nurses to communicate more appropriately and to support health independence by providing education that is specific to individual linguistic or learning needs (Coombs, Porter & Beauchamp 2016). This leads to appropriate, targeted care being provided, enabling clients to return to their normal lives as quickly as possible. They are seen as people, not just clients, so maintaining their dignity, sense of self and normal routines and activities should occur despite any nursing assistance that may be required. Judgement about the quality of nursing practice clients receive is usually made by the empowerment and respect that is offered through PCP (Edvardsson, Watt & Pearce 2016).

PCP can be just as **empowering** and rewarding for nurses as it can be for clients. Nurses facilitate and use their knowledge, skills and expertise to empower clients wherever possible, providing care in partnership with them, rather than just doing things *to* them or following a process. Providing PCP is not a new skill; rather, it takes a different approach, critically thinking about how we use our knowledge and skills in order to meet healthcare needs for clients while taking into account the individual's preferences and beliefs. PCP also influences the effort required to provide care, as there is often less resistance to, or fear or confusion about, treatment when decisions are made collaboratively (Clay & Parsh 2016).

Challenges of using person-centred practice

Logistically, it is sometimes challenging to accommodate every desire of the clients within our health services. Although many healthcare facilities mandate PCP (Richards, Coulter & Wicks 2015) and strive to use it effectively, it is not always easy in structured, multifaceted facilities. Nurses often struggle to find sufficient time in a busy day to sit with clients and listen to their concerns about procedures, tests and treatments, and then provide relevant information to enable them to make an informed choice.

Nursing is recognised as a service profession, driven by compassion and empathy. To be empathetic, we must 'walk in the shoes of others', truly understanding the person's feelings, expectations and needs (Cambridge Dictionary 2020). Once you do this, thus putting the person at the centre of the care you provide, you will discover the real joy of nursing – being welcomed into the world of our clients, forming therapeutic relationships built on respect and trust, and finding you are met with compliance and acceptance, which enables the most appropriate care to be provided for that individual. That is quality nursing.

NURSING PERSPECTIVE

We learned about PCP in class but it seemed a bit 'airy-fairy' to me. Of course, the client should influence their care – that is only right. So why spend time talking about it? It did not sink in for me until I went out on clinical placement and met Garry. Garry was a man in his mid-fifties who had decided to cease cancer treatment. I was shocked: this man was still young and had lots to live for. His first grandchild was only four months old. How could he give up now? After a few days of struggling with my own feelings, I heard Garry's full story. He was a tradie, having spent every day on work sites, and playing footy, camping and water skiing whenever he could. All of that stopped with the diagnosis. He felt he would lose his identity becaue he was unable to do all the things he loved – even to hold his grandchild. He knew his time was limited, regardless of the treatment, and he wanted to spend whatever time he had left at home, without the dreadful side-effects from the medication. Hearing that, I felt the full weight of my judgement hitting me. This man's reality was not what

I had thought, and I felt terrible to have thought of him as a quitter. He was in pain, suffering more from the treatments than the disease itself. Garry knew within himself that life would be better if he stopped the fight and embraced the time he had left in a positive way. Through this experience, I learned the power of supporting the client's autonomy. Knowing that you are supporting the person in the life they wish to lead and the decisions they wish to make, and respecting their values and beliefs, is just as powerful for providing quality health care as being able to clinically perform the administration of chemotherapy.

Video: PCP

Communication and interpersonal skills

Communication skills provide a powerful therapeutic tool to help build trust in a helping relationship. The ability to communicate effectively with others is a graduate attribute that is crucial in health professionals. In nursing, effective communication is needed to deliver safe, quality nursing care. It facilitates person-centred, EBP, reduces risk and harm to clients, improves clinical outcomes and enhances reflective practice (NMBA 2016).

What is communication?

Communication is the process of imparting or exchanging information by verbal, non-verbal, written or digital means (Arnold & Boggs 2020). The aim is to share information effectively and efficiently, using verbal, non-verbal and writing skills, and this is vital no matter what health setting you work in. As it is such an important skill, communication is embedded in the professional frameworks of nursing: National Safety and Quality Health Service Standards (Australian Commission on Safety and Quality in Health Care 2017), Aged Care Quality Standards (Aged Care Quality and Safety Commission 2019) and Registered Nurse Standards for Practice (NMBA 2016).

Each interaction in nursing involves communication, be it interprofessional, interpersonal or therapeutic communication. Effective communication includes being able to interact with colleagues, clients, family members and the public. Your communication strategies should focus on who you are communicating with, and be influenced by their age, ability to understand, literacy level, culture and language.

Therapeutic communication is the use of all elements of person-centred communication – verbal, non-verbal and active listening – to share information for the purposes of health improvement. Effective therapeutic communication can have a positive effect on client outcomes by improving education, empowering client involvement and control of their own health care, and ultimately increasing client satisfaction (Abdolrahimi et al. 2017).

The power of communication in nursing practice cannot be overstated, with clients identifying this as the key measure of quality nursing care (O'Toole 2016). Consider the effect of communicating with a client prior to, during and after procedures. By talking to the client and explaining what you are about to do, why you are doing it and what to expect, the client can prepare themselves for what is to come. Continuing this

therapeutic communication
a helping relationship process using verbal or non-verbal communication skills, whereby the nurse consciously influences or helps the client by promoting physical, mental and emotional wellbeing for improved health outcomes

open communication as you complete the procedure and at its conclusion enables clients to connect with you, trust in your competence and understand each step of the procedure. This improves coping mechanisms, reduces anxiety and increases adherence with treatments (Lavender 2017).

Person-centred communication is **interpersonal communication** that focuses on the unique person and is embedded in being genuine, empathetic and accepting of the individual (Arnold & Boggs 2020). Being genuine means that you are yourself, dropping all pretence of being what you think others want you to be. Acceptance means having unqualified, unconditional positive regard for others. To get the most out of your person-centred communication, you need to actively listen, allow time to speak and be heard, then respond with compassion.

Interpersonal communication skills are fundamental in the everyday interactions that occur in nursing practice. You will need to work hard to develop these throughout your nursing education, to ensure you can meet your responsibilities once you graduate and become a registered nurse. To develop effective interpersonal communication skills, nurses need to identify and acknowledge personal beliefs and values, prejudices and attitudes that can influence their thoughts and actions, and potentially are revealed in both verbal or written responses. Reflective practice promotes a self-awareness that helps you to identify gaps in communication and recognise your own learning needs to improve practice.

Person-centred communication theories and strategies can also be applied to communication between health professionals, which is the foundation for developing a rapport and relationship of trust and collegiality within the healthcare team. Sharing information with each other is how we learn, and learning from different professional perspectives makes our caregiving more complete. **Interprofessional communication** provides opportunity for growth in knowledge and skills, where we share different information that contributes to a joint cause. For example, a nurse might learn from a physiotherapist how to fit crutches to a client, then take these new skills into their own practice. **Intraprofessional communication** is the information we might share among our nursing colleagues to ensure continuity of care, such as client handover. Without these different methods of communication, it would be impossible to provide safe, holistic, person-centred care. Developing a good working relationship with the entire healthcare team also increases your sense of enjoyment and job satisfaction.

Strategies for effective communication

Communication strategies are blueprints for how information can be transmitted and exchanged. A variety of elements come into play and can influence the ability of the client or colleague to receive the information. These elements can vary from the volume, tone or even the amount of information provided, to the structure or order in which the information is delivered. Remembering that communication is a two-way process, be mindful of the manner in which you express confidence, empathy and respect to the client or colleague, but also be open-minded, patient and attentive to demonstrate that the information is being received and understood. Be aware of emotions and how they may influence misunderstandings. Ensure you take time to confirm your understanding and be prepared to receive or give constructive feedback. Simply presenting a friendly and respectful manner when establishing a therapeutic relationship can help to ensure engaging and encouraging communication can occur.

Within Australian hospitals, the AIDET mnemonic is frequently used to guide communication between nurses and clients. Devised by the Studer Group (2021), the AIDET framework is a step-by-step guide intended to ensure that appropriate interactions and effective communication with clients occur by adhering to the following five principles:

A *Acknowledge* – by acknowledging the client by name, be attentive and demonstrate a warm and friendly manner.
I *Introduce* yourself – by giving the client your name and position, state the purpose of the encounter and orient the client to the surroundings.
D *Duration* – establish the timing by stating how long you will be with them and address times relevant to the care process.
E *Explanation* – by educating the client, justifying your actions and ensuring that the client understands your explanation.
T *Thank* – appreciate the client by closing off the interaction.

ISBAR is another framework that is commonly used in the nursing and healthcare environment (Aldrich et al. 2009). This framework is used to facilitate communication between health professionals. ISBAR stands for:

I *Identify* – let the other person know who you are and who, or what, you need to talk about.
S *Situation* – relate the event and explain why another clinician has been contacted.
B *Background* – provide a history of what has happened and what actions were taken.
A *Assessment* – conduct an accurate assessment and report it in a systematic way.
R *Recommend* – suggest what actions you want from the clinician.

Verbal communication

Verbal communication involves speaking with others – whether that is the client, their family, friends or other health professionals. You need to be able to communicate clearly, articulating your message in language that can be understood by the recipient. This needs to take into account the language the client speaks as well as the complexity of the message and how you phrase the information to ensure you are understood. Depending on who you are communicating with, be aware of using jargon or medical terminology as this may make your message unclear. Diverse levels of understanding will also be conditional to age, cognition and level of education. This is known as health literacy, and should be assessed accordingly to provide adequate information in a way that is appropriate for the individual (Clouston, Manganello & Richards 2017).

While verbal communication does imply that you need to engage in speaking, it is just as important to listen. Active listening means you pay attention to what is being said as well as to how it is being conveyed; what is the context of the communication and the tone or tenor of the message being delivered? These cues can hint at the emotion behind the message and can change the entire meaning, if we are perceptive enough to identify them. One way to check is to ask clarifying questions, rephrase and repeat what you have heard to ensure the message has been interpreted correctly.

Non-verbal communication

You also need to develop skills in reading other people: their use of eye contact (or not), facial expressions, physical distancing and personal space (Lawrence, Perrin & Kiernan 2015). This will help you to interpret the real meaning behind what they are saying. This is known as non-verbal communication, or more commonly 'body language', and it is an important aspect of communication. These skills are inexact but it is essential as a nurse that you become attuned to emotions and any disharmony in communication so that you can practice safely, establish a positive rapport with the client and build trust.

Emotions have a huge influence on the way we respond to the environment around us and our ability to relate to other people. They can interfere with our ability to be open-minded, empathetic and unbiased, and to communicate effectively. The effects of emotions will not stop simply because you become a nurse. What *does* change is the ability to recognise the influence of emotions and how you train yourself to moderate these responses. This can be difficult, but you will start this work as a nursing student and develop it throughout your career. One of the best techniques is to engage in reflective practice, so that you gain insight into your own beliefs, opinions and world-views, thereby earning your unique triggers and developing the skills you need to moderate your behaviour.

Emotions also influence the ways in which others respond to us as nurses, as individuals and to their circumstances. This is especially true in health care, since being a recipient of care can cause people to feel incredibly vulnerable and exposed, making it difficult to communicate effectively. One of the most valuable tools we can have in our communication toolkit is silence. Allowing time for a client to gather their thoughts and find the right words, or to have an emotional reaction, whether internal or visible, shows respect for the individual. It acknowledges their unique experience, shows that we are present in the moment with them and makes them feel valued. It also gives us time to observe non-verbal communication as well as the environment, to ensure it is safe and appropriate for communication to occur effectively.

An important consideration in non-verbal communication is the influence of culture. There are incredibly rich, wide and diverse cultural groups within the Australian population, each with its own unique customs and accepted behaviours, which may not be consistent with your own **cultural norms** (Encyclopedia of Public Health 2019). It is crucial that you do not dismiss a person as not being engaged with you or the health service when in fact there are cultural considerations at play. For example, in many cultures – including some Aboriginal and Torres Strait Islander groups – direct eye contact is considered disrespectful and can be uncomfortable. Other groups consider physical touch between certain categories of people to be inappropriate, such as people of Japanese descent or people of the Islamic faith.

While there are accepted cultural norms in all cultures around the world, every person has a different interpretation and personal preference regarding how they wish to conduct themselves. We must never stereotype the people with whom we

cultural norm a set of behaviours, attitudes and traits considered normal to a specific group; these can be passed down from generation to generation as a guide for daily life and are often related to moral values, safety and belonging (Encyclopedia of Public Health 2019)

interact, or expect a certain style of behaviour based on their cultural background. We must use our communication skills and critical thinking to analyse each situation and modify our communication approach to best suit the individual with whom we are working.

Visual communication

As a nursing student, you are being assessed on your ability to communicate using the written word by completing essays, case studies and reports. These assessments are not just there to stress you out; they mimic the need for nurses to communicate through the written word in healthcare documentation and in articulating procedures, experiences and outcomes. In clinical practice, you will be required to write up care plans, handovers, referral letters, policies and procedures, and professional email communications. With the development of PCP and multidisciplinary care, the requirements for written communication are increasing.

Recording accurate documentation has long been a vital role of the nurse. Contemporary practices now include the use of medical information platforms for digital data collection, more commonly referred to as paperless or electronic medical records (EMR). The use of computerised record systems and documentation of personal information have developed into a specialised area of healthcare practice known as health **informatics** (Kluge 2017). These systems also often link with other platforms to access test results, share information across disciplines, report incidents and collect data and statistics. It is expected that nurses become familiar with and use these systems in all aspects of their practice, to maintain a quality healthcare system.

Digital health records are also providing a convenient way for medical records to be available to and about clients as our highly transient population moves around the country. No longer do people need to transfer paper-based records between health providers; their entire medical history is available to the authorised practitioner at the click of a button.

The geographic restrictions of Australia have long been a key factor in the provision of health care, especially beyond the boundaries of metropolitan populations. It is in this area that technological advancements have provided arguably the most significant effect on the regional and rural populations of Australia. Tele-medicine and digital health technology resources are now being used for medical consultations in metropolitan, rural and remote health services, enabling health practitioners to communicate with clients and other health professionals across different locations (Australian Institute of Health and Welfare 2020). Rapid technological advances are also being seen in national medical record management systems such as My Health Record, electronic prescriptions and discharge communications. Digital health is also evolving and growing in the consumer market, with personal health devices such as fitness and sleep trackers, and smartphone applications being used to monitor wellbeing data for improved personal health outcomes.

Despite the advances of technology in aiding communication between the client and the health system, challenges can still arise. Barriers include specific items or events that can distort or prevent effective communication, either from the nurse or the client. These might include physical, psychosocial or environmental obstacles (Birks, Chapman & Davis 2015), which may interfere with being able to determine what the client values or requires from their health care.

informatics the science of turning data into information

Tips to help you get the most from your communication

- Be clear and concise. Rambling conversation leads to confusion and uncertainty regarding the message being conveyed.
- Take time to communicate in the dynamic, fast-paced workplace. Rushed communication can result in miscommunication and misunderstandings, and these can have adverse effects on client care.
- Never underestimate the value of silence.
- Communicate openly to maintain a free flow of messages and exchange of ideas, views and engagement, to advocate for clients or improved practice. Open-minded conversations and being flexible ensure effective communication and respect for others.
- Be friendly and confident in your interaction when communicating. A friendly tone, smile and approachable manner will encourage engagement in honest and open communication. Being confident ensures that others believe in what you are saying.
- Be diligent in the use of digital technologies and their application to health communication.
- Environmental barriers may interfere with the transmission and reception of messages. Examples are temperature, distracting stimuli, equipment and background noise.
- Physical barriers, including ill-health, poor eyesight, hearing deficits and pain, are obstacles to effective communication.

Short-answer questions

CASE STUDY

Communication, person-centred care and evidence in practice

Michelle is a 36-year-old mother of two. Her husband, Ben, works for a fly in/fly out (FIFO) company as an electrician and is currently away from home. The family lives on several acres, and Michelle likes to ride horses competitively when she is able. After dropping off her two children at school today, Michelle returned home and was riding her horse when the horse stumbled in its approach to a jump and the two of them crashed through the set-up. Michelle hit her face on the poles and injured her right hand, possibly also breaking her ring finger. She has an open laceration on her right cheek that just breaks the vermilion border of her upper lip. Her hand is grazed and swollen, with an obvious disfiguration of the ring finger. She is in a lot of pain.

Having asked a neighbour to attend to her horse and drive her to the local hospital, Michelle is being attended by the doctor in the emergency department. He orders an x-ray for Michelle's hand and face and contacts the facial surgeon at another nearby hospital. Michelle is also prescribed analgesia and the nurse attends to cleaning her wounds.

QUESTIONS

1   Using PCP, what considerations do we, as nurses, need to think about while caring for Michelle?

2   What type of communication is needed while dealing with Michelle? Who else needs to be involved with the communication?

3   How can technology be used throughout this scenario? Consider the various locations: in the emergency department, outside the department or perhaps between departments.

4   What EBP is relevant to Michelle's treatment and care?

REFLECTION 11.2

One of the best ways to develop your communication skills is to consciously observe the interactions and communications that are going on around you. Pay close attention to the facial expressions, stance and overall attitude of those interacting, as these can communicate just as much information as the words being used. While observing, consider the following:

- Where are the people looking during the interaction?
- What are they doing with their arms and hands?
- How are they holding their body posture?

SUMMARY

- The provision of quality and safety in nursing practice is a critical role of the nurse. This role changes and progresses with the advancements of technology and the evolution of health care but the fundamentals remain the same: follow the principles of *evidence-based practice* and *person-centred care* to inform healthcare provision.
- EBP is the process of making clinical decisions with consideration of the most reliable evidence, the nurse's clinical experience and the context of the healthcare setting. The principles of EBP are very strongly related to PCP, and it is necessary to consider both in the provision of optimal nursing care.
- Sources of evidence are not all the same. It is important for nurses to identify, critically analyse and evaluate the quality of available evidence and then apply the best available evidence to the individual client's circumstances and the context of practice to provide safe and quality nursing care.
- PCP is the acknowledgement of the client as a person first and foremost, with a unique life experience. The client is an integral partner in the planning and implementation of their own health care, and nurses should recognise this in the provision of nursing care.

- PCP is beneficial for clients and nurses alike. The clients are more likely to feel empowered, and therefore to be comfortable with and willing to comply with the nursing care plan. Nurses are more likely to feel satisfied in their profession when they work *with* the clients, instead of simply doing interventions *to* the clients.
- Communication is a crucial skill for nurses. We, as nurses, use communication in every interaction, be it verbal, non-verbal or visual communication. Therapeutic communication facilitates growth, development and improved health outcomes. The interpersonal relationship is our interaction with other professionals, the clients, their families and the general public, to provide effective, safe, high-quality nursing care.
- Understanding and developing the two most commonly used communication frameworks and strategies, as well as knowledge and skills about barriers in communication, are key to improving your communication skills.

REVIEW QUESTIONS

Suggested responses

1 Outline the different facets of quality and safety in nursing care.
2 In evidence-based practice, why is it important to consider not only what the evidence says but how the information was obtained, who put the information together and where the information came from?
3 What are the potential benefits of employing person-centred practice?
4 What is the difference between the AIDET and ISBAR communication frameworks? Give examples of when you would use each one.
5 What types of health informatics and technologies have you seen employed in health care? What benefits do these bring to the provision of nursing care?

RESEARCH TOPIC

In addition to nurses using informatics in their practice, a recent Australian government incentive, known as e-health, is now using technology to securely connect all Australians to the healthcare system. Digital medical records allow for the sharing of medical information with different authorised practitioners, linking general practice with specialist services, electronic prescriptions and dispensing records. All are part of the e-health concept. This national program aims to provide equitable provision of service through effective and secure communication for every individual client around the country. The service holds personal information and is individually identified and linked to Medicare. Any authorised health practitioner around the country can access their medical history, test results, medication history and so on.

How are e-health and informatics affecting health outcomes for all Australians? Start your search by exploring the Australian Digital Health Agency's website at: http://www .digitalhealth.gov.au.

FURTHER READING

Birks, M., Chapman, Y.B. & Davis, J. (2015). *Professional and therapeutic communication.* Melbourne: Oxford University Press.

Caldwell, L. & Grobbel, C. (2013). The importance of reflective practice in nursing. *International Journal of Caring Sciences*, 6(3), 319–26.

Grant, A. & Goodman, B. (2019). *Communication and interpersonal skills in nursing*, 4th edn. London: Learning Matters.

Jirojwong, S., Johnson, M. & Welch, A.J. (eds) (2014). *Research methods in nursing and midwifery: Pathways to evidence-based practice*, 2nd edn. Melbourne: Oxford University Press.

Lawrence, J., Perrin, C. & Kiernan, E. (2015). *Building professional nursing communication*. Melbourne: Cambridge University Press.

McCormack, B. & McCance, T. (eds) (2017). *Person-centred practice in nursing and health care: Theory and practice*. 2nd edn. Oxford: Wiley Blackwell.

O'Toole, G. (2016). *Communication: Core interpersonal skills for health professionals*. Sydney: Elsevier.

REFERENCES

Abdolrahimi, M., Ghiyasvandian, S., Zakerimoghadam, M. & Ebadi, A. (2017). Therapeutic communication in nursing students: A Walker & Avant concept analysis. *Electronic Physician*, 9(8), 4968–77.

Aged Care Quality and Safety Commission (2019). *Guidance and resources for providers to support the Aged Care Quality Standards*. Retrieved from https://www .agedcarequality.gov.au/providers/standards.

Aldrich, R., Duggan, A., Lane, K., Nair, K. & Hill, K.N. (2009). *ISBAR revisited: Identifying and solving barriers to effective clinical handover in inter-hospital transfer: final project report*. Newcastle: Hunter New England Health. Retrieved from https://www.safetyandquality.gov.au/publications-and-resources/resource-library/ isbar-revisited-identifying-and-solving-barriers-effective-clinical-handover-project- toolkit.

Arnold, E.C. & Boggs, K.U. (2020). *Interpersonal relationships: Professional communication skills for nurses*, 8th edn. St Louis, MO: Elsevier.

Australian College of Nursing (ACN) (2019). Person-centred care (position statement, ACN, Canberra). Retrieved from; https://www.acn.edu.au/wp-content/uploads/ position-statement-person-centred-care.pdf.

Australian Commission on Safety and Quality in Health Care (ACSQHC) (2017). *National Safety and Quality Health Service Standards*, 2nd edn. Sydney: ACSQHC. Retrieved from https://www.safetyandquality.gov.au/standards/nsqhs-standards.

Australian Institute of Health and Welfare (2020). *Digital Health*. Retrieved from https://www.aihw.gov.au/reports/australias-health/digital-health.

Australian Nursing and Midwifery Accreditation Council (2019). *Registered nurse accreditation standards 2019*. Canberra: Australian Nursing and Midwifery Accreditation Council. Retrieved from https://www.anmac.org.au/sites/default/ files/documents/registerednurseaccreditationstandards2019.pdf.

Birks, M., Chapman, Y.B. & Davis, J. (2015). *Professional and therapeutic communication*. Melbourne: Oxford University Press.

Cambridge Dictionary (2020). *Empathy*. Cambridge University Press. Retrieved from https://dictionary.cambridge.org/dictionary/english/empathy.

Clay, A.M. & Parsh, B. (2016). Patient- and family-centered care: It's not just for paediatrics anymore. *AMA Journal of Ethics*, 18(1), 40–4.

Clouston, S.A., Manganello, J.A. & Richards, M. (2017). A life course approach to health literacy: The role of gender, educational attainment and lifetime cognitive capability. *Age and Ageing*, 46(3), 493–9.

Coombs, N.M., Porter, J.E. & Beauchamp, A. (2016). ED-HOME: Improving educator confidence and patient education in the emergency department. *Australasian Emergency Nursing Journal*, 19(3), 133–7.

Department of Health (2013). Appendix iv: History of Commonwealth involvement in the nursing and midwifery workforce. In Australian Government, *Review of Australian government health workforce programs*. Retrieved from https://www1 .health.gov.au/internet/publications/publishing.nsf/Content/work-review-australian- government-health-workforce-programs-toc~appendices~appendix-iv-history- commonwealth-involvement-nursing-midwifery-workforce.

Edvardsson, D., Watt, E. & Pearce, F. (2016). Patient experiences of caring and person- centredness are associated with perceived nursing care quality. *Journal of Advanced Nursing*, 73(1), 217–27.

Ellis, P. (2019). *Evidence-based practice in nursing*, 4th edn. London: Sage.

Encyclopedia of Public Health (2019). Cultural norms (entry). Retrieved from https://www.encyclopedia.com/education/encyclopedias-almanacs-transcripts- and-maps/cultural-norms.

Kang, M.-J., Jin, Y., Jin, T. & Lee, S.-M. (2018). Automated medication error risk assessment system (Auto-MERAS). *Journal of Nursing Care Quality*, 33(1), 86–93.

Kim, M.J., Mallory, C. & Valerio, T. (2020). *Statistics for evidence-based practice in nursing*, 3rd edn. Burlington, MA: Jones and Bartlett Learning.

Kluge, E.W. (2017). Health information professionals in a global e-health world: Ethical and legal arguments for the international certification and accreditation of health information professionals. *International Journal of Medical Informatics*, 97, 261–5.

Lavender, V. (2017). Communication and interpersonal skills. In D. Sellman & P. Snelling (eds), *Becoming a nurse: Fundamentals of professional practice for nursing*. London: Routledge, pp. 350–76.

Lawrence, J., Perrin, C. & Kiernan, E. (2015). *Building professional nursing communication*. Melbourne: Cambridge University Press.

McCormack, B. & McCance, T. (eds) (2017). *Person-centred practice in nursing and health care: Theory and practice*, 2nd edn. Oxford: Wiley Blackwell.

Moss, L., Shaw, M., Piper, I., Hawthorne, C. & Kinsella, J. (2017). Sharing of big data in healthcare: Public opinion, trust, and privacy considerations for health informatics researchers. In *Proceedings of the 10th International Joint Conference on Biomedical Engineering Systems and Technologies – Volume 5 (BIOSTEC 2017)*, pp. 463–8.

Nursing and Midwifery Board of Australia (2016). *Registered nurse standards for practice*. Retrieved from http://www.nursingmidwiferyboard.gov.au/Codes- Guidelines-Statements/Professional-standards/registered-nurse-standards-for- practice.aspx.

O'Toole, G. (2016). *Communication: Core interpersonal skills for health professionals*. Sydney: Elsevier.

Richards, T., Coulter, A. & Wicks, P. (2015). Time to deliver patient centred care. *British Medical Journal*, 350, h530.

Risor, B., Lisby, M. & Sorensen, J. (2017). PS-022 Complex automated medication systems reduce medication administration error rates in an acute medical ward. *European Journal of Hospital Pharmacy*, 24, A236–7.

SCONUL Working Group on Information Literacy (2011). *The SCONUL seven pillars of information literacy: Core model for higher education*. Society of College, National and University Libraries. Retrieved from https://www.sconul.ac.uk/sites/default/files/documents/coremodel.pdf.

Sherwood, G. & Barnsteiner, J (eds) (2017). *Quality and safety in nursing: A competency approach to improving outcomes*. Hoboken, NJ: John Wiley & Sons.

Studer Group (2021). AIDET patient communication. Retrieved from http://www.studergroup.com/aidet.

World Health Organization (WHO) (2017). *Patient safety: Making healthcare safer*. Geneva: WHO. Retrieved from https://apps.who.int/iris/handle/10665/255507.

12 Nursing as a profession: Legislation and regulation

Judith Lyons and Suzanne Bliss

LEARNING OBJECTIVES

At the completion of this chapter, you should be able to:

1 Discuss the legal and regulatory requirements and frameworks of nurses' and midwives' work as health professionals.
2 Outline the main features of the NMBA's Professional Practice Framework and explain its rationale.
3 Describe and explain the Standards for Practice as they apply to your field of nursing (registered or enrolled nurse).
4 Differentiate the scope of practice and professional boundaries of practice, including codes of ethics and conduct for nurses and midwives in Australia.

Introduction

All regulated health practitioners need to be aware of the standards imposed on them by their regulatory body so that they develop a practice that helps to keep the public safe. In Australia, the standards for nurses and midwives have been developed by the Australian Health Practitioner Regulation Agency (AHPRA), which regulates the Australian workforce through the Nursing and Midwifery Board of Australia (NMBA). The NMBA regulates registered nurses, enrolled nurses, midwives and nurse practitioners.

This chapter focuses on the professional standards of nursing and midwifery. It is intended to assist you in understanding your obligations, which include obtaining and maintaining your nursing or midwifery registration, as well your legal, regulatory and moral responsibilities, both as a nursing or midwifery professional and as an individual. It also differentiates the scope of practice for the registered nurse, enrolled nurse and midwife, as we are responsible for providing safe, quality care for clients.

The first section discusses the general legal and regulatory requirements of nurses. Next, we turn to the Professional Practice Framework, which constitutes an important part of nurses' legal and regulatory obligations. This framework forms the overarching statement of nursing's values, which are articulated in the Code of Ethics and Code of Conduct as well as the Standards for Practice for Registered and Enrolled Nurses (NMBA 2016a, 2016c) and the Midwife Standards for Practice (NMBA 2018a). We explain the registration standards first, then examine the Standards for Practice. These standards replaced the Competency Standards on 1 July 2016 and were developed to better reflect contemporary practice in nursing. The third section provides information on setting and maintaining professional boundaries, including the recently updated codes of ethics and conduct. Finally, we make some brief remarks relating to scope of practice.

Legal and regulatory requirements

It is essential that you have a thorough understanding of the professional, legal and ethical frameworks for nursing and midwifery practice. The professional and legal frameworks are complementary and establish the standards expected of nursing and midwifery in Australia. The national registration and accreditation scheme (NRAS) became operational in 2010 and is administered by AHPRA. This was a significant development, as it was the first time a range of health professions had been regulated by nationally consistent legislation in Australia. The regulation of health professionals focuses on public safety, and AHPRA regulates 15 health disciplines through its professional boards. The NMBA is the authority established under the *Health Practitioner Regulation National Law Act 2009*, which has been charged with regulating nursing and midwifery in Australia. The NMBA's functions include:

- registering nursing and midwifery practitioners and students;
- developing standards, codes and guidelines for the nursing and midwifery profession;

- handling notifications, complaints, investigations and disciplinary hearings;
- assessing overseas-trained practitioners who wish to practise in Australia; and
- approving accreditation standards and accredited courses of study (NMBA 2019a).

Australian Nursing and Midwifery Accreditation Council (ANMAC) the independent accrediting authority for the NMBA under the NRAS (ANMAC 2015, p. 4); it develops standards for accreditation and accredits nursing and midwifery programs and providers

The **Australian Nursing and Midwifery Accreditation Council (ANMAC)** is a peak body established in 1992 to facilitate a national approach to nursing and midwifery education by setting standards for accreditation and overseeing their implementation. The most recent registered nurse accreditation standards (ANMAC 2019) guide the accreditation of all nursing education programs, and the midwifery accreditation standards (ANMAC 2021) guide the accreditation of midwifery programs.

nurse includes enrolled nurses, registered nurses, nurse practitioners and any registered nurses with a scheduled medicines endorsement (NMBA 2019b)

All **nurses** and midwives need to register with the NMBA to practise as a nurse or midwife in this country. As regulated health professionals, nurses and midwives are responsible and accountable to the Nursing and Midwifery Board of Australia (NMBA 2016c, 2018a). Nurse or midwife registration means that you are required to practise as an individual within boundaries of practice and agreed standards of practice (Bryant 2005). You will need to access relevant information from the NMBA to understand your obligations under the law and in relation to nursing registration, standards, codes and guidelines. These are the Registered Nurse Standards for Practice (NMBA 2016c), the Enrolled Nurse Standards for Practice (NMBA 2016a) and the Midwife Standards for Practice (NMBA 2018a). The codes include the International Confederation of Nurses (ICN) Code of Ethics for Nurses, which were adopted by the NMBA in 2018, and the International Confederation of Midwives (ICM) International Code of Ethics for Midwives 2014 (also adopted by the NMBA in 2018). Codes also include the Code of Conduct for Nurses (NMBA 2018b) and Code of Conduct for Midwives (NMBA 2018c). The guidelines include **professional boundaries** for nurses and professional boundaries for midwives. Maintaining appropriate boundaries safeguards the public, the client and the nurse by controlling or limiting this power differential. This boundary setting enables a safe connection between the nurse and the client, based on the client's needs (NMBA 2010, Holder & Schenthal 2007).

professional boundaries limits that protect the space between the professional's power and the client's vulnerability

Midwifery is included in these guidelines as many nursing students undertake double degrees to practise as both nurses and midwives. As a nursing and/or midwifery student, you are registered with the NMBA on enrolment in your course and are expected to abide by all relevant standards, guidelines and frameworks.

Professional practice framework

A single Act of Parliament, the *Health Practitioner Regulation National Law Act 2009*, covers the full operation and implementation of the NRAS for all the selected health professions, including nursing. The main purpose of professional regulation has always been to protect the public. However, having a national scheme also provides scope for workforce mobility and flexibility, which reflects current trends in work patterns (Cashin et al. 2017). For example, under the NRAS, registered practitioners may practice across and between states and territories with their single national registration, whereas until 2010 nurses and midwives were required to register separately to practise in each jurisdiction.

The model of regulation for health professionals has moved away from self-regulation and is now cooperatively regulated by the profession itself and the government (or government agencies). In this chapter, we focus mainly on the function of developing codes, standards and guidelines; taken together, they constitute the NMBA's Professional Practice Framework (NMBA 2016f). This framework, which was substantially updated in 2016, is itself made up of several elements. The Professional Practice Framework incorporates many important professional values and articulates how they should (or could) be upheld. It also stipulates the **scope of practice** of registered nurses, enrolled nurses, midwives and nurse practitioners, alongside risk-management strategies and quality, health and safety guidelines. The overarching aim of the framework is to protect the public by establishing a minimum standard for the professional and safe practice of nurses and midwives in Australia (NMBA 2016f).

scope of practice the complete range of roles, functions, responsibilities, activities and decision-making abilities that a health practitioner is qualified, competent and authorised by legislation, regulation and employers to perform

The Professional Practice Framework consists of:

- standards for practice;
- various frameworks that are more limited in their scope, including:
  - a decision-making framework
  - a safety and quality framework for private midwives
  - a framework for assessing standards of practice for RNs, ENs and midwives
  - a framework for assessing supervised practice re-entry;
- codes of ethics (registered nurses and midwives);
- codes of conduct (registered nurses and midwives); and
- registration standards, including:
  - criminal history
  - English-language skills
  - continuing professional development
  - recency of practice
  - professional indemnity insurance arrangements
  - endorsement as a nurse practitioner
  - endorsement for scheduled medicines for midwives
  - endorsement for scheduled medicines for RNs (ANMF 2019).

The rest of this chapter examines some of the elements of the Professional Practice Framework in more detail. We begin with the registration standards.

Short-answer question
Video: Codes of conduct
Multiple-choice questions

Connecting with practice:
Professional policies
Multiple-choice questions

The registration standards

Registration standards define the minimum requirements you must meet to obtain and maintain nursing and/or midwifery registration. You must meet a range of requirements to become eligible for registration and you must declare this annually to the Nursing and Midwifery Board of Australia (NMBA). As nurses and/or midwives, you must meet the first five requirements of the mandatory registration standards, noted above. Let us examine each of these standards in more detail.

Criminal history registration standard

All healthcare agencies and education providers require applicants to undertake police checks to ensure they do not have a criminal history that may affect their ability to practise safely and ethically. Your university will require you to undertake fit-to-work police checks every year prior to undertaking clinical placements. Once you have completed your nursing or midwifery degree, and when applying for jobs, the criminal history registration standard forms part of your application process. AHPRA, on behalf of the NMBA, will check your 'criminal history during the registration process to ensure only those nurses and midwives who are suitable and safe to practise are granted registration in Australia' (NMBA 2017a). The NMBA Registration Standard: Criminal History has ten standards that assess your suitability as a safe health professional to ensure the safety of the public.

When you renew your registration, you must disclose any changes to your criminal history. You must inform the NMBA if you are:

- charged with an offence punishable by 12 months' imprisonment or more, or
- convicted or found guilty of an offence punishable by imprisonment in Australia and/or overseas (NMBA 2017a).

A criminal past may prohibit you from practising as a nurse or a midwife under the health practitioner regulation national law in force in each state and territory (the national law).

A Working with Children Check is also required for public safety, and you are required to provide evidence of this before undertaking clinical placement. Health professionals are also required to comply with mandatory notification (NMBA 2020) if there is concern about impairment, intoxication or working outside the scope of practice that can harm the public.

REFLECTION 12.1

Mandatory notification to AHPRA can be by any health professional or education provider, or by self-notification. What aspects could you self-report to keep the public safe?

English-language registration standard

The English Language Skills registration standard (NMBA 2019c) is relevant to every nurse and midwife applying for their initial registration, and is required whether they gained their qualification in Australia or overseas. It outlines the NMBA's requirements for English-language skills necessary for registration and provides the accepted pathways for demonstration of English-language competency. This includes having studied in Australia for five years, where the teaching and assessment was conducted in English. International students must demonstrate proficiency in English by passing an International English Language Testing System (IELTS) with a minimum score of seven, or an approved equivalent language test, to be registered to practise in Australia. Applicants are required to make a written declaration of English language proficiency in order to be registered with the NMBA, and thus universities also require this declaration on enrolment into the program.

Continuing professional development registration standard

The continuing professional development (CPD) registration standard outlines 'how nurses and midwives maintain, improve and broaden their knowledge, expertise and **competence**, and develop the personal and professional qualities required throughout their professional lives' (NMBA 2021a). In fact, the requirement for CPD is not only a registration standard; it is also Standard 3 in the Registered Nurse Standards for Practice (NMBA 2016c). The CPD standard requires nurses and midwives to complete a minimum of 20 hours of CPD directly relevant to their area of nursing practice each year, or 40 hours of CPD if practising as both a nurse and a midwife.

Nurses must ensure that they are fit to practise in two main areas. These are: (1) keeping up with the latest research and knowledge that relates to their sphere of practice; and (2) ensuring that their behaviours and attitudes are consistent with the standards and other codes, in terms of ethical and professional attributes. Being fit to practise in the second area necessitates a willingness to engage in reflection on practice and to critically self-reflect. This process may require you to adjust your behaviours or attitudes if they are inconsistent with the mandated professional attributes. Professional development is required in both main spheres of practice, and the NMBA sets out CPD requirements in its Guidelines for Continuing Professional Development (2016e).

CPD assists nurses to evaluate and to improve, if necessary, their practice standards, and to identify any gaps in knowledge or skills, so as to provide ethical, safe client care. The NMBA recommends that CPD (e.g. self-learning, attending workshops, seminars or conferences) is undertaken across each year through a variety of activities, rather than scrambling to do everything in a short period of time. The aim is to broaden and deepen your knowledge and skill base with respect to your area of professional practice.

Professional indemnity insurance registration standard

Under the national law, you are not allowed to practise unless you hold appropriate professional indemnity insurance (PII), which addresses the risks posed by uninsured practitioners (NMBA 2017b). PII secures your professional practice, and provides insurance against civil liability incurred by, or is due to loss from, an error or omission in the conduct of the nurse and/or midwife and a claim of negligence (NMBA 2017b; Nursing and Midwifery Council of New South Wales 2018). You may take out your own PII or have a third party's insurance arrangement through a professional organisation, employer, education provider or union (NMBA 2017b).

Recency of practice registration standard

A nurse or midwife is considered to have recency if they have maintained an adequate connection with, and recent practice in, clinical or non-clinical nursing and/or midwifery since qualifying for or obtaining registration (Nursing and Midwifery Council of New South Wales 2018). You will be required to undertake further studies, known as return to work studies, if you have not maintained your registration for between five and ten years. If it has been more than ten years since your practice lapsed, you cannot practise as a nurse unless you undertake and complete your degree or certification again (NMBA 2019d).

REFLECTION 12.2

The registration standards guide your safe practice. Think about what requirements you met prior to undertaking your first clinical placement. Which of these requirements were from your regulatory framework and why are they mandatory?

Professionalism in nursing

Professionalism refers to the expression of the knowledge, values, behaviours and relationships that underpin the trust and confidence that society has in, or can expect of, nurses and other health professionals. This relationship of trust that exists (or should exist) with the community is based on a set of principles that are sometimes described as a social contract. The use of the term 'contract' is an important reminder of the responsibilities, obligations and expectations that are paramount in these professional relationships. Through this social contract, the community can expect nurses (and the profession as a whole) to:

- Always act in the interests of clients, residents or consumers.
- Demonstrate an altruistic motivation concerned with the wellbeing of others and the good of society.
- Ensure that practice is based on intellectual action (use of disciplinary knowledge and critical thinking), combined with personal responsibility and ethical conduct.
- Respect individual diversity and dignity, and to practise with empathy and compassion.
- Adopt transparent, inclusive and person-centred approaches to practice, which empower people to determine their own needs and participate in the decisions and actions that affect their lives (and their care and support).
- Practice with integrity and transparency, demonstrating consistent adherence to strong moral and ethical principles that are consistent with community expectations, the profession's (and the organisation's) values, and applicable standards, codes and regulations.
- Practice with the spirit of collegiality and collaboration ('together we do better').
- Maintain a focus on CPD and improvement.
- Ensure that those who practice or behave unethically, incompetently or unprofessionally are identified, reported and held to account (e.g. investigated, disciplined, sanctioned).

According to Poorchangizi et al. (2019), professional standards and codes are a way of evaluating the profession.

Professional standards

Professional standards describe the *acceptable level of practice or care* that covers the broad range of nursing tasks and individual qualities required of every nurse to fulfil these tasks to an acceptable standard. They therefore reflect a recommended and attainable level of performance to which a nurse's actual performance can be compared. They can be used as both a self-assessment tool when you reflect on your own practice and as a tool with which employers can evaluate your practice. Standards also assist managers and administrators to develop and evaluate the policies, procedures and continuous quality improvement plans that apply to their institution or business.

Since 1 March 2018, the various professional standards for nurses and midwives have been consolidated into three groups: (1) Standards for Practice; (2) Codes of Conduct; and (3) Codes of Ethics. We discuss each of these in turn, beginning with the Standards for Practice.

The Standards for Practice constitute mandatory practice criteria, as well as statements about the appropriate personal qualities that nurses must possess, such as compassion and responsiveness.

The Registered Nurse Standards for Practice came into effect on 1 June 2016, while the new Enrolled Nurse Standards for Practice were implemented on 1 January 2016. The standards for practice go beyond the competencies; they constitute a statement that communicates the level of quality and attainment of practice required of nurses to the government, the public and the profession (Cashin et al. 2017).

The standards were developed through extensive literature reviews, research and stakeholder (including nurses) consultation, such that they reflect current nursing practice in all contexts and provide clear national guidelines. In particular, the guidelines inform the public about the standards that can be expected of both registered nurses and enrolled nurses. They are also used to assess registered nurses and enrolled nurses returning to work after a lengthy absence, or who have trained abroad. Finally, the standards are meant to improve usability for all nurses (NMBA 2016b, 2016d). Nevertheless, there is a substantive overlap with the previous competencies, although the standards themselves have been streamlined and simplified to some extent. We discuss the standards for the registered nurse first and then briefly turn our attention to the enrolled nurse standards.

Registered Nurse Standards for Practice

There are seven standards for the registered nurse that require them to:

1 Think critically and analyse nursing practice.
2 Engage in therapeutic and professional relationships.
3 Maintain the capability for practice.
4 Comprehensively conduct assessments.
5 Develop a plan for nursing practice.
6 Provide safe, appropriate and responsive quality nursing practice.
7 Evaluate outcomes to inform nursing practice (NMBA 2016c).

The NMBA has helpfully represented the standards diagrammatically (see Figure 12.1). We can see that these standards interconnect along two axes: horizontal and vertical. Essentially, the first three (horizontal) standards constitute what we call 'professional' requirements, while the last four constitute 'practice' requirements. This way of representing the standards diagrammatically captures the idea that the standards are interconnected (NMBA 2016c). This means that fulfilling each practice standard requires the satisfactory fulfilment of each professional standard. For example, Standard 6 – Provides safe, appropriate and responsive quality nursing practice will demand that the nurse: (1) thinks critically and reflects on their practice; (2) engages in therapeutic and professional relationships; and (3) has maintained their capability for practice (NMBA 2016c). But the reverse is also true: fulfilling each professional standard requires the nurse to also have the capacity to fulfil each practice standard. Let us now consider a specific example.

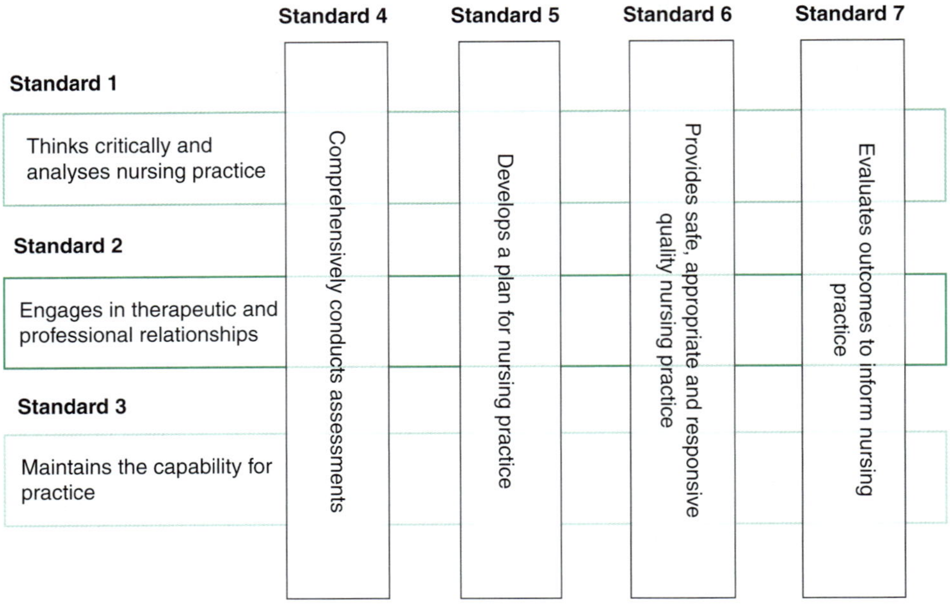

Standard 4 — Comprehensively conducts assessments

Standard 5 — Develops a plan for nursing practice

Standard 6 — Provides safe, appropriate and responsive quality nursing practice

Standard 7 — Evaluates outcomes to inform nursing practice

Standard 1 — Thinks critically and analyses nursing practice

Standard 2 — Engages in therapeutic and professional relationships

Standard 3 — Maintains the capability for practice

Figure 12.1   Registered Nurse Standards for Practice

Source: NMBA (2016c).

NURSING PERSPECTIVE

It is 1.45 pm and registered nurse Harry has just started the afternoon shift at a busy hospital. One of his assigned clients is Gwen, an 83-year-old woman who was transferred from the emergency department earlier that day. She has moderately advanced dementia and was admitted to hospital because she has been febrile for the last couple of days. The nurse doing the handover described Gwen as 'time-consuming', 'quieter than she was' but 'difficult to do anything with'. She suggests that whoever is assigned to Gwen should just 'leave her alone in the bed to rest, and 'if they do this, they should have a trouble-free shift'.

Harry considers checking Gwen last so that he does not get behind with his other clients but decides against this. Instead, he goes to see Gwen first and finds her lunch tray untouched at the end of the bed and the curtains drawn. Harry can see she is breathing rapidly and when he touches her brow she feels hot. Gwen is grimacing, and she is lying sideways on the bed, talking to herself. Checking the medication order chart, Harry observes that the IV antibiotics have been given for a chest infection, but no analgesia. Antibiotics for a urinary tract infection have been ceased.

Harry takes Gwen's hand and introduces himself. She shakes his hand and asks when her mother will come to collect her, and they chat for a little while about her mother. Harry explains that he needs to take care of her arm and asks permission to unwrap her bandage. Although Gwen appears reluctant, she eventually offers her arm and he is able to unwrap the bandage around her intravenous cannula site. Harry continues to chat and carefully asks her another question or suggests she tell him more when Gwen begins to show concern at what he is doing. Once the bandage is removed, Harry finds the inner layer is quite wet and the cannula is clearly no longer working. It seems that the IV antibiotics have just leaked out onto the bandage. Above the cannula site, Gwen's arm is swollen and inflamed.

Harry contacts the medical intern to explain what has happened and asks her to review the need for analgesia and to re-site the intravenous cannula. He is then able to help Gwen sit up and, after checking on his other clients, assists her to eat a little of her lunch. There is also some personal information about Gwen in the care plan. Harry reads that she had been a prominent council member in the area and had an interest in showing cats. Harry is able to give Gwen her familiar crochet rug and chat about cats to help relax her while taking her vital signs before the intern arrives.

Later on, Harry assists Gwen to take her medication. Reading the care plan, Harry discovers Gwen prefers her tablets with yoghurt. When he gives her the tablets he notices that Gwen swallows the tablets one by one and requires much explanation and encouragement from him. If he tries to hurry Gwen, she becomes flustered and refuses to take the medication. Harry documents these details in his notes, flagging that he must pass this information on when handing over to the nurses on the next shift.

We can see from this example that the connection and interrelation between the different standards is much clearer than was the case with the competencies. Harry has cared for Gwen in a safe, person-centred manner that is consistent with the seven standards. He has fulfilled the professional standards by thinking critically (Standard 1) when declining to take the previous nurse's instructions at face value, and by initiating a therapeutic relationship with Gwen (Standard 2), managing her care in a way with which she feels comfortable. Harry is also on his way to fulfilling his practice standards. He has comprehensively conducted Gwen's assessments (Standard 4) and notified the relevant person when he realised there were problems. He clearly provided safe, appropriate, quality and responsive care (Standard 6) when he recognised and responded to the issue with the cannula, assisting Gwen with her medication and helping her to eat. He also contributed to Gwen's nursing care plan (Standard 5) by documenting strategies to encourage her to take her medications, and by suggesting that the intern review her treatment plan. Assuming Harry has completed his other requirements for registration, such as maintaining his capability for practice (Standard 3), and that he is a reflective practitioner (Standard 7), we can see that he is upholding the Registered Nurse Standards for Practice to the appropriate level.

The new standards give nurses a more holistic way of understanding their professional requirements and how they might work in practice. While you will no doubt receive more specific instruction on each of these standards across your degree, it is worth discussing in more detail the first three standards given, which are, in some sense, foundational for your *professional* development (according to the aims of this chapter).

Standard 1: Thinks critically and analyses nursing practice

The term 'critical thinking' is somewhat abstract and can be understood in several ways. It is a philosophical term that refers to the capacity to *reason well* in the broadest sense (see Chapter 9). This includes, among other things, the ability to develop an argument by supporting your claims with appropriate reasons or evidence. It also refers to the capacity to evaluate the claims of others and to distinguish between claims that are well supported and those that are spurious. Although these features of critical thinking are taken for granted in the context of the standards, there are more specific definitions relevant to nurses. In the nursing context, critical thinking specifically refers to (1) the complex thinking process associated with clinical reasoning and (2) reflection on one's practice. Let us discuss each of these in turn.

The clinical reasoning cycle (see Figure 12.2) represents the complex process that nurses navigate when caring for clients. We should emphasise, however, that this process is not linear: we can think of it as a series or spiral of interlinked clinical encounters in which the context will change over time. Nurses must be able to gather information by collecting cues; mentally process the information; form a judgement

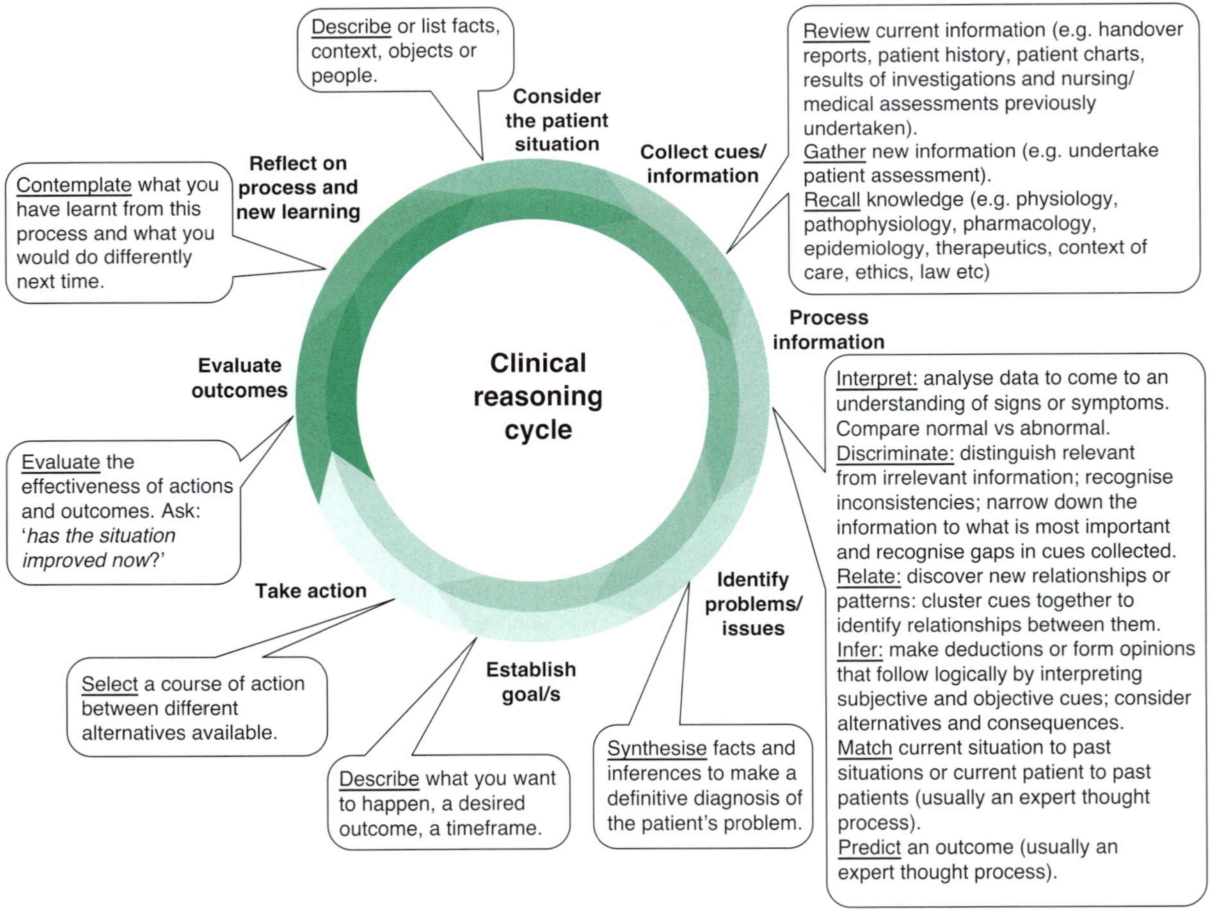

Figure 12.2   The clinical reasoning cycle
Source: University of Newcastle (2009, p. 6).

about the client's situation; plan and implement interventions; evaluate outcomes; and both reflect on and learn from the process (University of Newcastle 2009). This reasoning process depends on a disposition to think critically (Scheffer & Rubenfeld 2000), and is influenced by one's attitudes, perspectives, values and preconceptions (McCarthy 2003). Critical thinking is particularly important for nurses when they interpret client data and choose their intervention (Cruz, Pimenta & Lunney 2009), as these phases in the cycle carry higher risk. Registered nurses are required to consciously cultivate the disposition to think critically (see Chapters 7 and 9) and reflect on their own practice so they can identify areas for improvement. The capacity to think critically develops with practice, and you will start to gain critical thinking skills throughout your university degree program. There are many ways to improve your critical thinking capacities, and the readings and assignments you are set at university are designed to develop your critical thinking skills. Specific examples of thinking critically in the nursing context include the questioning of colleagues and other health professionals (when appropriate) instead of blindly following orders, a willingness to consider and see things from the perspectives of others, thinking up new or more effective ways of doing things (within your scope of practice) and taking responsibility for addressing problems (rather than assuming that someone else will).

Reflection on practice is also a rather vague concept. While there are 'reflective models' that can be followed – for example, Driscoll's reflective cycle (see Chapter 9 for an overview of various reflective models) – a necessary precondition for reflecting on practice is the development of *self-awareness* (see Chapters 7, 9 and 10). This is only possible by forming an intention to understand your own values, beliefs, attitudes and assumptions over time. Critical self-reflection requires humility; this in turn requires an openness to working on, or adjusting, your values and attitudes if they are proving a barrier to providing excellent person-centred care – or indeed if your personal life is in turmoil. This process requires emotional intelligence, especially with respect to managing your own emotions appropriately (see Chapter 10). Reflective models can be a useful aid when it comes to supporting your reflective capacities but they are not a substitute for self-awareness. Nevertheless, reflecting on your own practice is one way of analysing nursing practice – the other requirement in Standard 1.

Standard 2: Engages in therapeutic and professional relationships

The term 'therapeutic relationship' is used frequently in the nursing literature, yet specific accounts or analyses of what this might involve are scarce. Two components of a therapeutic relationship that most nurses recognise from their first year of study onwards are the importance of appropriate communication and appropriate professional boundaries. This is not surprising, considering these two components are emphasised in the criteria that specify how this standard is demonstrated in practice (NMBA 2016b). Although these two components are important, they do not really capture the essence of the therapeutic relationship *in a way that is meaningful to clients.* So, rather than discussing each criterion under this standard, we provide an account of the elements we think are important for successfully developing a therapeutic relationship. In what follows, we appeal to Muetzel's (1988) simple yet powerful account of the nature of therapeutic relationships that captures the elements that both nurses and clients believe to be important. Crucially, Muetzel's suggestions are borne out through empirical research in terms of improved client outcomes (Richardson, Percy & Hughes 2015). While Muetzel's model contains just three components, these express in a more profound way the elements of the nurse–client relationship that function as **therapeutic interventions**, because they actually assist the process of recovery. We discuss each of these elements in turn.

The first element in Muetzel's model is *partnership*. The idea of partnership implies that the decision-making process is shared, thereby conforming to the ethical principle of autonomy ('self-rule'), where the client's wishes in relation to their healthcare plan are paramount (Beauchamp & Childress 2013). It also suggests that the nurse and client are collaborating in the goal of recovery or amelioration of symptoms, such as pain. These factors underscore the importance of trust in the therapeutic relationship: the client must believe that the nurse has the client's best interests at heart and will uphold their fiduciary duty to the client. This element reflects the fact that clients, for the most part, do not want paternalistic treatment; rather, they need to feel that they are equal players in developing their care and treatment program.

The second element is *intimacy*. This might seem strange at first, as intimacy is often associated with romantic or sexual relationships. In the nursing context, however, it refers to a 'professional intimacy', and perhaps also 'emotional intimacy'. In practice, this means that the nurse recognises the client *as a person* rather than simply as a 'diagnosis' or a 'task to carry out'. Persons are multidimensional human beings (physical, intellectual, emotional, social, spiritual and interpersonal) whose characteristics relate in complex ways and whose personality and values are shaped by their history and other relationships (Atkins et al. 2020). Essentially, we become persons only as a result of our social context, and there is a universal need among humans to value others and *be valued by them.* In his research on dignity, Chochinov (2007) showed that, as he put it, health professionals (especially doctors and nurses) function as a 'mirror' to the client, with the client reflecting a view of themselves *as they are regarded by the health professional* (in Atkins et al. 2020). This means that if a nurse's actions suggest indifference or annoyance, clients can come to see themselves as a problem. The nurse's attitude therefore has the potential to influence the client's recovery, for better or worse. On the other hand, if the nurse recognises the client as a person and shows genuine concern and interest in their recovery, the client is likely to find it easier to maintain their self-esteem and their motivation to recover.

As with partnership, being intimate is inherently *relational*; thus, the qualities nurses need to demonstrate intimacy include authenticity, openness and sincerity. Developing intimacy also requires self-disclosure on the part of the nurse (Richardson, Percy & Hughes 2015). This means that, where possible, nurses would do well to talk a little about themselves and share their feelings in a considered and genuine way. Sharing in this way helps the client to develop trust in the nurse and to feel recognised as a person. The fact that intimacy can flourish in the nurse–client relationship certainly makes the possibility of partnership more viable.

The final element of Muetzel's model is *reciprocity*. While there are certainly connections between reciprocity and partnership, there are subtle, yet important differences in focus. The idea of reciprocity suggests that the therapeutic relationship is one that benefits both client and nurse – counter-intuitive as that might seem. If we think back to the notion of virtue discussed in Chapter 7, we can understand reciprocity on the part of the nurse as being a virtuous act that steers a middle path between selfishness and extreme selflessness (altruism). Thus, nurses need to balance their own interests against those of the client, and must adjust their care to the requirements of particular situations (Hem & Petterson 2011). Like the other two elements, reciprocity underscores the relational aspect of the nurse–client encounter, to which mutuality, collaboration and the sharing of values and beliefs are central (Richardson et al. 2015).

The capacity to engage in partnership, intimacy and reciprocity requires nurses to develop several personal attributes. Emotional intelligence, along with the capacity for critical self-reflection, is particularly important (see Chapters 7 and 10). It is important for you, as a student nurse, to form an intention to cultivate these qualities in yourself, as you will have the ability to influence your clients' health for better or worse, based on the quality of your relationship with them.

Standard 3: Maintains the capability for practice

We touched on this standard earlier in this chapter – see 'Continuing professional development registration standard'.

Enrolled Nurse Standards for Practice

The rationale behind the Enrolled Nurse Standards for Practice is the same as for the registered nurse standards. However, the content of the standards, while similar in certain ways, is pitched rather differently. There are three domains under which the various standards fall: (1) professional and collaborative practice; (2) provision of care; and (3) reflective and analytical practice (Townsville Hospital and Health Service 2016, p. 9). We do not discuss each of these domains and their respective standards here; however, if you are, or are intending to become, an enrolled nurse, you must familiarise yourself with all these requirements, which are available on the NMBA's website (NMBA 2016a). Instead, we focus on one of the standards that falls within the scope of the first domain: the requirement to 'accept accountability and responsibility for own actions'.

One notable modification to the Standards for the Enrolled Nurse was the highlighting of the requirement that enrolled nurses be supervised by a registered nurse at all times, either directly (where the registered nurse is physically present and works alongside the enrolled nurse) (ANMF 2014, p. 11) or indirectly (where the registered nurse is not physically present but must be immediately contactable). The duties and scope of practice of enrolled nurses therefore differ in a few ways from those of the registered nurse. It is crucial that enrolled nurses have personal qualities that enable them to accept instructions from registered nurses, even when the registered nurse may have far less experience and/or be much younger. A strong sense of collegiality and a good dose of humility are required to ensure that this relationship remains constructive. This does not, however, mean that an enrolled nurse should stand back when they believe the registered nurse is making a poor decision. An enrolled nurse with more experience is likely to have greater clinical reasoning skills than a newly graduated registered nurse, and thus should speak up if they believe the registered nurse has made a decision that is not in the client's best interests or is likely to lead to a poor outcome in some way (such as breaching safety and quality guidelines). This means that a sense of responsibility for client outcomes is needed, along with sound relational skills, so that they have the ability to voice concerns in a helpful, non-accusatory manner. It is not good enough to cede all responsibility to the registered nurse.

The term 'responsibility' can be understood in at least two different ways (de Ruyter 2002). The first sense refers to the idea of being accountable – either to oneself or to others – for one's own actions. The standards certainly emphasise this sense of responsibility in their statement that enrolled nurses must be accountable not only for their own care but also for the delegated care they provide (Keast 2016). Thus, we can say that enrolled nurses, like registered nurses, have a non-delegable duty of care to clients, families and colleagues, and must accept this responsibility for each and every shift they work. The second sense of 'responsibility' involves being sensitive to the needs of others and responding to those needs appropriately (de Ruyter 2002). We suggest that this sense of being responsible is just as important for enrolled nurses as it is for registered nurses. Obviously, the two senses of responsibility are connected – for instance, if we expect someone to respond to the needs of others, we assume that they can *take responsibility* for doing so (de Ruyter 2002). Moreover, by praising them for their responsiveness, we presume that they are *accountable* (morally responsible) for their actions. We can think of the difference between the two like this: a person who takes responsibility for another person is aiming to act responsively in future situations, whereas a person who is responsible for their actions is accountable for something they have already done (or should have done). A nurse should take responsibility for the wellbeing of others, not only because it is the right thing to do, but because they are morally responsible for harms caused *as a result of failing to do something they should have done* (Forrester & Griffiths 2015). This principle is enshrined in the Civil Liability Acts of the various states and territories in Australia. In the course of their work, all nurses have a duty of care to their clients. If they fail to carry out a particular task that they should have performed as part of the care plan, they can be deemed negligent if the client suffers harm as a direct result of that omission.

CASE STUDY

Tribunal suspends nurse for three months for professional misconduct

Registered nurse Ms T had her registration suspended for three months from 4 December 2017 for professional misconduct.

Ms T had been working at an aged-care facility in Queensland, where she was accused of acting unprofessionally. An allegation was made that she took 7 mL of morphine belonging to the facility, administered it to herself and replaced the morphine she had taken with water. Additionally, Ms T tried to persuade another registered nurse not to report the matter when they detected the inconsistency in the documentation.

The NMBA was notified of the incident and referred Ms T to the Queensland Civil and Administrative Tribunal. The tribunal upheld the allegations, although it determined that the accusation Ms T had taken the morphine herself was not proven. Nevertheless, the Tribunal found that Ms T had behaved in a manner that constituted professional misconduct, and duly suspended her registration for three months. She was also required to undertake further education on Schedule 8 medications.

QUESTION
How has this nurse breached the standards for practice?

Short-answer question
Video: CPD

What are professional boundaries?

We suggest that the term 'professional boundaries' can be understood in two different, yet interrelated, ways. Specifically, a professional boundary refers to a hypothetical line between a professional and personal relationship that nurses should not cross. When clients entrust themselves to the care of a nurse, they place themselves in a position of vulnerability; the relationship between nurse and client is one in which the power imbalance is in the nurse's favour. Nurses therefore have a weighty responsibility to respect the trust placed on them, and to not abuse or exploit the power relationship in the nurse–client interaction. If nurses cross the boundary of unprofessional behaviour or misuse their power, they endanger the safety (physical, emotional, cultural or spiritual) of their clients. Nurses can be deemed unprofessional if they are disinterested, neglectful or not adequately involved in the care they provide, or if they are over-involved. Over-involvement with clients occurs when professional and therapeutic boundaries are violated by engaging in inappropriate relationships with the client (or their family) in their care. For example, there have been cases where nurses have had sexual relationships with their clients or have given special attention to clients they knew at the expense of other clients. Such *conflicts of interests* should be avoided at all costs, in line with your professional responsibilities as a nurse.

When working as a student or professional nurse, it is important that you recognise and maintain boundaries that establish appropriate limits to personal and therapeutic relationships. This is a complex area of your practice, and the guidance on boundaries does not provide specific advice about what to do or how to act in difficult situations. Nevertheless, there are general rules relating to professional boundaries in the codes of conduct for nurses and midwives, with which you must familiarise yourself.

The codes and professional boundaries

The second, and more general, sense of the term 'professional boundaries' refers to the frameworks for ethical and professional conduct stipulated by nursing codes. Professional boundaries are intended to safeguard the public and clients in our care whose treatment and safety may be affected by the incompetent, unethical or illegal conduct of nurses. The Code of Conduct and Code of Ethics articulate what we might call 'boundary standards' for nurses. These codes set *minimum standards* that nurses are expected to uphold, both within and outside of professional domains, to ensure the 'good standing' of the profession in Australia. These codes provide a framework for legal, professionally accountable and responsible nursing practice in clinical, educational, administration and research areas of nursing. In this way, they specify certain values that inform the public about what they can expect of nurses when providing care. Nurses must abide by the various codes, and doing so ensures that the public and community are protected from unwarranted distress, confusion or harm, and that clients are not abused by the nurses who care for them. These codes are:

- the Code of Conduct for Nurses in Australia
- the Code of Ethics for Nurses in Australia.

Code of Conduct for Nurses

The Code of Conduct for Nurses in Australia (NMBA 2018b) was reviewed and updated in 2018. The Code of Conduct has four domains, with each domain representing overarching principles with which nurses must conform. These domains are concerned with legal compliance; person-centred, safe and collaborative practice; practising with integrity; and promoting health and wellbeing. If you are undertaking a double degree in nursing and midwifery, you will need to understand and abide by the professional codes and frameworks for both nursing and midwifery.

We do not discuss all aspects of the Code of Conduct here, and we strongly recommend you visit the NMBA's website and download a copy so you can study it in detail (NMBA 2018b). However, we would like to briefly highlight one of the principles in the code that may not be particularly clear to student nurses. This principle is 'cultural practice and respectful relationships', which falls under the domain of practising safely, effectively and collaboratively. The fact that this principle is also emphasised in the Code of Ethics makes it a particularly good example for discussion here.

Cultural safety and respectful relationships

The notion of cultural safety originated in New Zealand in the 1990s, advocated by Irihapeti Ramsden (1993) in response to challenges Māori experienced with Western-based models of health care. The concept has been refined further to encompass the notion of cultural appropriateness in healthcare practice. The codes and standards for nurses share a common theme of fairness, respect and tolerance for those from culturally and linguistically diverse backgrounds, consistent with the international covenants to which Australia is a signatory.

The assumption that underlies the concept of cultural safety is that there exists a power differential between the health professional and the client or community. The subsequent discussion of cultural safety also presupposes that those who wield most power in these relationships have a choice of either perpetuating or challenging their own oppressive practices. Clear (2008) points out that 'unsafe' cultural practice has the capacity to 'diminish, demean or disempower the cultural identity and wellbeing of an individual' (p. 2). Being culturally safe therefore means practising nursing in ways that do not diminish individual and community cultural identity.

Regrettably, it is not always clear how to practise in ways that support individual and community identity. Even those of us who think we are culturally inclusive can harbour cognitive biases that cloud our judgement and drive unhelpful behaviours. Indeed, research in social psychology shows that people tend to judge others more harshly than they judge themselves (Gilovich & Eibach 2001). If we are called upon to explain our own behaviour, we tend to appeal to situational factors that have affected our performance, rather than pointing to our own (undesirable]) values or character traits. When we explain others' behaviour to ourselves, however, we tend to invoke character traits, attitudes or values rather than considering possible situational factors (Paley 2015). This bias is known as the 'fundamental attribution error'. Like other types of cognitive biases, the fundamental attribution error involves spontaneous, largely unconscious judgements. Let us imagine that I am driving on a busy road when a car cuts in front of me, dodging in and out of the traffic. My first thought is 'What an idiot!' – I attribute arrogant or aggressive traits to the driver instead of thinking 'Oh, that poor person must be in a hurry'. On the other hand, if I am in a desperate hurry to reach my mother who has been taken to hospital, I justify my aggressive driving behaviour by appealing to a 'family emergency'.

Attribution biases are not confined to judgements about individuals; they also occur at the level of groups. Group-serving bias is observed between the attributions we would make for the group one belongs to (the 'in-group') and the sorts of attributions we are likely to make for members not considered part of our group (the 'out-group'). While Australia is a multicultural country, some of us think of the in-group as people of British and northern European heritage, as these individuals tend to wield the most social and political power. The out-group, in this context, is peoples from cultures other than those, with certain cultures – such as Aboriginal and Torres Strait Islander peoples, or those of the Muslim faith – being especially marginalised. When judging our own group, we tend to internalise positive qualities or outcomes, and externalise negatives. However, when judging the out-group, positives are externalised and negatives are internalised. Thus, if people in the out-group fail or fall short in some way, this is thought to stem from an internal trait (such as a character flaw or lack of ability). On the other hand, if they do well, it is explained by situational (external) factors. For example, if 'our' football team wins, we tend to attribute its success to 'internal' factors such as having especially talented players who have trained tirelessly, whereas if the other team wins, we tend to attribute its success to 'external' factors, such as an incompetent referee.

Because we are usually unaware of making these attributions, these biases are likely to have a significant influence on the way nurses make assumptions about, and relate to, clients from culturally marginalised groups. Thus, these types of cognitive biases undermine fair judgement. A recent example was reported on SBS (Morelli 2017), where an Aboriginal woman reported that she was frightened of returning to Broome for crucial medical treatment after she was told she was 'too drunk' to catch a bus. The woman alleged the driver had threatened to kick her off the bus during the nine-hour journey back to her community of Mulan. In fact, she was suffering from hypoglycaemia, the symptoms of which resemble alcohol intoxication.

At the time of the incident, this woman was in her sixties and had both heart and kidney problems, as well as diabetes that required ongoing management (Morelli 2017). While waiting for several hours for the night bus at the Broome Tourist Bureau, she went into a state of hypoglycaemia and required urgent medical attention. Her husband stated that she may have died but for the help of a kind stranger. Nurses and

midwives, therefore, would do well to recognise their own cognitive biases and make a conscious effort to mitigate them. Indeed, this is one way of being a 'critical thinker' – a skill much emphasised by the various nursing bodies. We cannot avoid discrimination without being aware of how our shared values and meanings, which determine the way 'our group' understands the world, influence our reactions to individuals from other groups.

Code of Ethics for Nurses and Midwives in Australia

Nurses and midwives in Australia are required to abide by the ICN Code of Ethics for Nurses (ICN 2018b) and the ICM Code of Ethics for Midwives (ICN 2018a). In the second element of the ICN code, 'Nurses and practice', there is a requirement to 'Monitor and promote the personal health of nursing staff in relation to their competence for practice' (ICN 2018b). This suggests that the ICN considers nurses to have an *ethical duty* to keep themselves healthy – physically and mentally or emotionally – and to reflect on the connection between keeping oneself healthy and other nursing values.

The third element of the ICN code, 'Nurses and the profession', exhorts nurses to 'Promote participation in national nurses' associations so as to create favourable socioeconomic conditions for nurses' (ICN 2018b). Thus, these codes encourage nurses to join their relevant professional association (such as the Australian College of Nursing) or a relevant trade union. In Australia, the main nursing union is the Australian Nursing and Midwifery Federation (ANMF). There are also state branches of the ANMF and state-based nursing unions, such as the New South Wales Nursing and Midwifery Association.

We strongly encourage you to go to the NMBA's website and download a copy of the ICN and ICM Code of Ethics relevant to your area, and familiarise yourself thoroughly with their content.

Scope of practice

The concept 'scope of practice' is interpreted in ways that are inconsistent, indicating that it is poorly understood, even by nurse academics (Birks et al. 2016). The scope of practice for nurses, midwives and enrolled nurses differs depending on the education, knowledge and skills application that come with the level of study and accreditation standards. In general, 'a profession's scope of practice is the full spectrum of roles, functions, responsibilities, activities and decision-making capacity that individuals within that profession are educated, competent and authorised to perform' (NMBA 2007).

These roles and responsibilities are outlined in documents such as the practice standards and codes. Nevertheless, they are defined too broadly to provide adequate guidance for nurses when trying to determine the legal and professional boundaries of their practice (Birks et al. 2016). International research has shown that local context influences the understanding of scope of practice, and that the general lack of clarity inhibits understanding and applying the notion in practice (Fealy 2014). The fact that some functions within the scope of practice of any profession may be shared with other professions, or other individuals or groups (NMBA 2010), also adds to the confusion.

Scope of practice is therefore characterised by a shifting set of parameters that change according to many different factors, including rapidly changing technology and healthcare needs. Birks and colleagues (2016) highlight the need for further research into scope of practice that considers the views of all stakeholders, including governments, service providers, clients and nurses. More research needs to be done in establishing the breadth and depth of nurses' roles, including the potential capacity of nurses. The relatively recent move to endorsing nurse practitioners in Australia is a good example of how the scope of practice for nurses can potentially be expanded. In the meantime, the best advice we can give to students and recently graduated nurses is to ensure that your practice is consistent with the standards and codes, and to seek advice from your superiors if you have any doubts.

SUMMARY

- The section on legal and regulatory framework describes the key aspects and requirements for registration and maintenance of registration to practise in Australia.
- The NMBA's Professional Practice Framework is one important element in the process of self-regulation. It incorporates many important professional values and articulates how they should (or could) be upheld. The Code of Conduct, for example, sets out how all nurses and midwives should comport themselves in relation to self, clients, colleagues and the broader community. The ICN Code of Ethics, on the other hand, articulates values that the profession holds. The framework also sets out registration standards and standards for practice of both nurses and midwives. It stipulates the scope of practice of registered nurses, enrolled nurses, midwives and nurse practitioners, alongside risk-management strategies and quality, health and safety guidelines. The overarching rationale of the framework is to protect the public by establishing the requirements for the safe and professional practice of nurses and midwives in Australia.
- There are seven Standards for Practice for the Registered Nurse. The first three address what we have called 'professional requirements': (1) thinks critically and analyses nursing practice; (2) engages in therapeutic and professional relationships; and (3) maintains the capability for practice. The last four may be called 'practice requirements': (4) comprehensively conducts assessments; (5) develops a plan for nursing practice; (6) provides safe, appropriate and responsive quality nursing practice; and (7) evaluates outcomes to inform nursing practice (NMBA 2016c). Fulfilling each standard requires an ongoing commitment from the nurse to develop and hone their skills in these areas. Taken together, these standards are essentially a summary of the clinical reasoning cycle, along with the skills needed to engage effectively in clinical care.
- The section on professional boundaries discusses the codes of conduct and ethics that apply to nurses and midwives. It highlights the domains and principles that these codes provide for nurses and midwives to provide safe competent quality care to people in their care and their clients' families.

Suggested responses

REVIEW QUESTIONS

1   Use the NMBA decision-making framework to assess the standards of practice for your level of professional qualification (registered nurse, enrolled nurse or midwife).
2   Use the NMBA professional boundaries decision-making flowchart, techniques and strategies to manage potential professional boundary breaches.
3   Based on your lived experience as a student nurse and using a specific example, identify ethical dilemmas and standards of conduct as outlined in the ICN Code of Ethics for Nurses.
4   Identify how you would resolve the dilemmas.
5   What is the difference between law and ethics?

RESEARCH TOPIC

Connecting with practice:
Complaints or concerns

Research the various categories under which a complaint about a nurse or midwife may be lodged by a client, member of the public or colleague. Describe these categories and outline the complaint or notification and follow-up process in your state or territory. Try to find some examples of complaints about nurses or midwives and identify the category under which that the complaint/s fell.

FURTHER READING

Allan, S. (2019). *Law and ethics for health practitioners-ebook*. Sydney: Elsevier.

Atkins, K., De Lacey, S., Ripperger, B. & Ripperger, R. (2020). *Ethics and law for Australian nurses*, 4th edn. Melbourne: Cambridge University Press.

Chiarella, M. & Adrian, A. (2014). Boundary violations, gender and the nature of nursing work. *Nursing Ethics*, 21(3), 267–77.

Johnstone, M.-J. (2015). *Bioethics: A nursing perspective*, 6th edn. Sydney: Elsevier.

Numminen, O., Repo, H. & Leino-Kilpi, H. (2017). Moral courage in nursing: A concept analysis. *Nursing Ethics*, 24(8), 878–91.

Starr, L. (2017). Disciplinary action for failing to report an error. *Australian Nursing and Midwifery Journal*, 25(2), 25.

Staunton, P. & Chiarella, M. (2017). *Law for nurses and midwives*, 8th edn. Sydney: Elsevier.

Tedesco-Schneck, M. (2013). Active learning as a path to critical thinking: Are competencies a roadblock? *Nurse Education in Practice*, 13(1), n58–60.

REFERENCES

Atkins, K., De Lacey, S., Ripperger, B. & Ripperger, R. (2020). *Ethics and law for Australian nurses*, 4th edn. Melbourne: Cambridge University Press.

Australian Nursing and Midwifery Accreditation Council (ANMAC) (2015). *Review of the Enrolled Nurse Accreditation Standards: First Consultation Paper*. Canberra: ANMAC.

———— (2019). *Registered Nurse Accreditation Standards*. Retrieved from https://www.anmac.org.au/sites/default/files/documents/registerednurseaccreditationstandards2019_0.pdf.

———— (2021). *Midwife Accreditation Standards 2021*. Retrieved from https://www.anmac.org.au/sites/default/files/documents/06920_anmac_midwife_std_2021_online_05_fa.pdf.

Australian Nursing and Midwifery Federation (ANMF) (2014). *National Practice Standards for Nurses in General Practice*. Retrieved from https://www.anmf.org.au/documents/National_Practice_Standards_for_Nurses_in_General_Practice.pdf.

———— (2019). *ANMF Position Statement: Professional practice framework for nurses and midwives*. Retrieved from https://anmf.org.au/documents/policies/PS_Professional_practice_framework_for_nurses_and_midwives.pdf.

Beauchamp, T.L. & Childress, J.F. (2013). *Principles of biomedical ethics*, 7th edn. New York: Oxford University Press.

Birks, M., Davis, J., Smithson, J. & Cant, R. (2016). Registered nurse scope of practice in Australia: An integrative review of the literature. *Contemporary Nurse*, 52(5), 522–43.

Bryant, R. (2005). *Issues paper: Regulation, roles and competency development*. Geneva: International Council of Nurses.

Cashin, A., Heartfield, M., Bryce, J., Devey, L., Buckley, T., Cox, D., Kerdo, E., Kelly, J., Thoms, D. & Fisher, M. (2017). Standards of practice for registered nurses in Australia. *Collegian*, 24, 255–66.

Chochinov, H.M. (2007). Dignity and the essence of medicine: The A, B, C, and D of dignity conserving care. *BMJ*, 335(7612), 184–7.

Clear, G. (2008). A re-examination of cultural safety: A national imperative. *Nursing Praxis in New Zealand*, 24(2), 2–4.

Cruz, D.M., Pimenta, C.M. & Lunney, M. (2009). Improving critical thinking and clinical reasoning with a continuing education course. *The Journal of Continuing Education in Nursing*, 40(3), 121–7.

de Ruyter, D. (2002). The virtue of taking responsibility. *Educational Philosophy and Theory*, 34(1), 25–35.

Fealy, G. (2014). *National review of the scope of nursing and midwifery practice framework: Final report*. Retrieved from http://www.lenus.ie/hse/handle/10147/323574.

Forrester, K. & Griffiths, D. (2015). *Essentials of law for health professionals*, 4th edn. Sydney: Elsevier.

Gilovich, T. & Eibach, R. (2001). The fundamental attribution error: Where it really counts. *Psychological Inquiry*, 12(1), 23–6.

Hem, M.H. & Petterson, T. (2011). Mature care and nursing in psychiatry: Notions regarding reciprocity in asymmetric professional relationships. *Health Care Analysis*, 19, 65–76.

Holder, K. & Schenthal, S.J. (2007). Watch your step: Nursing and professional boundaries. *Nursing Management*, 38(2), 24–9.

International Council of Nurses (ICN) (2018a). *Code of Ethics for Midwives*. Retrieved from https://www.internationalmidwives.org/assets/files/general-files/2019/10/eng-international-code-of-ethics-for-midwives.pdf.

———— (2018b). *Code of Ethics for Nurses*. Retrieved from http://www.icn.ch/who-we-are/code-of-ethics-for-nurses.

Keast, K. (2016). Taking enrolled nursing into a new era. *Australian Nursing and Midwifery Journal*, 23(8), 20–6.

McCarthy, M. (2003). Detecting acute confusion in older adults: Comparing clinical reasoning of nurses working in acute, long-term and community health care environments. *Research in Nursing and Health*, 26, 203–12.

Morelli, L. (2017). 'Just because I'm Indigenous doesn't mean I'm a drunk': Diabetic woman threatened with removal from bus. *SBS Online* (National Indigenous Television). Retrieved from https://www.sbs.com.au/nitv/article/2017/06/22/just-because-im-indigenous-doesnt-mean-im-drunk-diabetic-woman-threatened-removal.

Muetzel, P.A. (1988). Therapeutic nursing. In A. Pearson (ed.), *Primary nursing: Nursing in the Burford and Oxford Nursing Development Units*. Beckenham, UK: Croom Helm, pp. 89–116.

Nursing and Midwifery Board of Australia (NMBA) (2007). A national framework for the development of decision-making tools for nursing and midwifery practice. Retrieved from https://www.nursingmidwiferyboard.gov.au/codes-guidelines-statements/frameworks.aspx.

——— (2010). *A nurse's guide to professional boundaries*. Retrieved from http://www.nursingmidwiferyboard.gov.au/Codes-Guidelines-Statements/Professional-standards.aspx.

——— (2016a). *Enrolled Nurse Standards for Practice. Retrieved* from http://www.nursingmidwiferyboard.gov.au/Codes-Guidelines-Statements/Professional-standards/enrolled-nurse-standards-for-practice.aspx.

——— (2016b). *Fact sheet: Enrolled Nurse Standards for Practice*. Retrieved from http://www.nursingmid wiferyboard.gov.au/Codes-Guidelines-Statements/FAQ/Enrolled-nurse-standards-for-practice.aspx.

——— (2016c). *Registered Nurse Standards for Practice*. Retrieved from http://www.nursingmidwiferyboard.gov.au/Codes-Guidelines-Statements/Professional-standards/registered-nurse-standards-for-practice.aspx.

——— (2016d). *Fact sheet: Registered Nurse Standards for Practice*. Retrieved from http://www.nursingmidwiferyboard.gov.au/Codes-Guidelines-Statements/FAQ/fact-sheet-registered-nurse-standards-for-practice.aspx.

——— (2016e). *Guidelines for Continuing Professional Development*. Retrieved from http://www.nursingmidwiferyboard.gov.au/Codes-Guidelines-Statements/Codes-Guidelines/Guidelines-cpd.aspx.

——— (2016f). *Professional practice framework for nurses and midwives*. Retrieved from http://anf.org.au/documents/policies/PS_Professional_practice_framework_for_nurses_and_midwives.pdf.

——— (2017a). *Registration Standard: Criminal History*. Retrieved from https://www.nursingmidwiferyboard.gov.au/Registration-Standards/Criminal-history.aspx.

——— (2017b). *Registration Standard: Professional indemnity insurance standard*. Retrieved from https://www.nursingmidwiferyboard.gov.au/Registration-Standards/Professional-indemnity-insurance-arrangements.aspx.

——— (2018a). *Midwife Standards for Practice*. Retrieved from https://www.nursingmidwiferyboard.gov.au/Codes-Guidelines-Statements/Professional-standards/Midwife-standards-for-practice.aspx.

——— (2018b). *Code of Conduct for Nurses*. Retrieved from http://www.nursingmidwiferyboard.gov.au/Codes-Guidelines-Statements/Professional-standards.aspx.

———— (2018c). *Code of Conduct for Midwives*. Retrieved from http://www
.nursingmidwiferyboard.gov.au/Codes-Guidelines-Statements/Professional-
standards.aspx.

———— (2019a). *About*. Retrieved from https://www.nursingmidwiferyboard.gov.au/About
.aspx

———— (2019b). Fact sheet: Professional indemnity insurance arrangements. Retrieved
from https://www.nursingmidwiferyboard.gov.au/codes-guidelines-statements/
faq/fact-sheet-pii.aspx

———— (2019c). English Language Skills Registration Standards. Retrieved from
https://www.nursingmidwiferyboard.gov.au/Registration-Standards/English-
language-skills.aspx

———— (2019d). Policy: Re-entry to practice for nurses and midwives. Retrieved from
https://www.nursingmidwiferyboard.gov.au/Codes-Guidelines-Statements/
Policies/reentry-to-practice-policy.aspx

———— (2020). *Mandatory Reporting about registered health practitioners Guidelines*.
Retrieved from https://www.nursingmidwiferyboard.gov.au/search.aspx?q
=guidelines%20for%20mandatory%20notifications.

———— (2021a). Continuing Professional Development. Retrieved from https://www
.nursingmidwiferyboard.gov.au/registration-standards/continuing-professional-
development.aspx.

———— (2021b). *Nurse Practitioner Standards for Practice*. Retrieved from https://www
.ahpra.gov.au/documents/default.aspx?record=WD21%2f30761&dbid=AP&
chksum=xdi7RHeXbB7YyopbEfd6ag%3d%3d.

Nursing and Midwifery Council of New South Wales (2018) *Professional Standards*.
Retrieved from https://www.nursingandmidwiferycouncil.nsw.gov.au/professional-
standards.

Paley, J. (2015). Compassion and the fundamental attribution error: A reply to Rolfe &
Gardner. *Nurse Education Today*, 35(3), 474–9.

Poorchangizi, B., Borhani, F., Abbaszadeh, A., Mirzaee, M. & Farokhzadian, J. (2019).
The importance of professional values from nursing students' perspective. *BMC
Nursing*, 18(26).

Ramsden, I. (1993). Cultural safety in nursing education in Aotearoa (New Zealand),
Nursing Praxis in New Zealand, 8(3), 4–10.

Richardson, C., Percy, M. & Hughes, J. (2015). Nursing therapeutics: Teaching care,
compassion and empathy. *Nurse Education Today*, 35, e1–5.

Scheffer, B. & Rubenfeld, M. (2000). A consensus statement on critical thinking in
nursing. *Journal of Nursing Education*, 39, 352–9.

Townsville Hospital and Health Services (2016). *Practical guide for clinical partner nurses
and midwives*. Brisbane: Queensland Health.

University of Newcastle School of Nursing and Midwifery (2009). *Clinical reasoning:
Instructor resources*. Retrieved from https://www.newcastle.edu.au/__data/
assets/pdf_file/0010/86536/Clinical-Reasoning-Instructor-Resources.pdf.

13 Being a safe and ethical practitioner

Gina Richards, Joyce Hendricks and Elisabeth Jacob

LEARNING OBJECTIVES

At the completion of this chapter, you should be able to:

1 Explain the terms 'clinical governance' and 'clinical risk'.
2 Demonstrate an understanding of the legal and ethical implications of actions taken in nursing practice.
3 Explore how the registered nurse demonstrates professionalism.

Introduction

Being a safe and ethical nurse in the healthcare environment requires an understanding of various frameworks that underpin and guide nursing practice. A generalised healthcare safety system is implemented to ensure the wellbeing of all those in the healthcare system. This safety system is known as clinical governance. In the healthcare setting, a clinical governance framework ensures that the delivery of health care occurs in a safe environment.

In addition to a clinical governance framework, healthcare staff also work within ethical and legal frameworks that underpin and govern their practice. In a nurse's daily practice, every action is based on the need to make informed decisions, which are based on the nurse's moral and ethical principles, their knowledge and understanding of different clinical situations and the legal accountabilities underpinning nursing practice. To make informed decisions, nurses must be aware of their own personal ethical stance and consider this, together with legal and professional requirements such as the codes of ethics and professional conduct (ICN 2012; NMBA 2018) and the Registered Nurse Standards for Practice (NMBA 2016).

This chapter discusses the frameworks that guide practice. It introduces the concepts of quality and safety, clinical governance, clinical risk, ethical issues and the tenets of professionalism.

Clinical governance and clinical risk

The aim of **clinical governance** is to continuously improve the delivery of client care, ensuring the maintenance of high standards and quality services through systems and processes that minimise **clinical risk**. This occurs when nurses work within the legal boundaries set by state and federal legislation, together with organisational policies and procedures. These organisational policies and procedures are guides for nursing practice specific to an organisation. They contain up-to-date, client-centred information, developed to enable the application of evidence-based practice. Nurses are required to be accountable for their nursing actions and to meet their ethical responsibilities as outlined in the NMBA codes and standards. Through working within these frameworks, clinical risk is minimised.

Research shows that within a healthcare environment, clients may sustain an adverse event. In Australian hospitals, the issue of adverse events was first raised by Wilson and colleagues (1995) and is defined as 'an unintended injury or complication which results in disability, death or prolongation of hospital stay, and is caused by healthcare management issues rather than the patient's disease' (p. 37). Adverse events may include a nosocomial (hospital-acquired) infection such as pneumonia, a urinary tract infection, injuries resulting from a fall or incidents resulting from incorrect medication administration (Davis & Beale 2015; Zanetti et al. 2020). The Australian Institute of Health and Welfare (AIHW 2018, p. 423) reported on clients who had indicated that they had experienced an adverse event during their hospital stay: 'in 2015–2016 576,000 hospitalisations (5.4 per 100) reported one or more adverse events' (p. 423). As some adverse events are preventable, each incident is examined

clinical governance
a generalised safety system implemented to ensure the wellbeing of all people by ensuring that the delivery of health care occurs in a safe environment

clinical risk any variance from intended treatment, care, therapeutic intervention or diagnostic result, regardless of whether an unfortunate outcome occurs (Wilson and Tingle 1999)

to consider how processes and systems could be improved and changed to reduce the likelihood of such an event happening in the future.

Client safety is a broad subject, and here we use it to discuss safety in clinical care. Central to client safety is the commitment of individuals to practising safely and to being responsible and accountable for the care they deliver. Nurses are central to client care and have a professional responsibility to understand and participate in activities to improve client care.

In Australia, the National Safety and Quality Health Service Standards (NSQHS) (ACSQHC 2017) were developed by the Australian Commission on Safety and Quality in Healthcare (ACSQHC) in consultation with the Australian government, states and territories, private-sector providers, clinical experts, clients and carers. The aim of the standards is to protect the public from harm in the healthcare industry and to improve the quality of health services. The eight standards provide a benchmark for the level of care consumers can expect from Australian healthcare providers.

Through audit and accreditation of the eight standards within organisations, performance as an internal quality assurance mechanism is measured and assessed against known benchmarks (ACSQHC 2017). The standards provide evidence-based improvement strategies for healthcare organisations to deal with recognising any gaps in practice that may affect clients.

These eight standards cover:

1   Clinical governance
2   Partnering with consumers
3   Preventing and controlling healthcare- associated infection
4   Medication safety
5   Comprehensive care
6   Communicating for safety
7   Blood management
8   Recognising and responding to acute deterioration (ACSQHC 2017, p. 1).

Through the Australia-wide implementation in 2011 of the NSQHS standards, there have been resultant improvements in the safety and quality of client care, with decreases in the levels of the incidence of various adverse events.

This improvement in client safety and quality of care is achieved through the implementation of a clinical governance framework, utilising processes that identify clinical risk, implementing systems to minimise risk and a quality improvement cycle that is adopted by all staff. There is a public expectation that quality care client safety are central to the nurse's actions.

Clinical governance

Clinical governance is a systematic approach that aims to improve and maintain high standards of care within a healthcare setting. This framework helps all personnel working in a healthcare setting to understand how they can continuously improve the quality and standards of care and implement the principles of best practice for their clients. Initially in 2011, ACSQHC developed a mandatory accreditation system for all public and private health facilities nationally, together with a set of standards to gauge performance and guide improvement initiatives, and as a means to report on safety and quality in the healthcare setting. Nationally, clinical governance structures in health departments and services ensure that regular audits of safety and quality are undertaken. Risk management, with constant monitoring and surveillance of client care activities, provides a measure of assurance for the public and those working in the health industry that a high level of quality and safety will be maintained within healthcare organisations. While the ACSQHC standards emphasise hospital-based services, similar principles, standards and accreditation processes are applied across the healthcare system, including aged care, disability care and community care.

Clinical risk management

The definition provided by the Royal College of Nursing (2000) states that risk management aims to 'develop good practice and reduce the occurrence of harmful or adverse incidents' (p. 19). Risk management is concerned with all aspects of client safety. Any change in the expected outcomes of client care that affects the client negatively may be considered a clinical risk. Clinical risk-management strategies provide systems for the reporting and investigation of incidents, with a resultant understanding of their causes through examination of the errors and complaints. It is a process of investigating and analysing an incident or potential incident; applying evidence-based strategies to a situation to reduce the effect on client safety; evaluating the consequences; and assessing the likelihood that the situation will recur.

Clinical risk assessment is not about levelling blame on an individual, as people can make mistakes. It is about looking at systems and processes and identifying what went wrong and where the process failed. A 'no blame' policy is inherent to such processes. This policy means that the person who made or found the mistake does not have the finger pointed at them for either having made a mistake or reporting it. It is the client's safety that is the main concern, so examining the processes, factors and systems already in place may allow investigators to understand how the error occurred and could have been prevented, or to reduce the possibility of the same error occurring again. Reducing clinical risk is assisted by health professionals undertaking quality-improvement activities. The Western Australian Health Department's Clinical Risk Management Guidelines (2019) state that managing clinical risk is about minimising harm to clients by:

- identifying what can and does go wrong during care;
- understanding the factors that influence this;
- learning lessons from adverse events;
- ensuring action is taken to prevent recurrence; and
- putting systems in place to reduce risks (p. 2).

Risk-management process

Many areas of risk management can be handled at the ward level by staff, and all staff have a responsibility to identify risks and to report them to their manager. This ensures that there is continuous monitoring and improvement in the reduction of risks in the clinical area. This also forms a part of the quality improvement cycle, which results in the improvement of quality client care delivery.

Quality improvement is an important feature of health service management. It follows a basic cycle that includes four steps: (1) set the standards or expectations of performance; (2) audit current performance against these standards; (3) identify areas for improvement and formulate an improvement plan; and (4) implement the plan and re-audit to assess success. These steps facilitate the maintenance of safety and quality of health-service delivery for both clients and staff.

REFLECTION 13.1

Reflect on the following questions and record your responses in your reflective journal or professional portfolio.

- Client safety is important to nursing. Briefly describe an experience you have had in a healthcare setting where you could identify a risk to client safety.
- How could this risk have been avoided?

NURSING PERSPECTIVE

As a registered nurse with 25 years of experience, I can fully appreciate the importance of managing clinical risk. I have seen clients who have suffered due to nurses not maintaining correct standards of practice or trying to take short-cuts. I can remember one incident, when I went into a client's room and found her sleepy in the middle of the day. I had trouble waking her, as she was not responding to my voice. I knew she had diabetes and was on an insulin infusion, so I checked the infusion and noticed that it was on 100 mL/hr. I know that a rate of insulin that high should never be administered (it was ordered at 10 mL/hr), so I stopped the infusion and took the client's blood sugar. It was very low, so she was administered IV glucose to reverse the huge insulin dose she had received. I found the nurse caring for the client, who was a junior nurse and not familiar with insulin infusions. The policy at our hospital for insulin infusions is to have them checked by two registered nurses prior to administration. The ward was really busy, so only the nurse commencing the infusion had checked the rate. Having two people check the infusion may have prevented the potentially deadly incident. This is a clear example of why policies and procedures are implemented in hospitals. The incident caused extra work for the nurse looking after the client and the senior nurses on the ward, so trying to take a short-cut actually caused a lot more work. (Darren, emergency registered nurse)

Multiple-choice questions
Short-answer questions
Connecting with practice:
Clinical governance
Videos: Risks

Legal and ethical issues, strategies and dilemmas

Legal practice

legal requirements requirements from a higher source such as government, which are commands or orders that must be obeyed and are backed by punishments; these are binding, irrespective of personal beliefs

Legal and ethical practice are the cornerstone of professional nursing practice and behaviour. These principles are often intertwined, but they focus on different aspects of nursing practice. **Legal requirements** stem from a higher source, such as government, and consist of legislation, Acts or regulations that must be adhered to; if not, there are civil or criminal penalties. Legal rules are binding, irrespective of personal beliefs.

Nurses work within three tiers of regulation, which provide a regulatory framework for practice. These include federal and state/territory legal regulations; the NMBA codes, standards and guidelines for practice; and the healthcare organisation's policies and procedures. Each state or territory has its own legislation relating to the area of health – examples are the *Poisons and Therapeutic Goods Acts 1964* (NSW) and the *Privacy and Personal Information Protection Act 1988* (NSW) – as well as federal laws – for example, the *Health Practitioner Regulation National Law 2009* (Cth). It is important for nurses to understand that when working in different locations in Australia, the laws that apply in that state or territory may vary, so they need to be aware of the differences and how they apply to nursing practice.

The three tiers of regulation define the standard of care that a nurse should deliver. Nurses are expected to provide a level of care that ensures a client is not placed at risk of harm or injury. This applies to the areas of direct client care, clinical risk management and duty of care, as well as indirect client-care activities such as documentation in the client's notes and client confidentiality. The standard of nursing care delivered is determined by what would be deemed competent practice for a nurse in a similar situation, who has a similar level of skill and experience. Where this standard of care is compromised, consideration is given to the relevant circumstances surrounding a reported issue, examination of the institutional policies and procedures, relevant documentation and any specialist organisational standards. Ethical principles form the basis of legislation, standards and codes, and organisational policies and procedures.

Multiple-choice question

Ethical principles

Ethical principles are the basis for each person's manner of interacting and behaving with other people. Ethics form each person's sense of right and wrong, backed by their moral reasoning, and determine how a person will act in a given situation. Ethics are the rules or principles of conduct and behaviour that are derived from our personal experiences, religious and moral beliefs, cultural background, life experience and social status (Berglund 2019). Ethical nursing practice 'is based on critical, reflective thinking about one's duties and obligations as an individual nurse in relation to clients and as a member of a profession fulfilling a social contract' (Aroskar 1982, p. 23). The social contract is the relationship between the nursing profession and society 'to provide safe care' (Cusack et al. 2019, p. 25).

There are four main ethical principles applicable to nursing: non-maleficence, beneficence, respect for autonomy and justice (Haddad & Geiger 2020). *Non-maleficence* is an obligation 'above all to do no harm', and is the cornerstone of health care, upon which practices and legislation, duty of care, negligence and malpractice are all based. *Beneficence* means to do good or bring about a benefit for an individual. It is a balance of probable outcomes for an action against risk, costs and possible harm. *Respect for autonomy* relates to the individual having choice or the right to make their own decisions. A person may have diminished autonomy (such as with mental incapacitation or illness), and this issue needs to be recognised and considered when making decisions regarding client care. It relates to such areas as informed consent and refusal of treatment. *Justice* relates to being fair with all persons. This can be

ethical principles themes of conduct that are influenced by the personal experience of a person, such as religious beliefs, cultural experiences, life experience and social status

explained as ensuring that all clients are given the same opportunities for care, with one person not being given preferential treatment over another (Atkins et al. 2020; Haddad & Geiger 2020).

Nurses in Australia are required morally and by law to practise within the ethical standards stipulated by the NMBA. These include the Code of Conduct for Nurses (NMBA 2018) and Registered Nurse Standards for Practice (NMBA 2016). Until 2018 the NMBA published a Code of Ethics for Nurses, but these have since been replaced by the International Council of Nurses' Code of Ethics for Nurses (2012). These documents outline the ways in which nurses are expected to act within a nursing context and in clinical practice. These requirements for behaviour and practice are based on the universal human rights of people and the responsibility of nurses to maintain the dignity and worth of all people while in care.

The Australian Charter of Healthcare Rights outlines the human rights of individuals regarding the nature of their healthcare delivery, and is used in all Australian healthcare settings. The document outlines seven client rights: the right to access, safety, respect, partnership, information, privacy, and to give and receive feedback (ACSQHC 2019). While the charter is not legislated, it is an ACSQHC initiative, and sits under the clinical governance umbrella outlining the obligations health professionals are expected to uphold towards clients under existing law, professional codes of practice and employer policies. The document outlines health consumers' rights and gives information about where complaints can be lodged if health consumers feel their rights are not being met.

Ethical dilemmas

In day-to-day practice, nurses may find themselves in situations where their personal code of ethics may differ from the client's ethical values or the organisation's policy, procedures or expected practices. Often, in nursing practice, there is no clear-cut answer, with the available options perhaps resulting in an outcome that is not acceptable to the ethical standards of the nurse (Atkins et al. 2020; Lachman 2016). This is known as 'an ethical dilemma'. To be categorised as an ethical dilemma, a situation must fulfil three separate conditions: the first is a situation in which a person must make a decision about which course of action is best; the second is that there must be different courses of action to choose from; and the third is that, no matter what course of action is taken, there is no perfect solution (Ganz, Wagner & Toren 2014) – that is, at least one of the ethical principles may seem to be compromised. Ethical dilemmas may occur when the nurse feels that they are unable to provide the care they believe a client deserves. This may be due to lack of time, questionable or unsafe practices, or a lack of available resources, thus forcing the nurse to weigh and prioritise care, which may result in conflicting with their ethical values.

How to manage ethical challenges

Strategies for managing ethical challenges include ensuring that nurses are well informed about the ethical standards specified by the NMBA and that they understand how they are expected to practise within this framework. Being familiar with the Code of Ethics for Nurses (ICN 2012) will help nurses to make decisions in difficult situations by assisting them to reflect on their own conduct and that of others to determine whether the standards and values of the nursing profession are being upheld. Through considering the Code of Ethics for Nurses and understanding the health service's vision, values and expectations, decisions on care become clearer. Talking to other nurses about their experiences and how they have managed to reconcile ethical issues also assists nurses to make sense of any discordant ethical issues. If nurses are uncomfortable talking to their colleagues, the use of workplace counselling services may be an option.

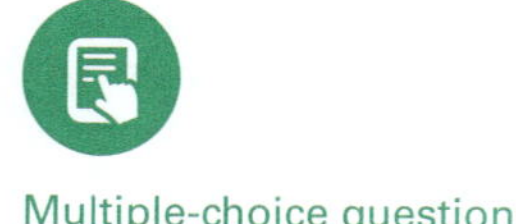

Multiple-choice question

CASE STUDY

An ethical dilemma

Mary is a registered nurse working in a busy surgical ward. She has been allocated the care of two post-operative clients who require analgesia via an intravenous infusion. When taking handover from the recovery nurse for one of her clients, Mary is told that there are not enough intravenous pumps on the ward and that she will have to calculate the infusion rate for the narcotic analgesia via the drip method. Although Mary understands how to use the drip method, she is aware that the hospital's policies and best practice guidelines for a narcotic infusion require the use of an intravenous pump for administration.

QUESTIONS

1 Which of the NMBA codes, standards and guidelines would be useful in determining what your responsibilities as a nurse are in this scenario?

2 What is the term used to discuss the nurse's obligation to work within the three tiers of regulation?

3 What should Mary do to resolve the ethical conflict?

4 To whom could you go if a similar situation occurred when you were out on clinical placement?

Short-answer questions
Video: Ethical issues
Connecting with practice:
Everyday ethics

REFLECTION 13.2

Can you think of ethical issues you may experience due to the culture in which you grew up or the values you hold? How will you manage difference between your ethical beliefs and those of your clients when on clinical placement?

Professionalism and being a professional

The profession of nursing has undergone significant change in Australia over the past three decades. Once viewed as a vocation or a calling that was believed to suit the caring nature of women, nursing has evolved into a gender-neutral profession that views a nurse as a significant, university educated professional in health care. Registered nurses are autonomous in their practice, with knowledge, skills and attitudes that promote client advocacy and client-centred care.

As members of a profession, nurses are expected to demonstrate a level of **professionalism** commensurate with the NMBA professional codes, **standards for practice** and guidelines to which they are accountable and responsible (see Chapter 12 for more details). The NMBA oversees the profession and is responsible for:

- setting criteria for the registration of nurses and midwives
- developing standards, codes, and guidelines for the nursing and midwifery profession
- handling notifications, complaints, investigations and disciplinary hearings
- assessing overseas-trained practitioners who wish to practise in Australia, and
- approving accreditation standards and accredited courses of study.

Since 1994, nurses have topped the Australian Roy Morgan Image of Professions survey as the most trusted profession (Roy Morgan 2021). This survey rates 30 professions according to their ethical and honesty standards. Members of the public view professionals as experts in their field and consider that they have high levels of integrity, abide by professional standards and demonstrate ethical practices. The registered nurse needs to portray professionalism at all times. Some ways in which professionalism can be portrayed are through showing respect for all persons, having excellent communication skills and possessing the requisite skills, knowledge and capability to undertake nursing practice within the frameworks, codes and guidelines described above.

As professionals, nurses are responsible and accountable for their actions to clients, their employer, the NMBA and common law. A nurse exhibits integrity and honesty by standing up and reporting it if they have done something wrong (or believe someone else has). It could be that they have given the wrong medication or forgotten to undertake a treatment; however, they need to be honest and own up to having made the error in the interests of the client's safety. Professor McCardle, the Chief Nursing Officer in Northern Ireland, summed up nursing professionalism by saying, 'Enabling professionalism means doing the right thing, every time, in every environment, regardless of who is or isn't watching' (NMC 2017). Professionalism consists of components that are both observable and non-observable by others.

The image of the nurse

The nurse's image has changed dramatically over time – particularly their attire and appearance (see Chapter 8).

Observable characteristics

Appearance

The first observable component of professionalism in nursing relates to appearance. Nurses no longer wear the white uniform and veil that was the norm in most countries in the past. Today, nurses working in the healthcare environment wear a variety of uniforms or other attire, depending on the dress code where a nurse works. What is expected by the public is a professional who is neat and clean, and who portrays

---

professionalism a demonstration by group members of the shared professional standards and ethical values required to maintain the quality of service the public expects to receive

standards for practice documents specifying the expected practice of a registered nurse; designed to ensure nursing care is delivered in a safe, reliable and consistent fashion

a demeanour of competence (Daigle 2018; Clavelle, Goodwin & Tivis 2013, Sutherland et al. 2013). Infection control, organisational policy and comfort are the primary considerations in the style of uniform adopted by nurses.

Organisational uniform policy considers staff comfort, which may be reflected by the choice of scrubs, or perhaps polo shirts and trousers, as such clothing enables ease of movement while performing nursing tasks. Shoes are generally closed in and made of an impermeable material for work safety. Hair that is shoulder length or longer is generally tied up as an infection-control measure. Jewellery may consist of a wedding band with a flat surface as the only finger jewellery worn. Bracelets may pose an infection risk or possible risk of injury for clients, and are discouraged for these reasons. Watches may be required to be removed when undertaking client care, unless it is a fob watch, which hangs on the nurse's chest out of the way. Necklaces and earrings are also discouraged as a safety risk, as a client in a disorientated state may be able to pull on them. This is also the case with other facial piercings. Infection control is the main principle behind uniform regulations, to ensure there is no compromise to client care. 'Scrubs' are a common choice of uniform in the healthcare setting. Although they may include different colours to delineate professions, it is often difficult for the client to easily discern who is attending them. The nurse needs to ensure that they wear their identification badge and verbally introduce themselves to the clients as a nurse (Clavelle et al. 2013; Sutherland et al. 2013).

Communication

A second observable component of professionalism is communication skills (see Chapter 11). This applies to both verbal and written documentation. The nurse needs to be able to clearly and articulately discuss with the client, their family and colleagues the daily aspects of nursing care, and to document this care appropriately. The nurse's communication skills need to demonstrate that they can change the way they interact with clients, showing consideration of any differences in age, culture and language. Nurses need to be cognisant of how their attitude, tone of voice and mannerisms may affect how the nurse is portrayed. Communicating with members of the interdisciplinary healthcare team in both verbal and written formats is an important aspect of the nurse's role. Nurses advocate for the client with their colleagues, and this is best achieved through respectful, knowledgeable communication with the other health professionals.

Non-observable characteristics

Integrity and honesty

Many professional attributes are not observable; rather, they are internal qualities, relating to the attitude and demeanour of the nurse. Examples are integrity and honesty, which are ethical principles that underpin each person's way of interacting with the world yet are observable only when they become actions. Nursing practice examples may include documenting accurately that client care has been attended to; reporting changes in the client's condition; or owning up to any errors that have been made or where treatment has been missed. These acts rely on the nurse's honesty and integrity. Through demonstrating such honesty and integrity, the nurse shows that they are a trustworthy, collegial team member and a professional. These non-observable internal attributes are very important aspects of a nurse's professionalism.

Respect

Another more intangible characteristic of a professional, visible only through action, is respect. Showing respect for each individual – be they a client or a colleague – no matter what their age, gender, religious beliefs, culture or race may be, is an important aspect of being a professional nurse. All nurses need to understand that other healthcare staff and clients may hold differing viewpoints from their own but that they need to respect the other person's viewpoint and needs. A self-aware nurse (see Chapter 10) who understands their own biases or values and ensures that these do not influence their nursing practice is demonstrating professionalism.

The Australian Charter of Healthcare Rights (ACSQHC 2019), the Registered Nurse Standards for Practice (NMBA 2016), the Code of Conduct for Nurses (NMBA 2018) and the International Council of Nurses Code of Ethics (ICN 2012) all stress the importance of respect for clients. They stipulate that nurses maintain respectful, professional relationships with clients and colleagues.

Professional boundaries

Respecting clients and one's self as a nurse means being aware of professional boundaries (see also Chapter 12). Professional boundary guidelines are established to protect both nurses and clients, as there is a power differential between the nurse and the more vulnerable client (NMBA 2016). If a nurse violates a professional boundary, they are acting in an unprofessional manner. Boundary crossing may cause the client to feel uncomfortable or threatened by the nurse. It may range from disclosing personal information about the nurse's personal life or finances through to sexual misconduct or stealing. The former may occur through a sense of familiarity and trust that has been built up with a client, the appeal of being in a helping role, or simply a general lack of understanding of relevant boundaries (Mendes 2017); in contrast, the latter is harmful – or potentially harmful – to the client because it establishes grounds for exploitation and manipulation of the client (Petosa 2018).

Professional organisation membership

Being a member of a professional nursing organisation, and supporting their profession through their membership and interaction, demonstrates a nurse's professionalism. Professional organisations provide a variety of benefits to nurses, including:

- advocating for the profession to the government regarding policy in healthcare and nursing matters;
- providing opportunities for continuing professional development through their online resources and workshops;
- holding nursing and research conferences, which provide opportunities for networking on a national and global platform; and
- enabling access for members to their journal repositories to help them remain updated with the latest evidence-based practice information.

At a local level, they provide:

- networking opportunities with other nurses through attendance at local events;
- continuing professional development hours available from the talks given by invited industry leaders; and

- personal growth and development through being involved on committees and with events.

In Australia, several professional nursing organisations are available for nurses to join for an annual fee (see Chapter 16). These include large organisations such as the Australian College of Nursing and Sigma Theta Tau. Many smaller, discipline-specific groups also exist, such as the Cancer Nurses Society of Australia and the Transplant Nurses Association. Supporting the profession of nursing is an important aspect of being a nurse. Being an active participant assists in shaping current and future practice and the face of the nursing profession.

REFLECTION 13.3

- Can you think of a nurse you believe is highly professional in the way they interact with clients, colleagues and/or students? Think of the reasons you consider they demonstrate professionalism.
- How can you, as a student nurse, demonstrate professionalism in the academic environment of the university?
- What behaviours or signs would lead you to think that a nurse or a student was overstepping their professional boundaries?

Multiple-choice questions
Short-answer question
Videos: Professionalism

SUMMARY

- Clinical governance is a generalised hospital safety system implemented to ensure the wellbeing of all people by ensuring that the delivery of health care occurs in a safe environment. Clinical governance aims to reduce clinical risk, which is any variance from intended treatment, care, therapeutic intervention or diagnostic result, regardless of whether an unfortunate outcome occurs.
- Legal and ethical practice is the foundation of professional nursing practice and behaviour. Legal implications apply around documentation of client notes, confidentiality and duty of care. Nurses are expected to provide a reasonable level of care in which the client is not put at risk of injury. Nurses in Australia are required to practise within the ethical standards stipulated by the NMBA. These include the International Code of Ethics (ICN 2012) the Code of Conduct for Nurses (NMBA 2018) and the Registered Nurse Standards for Practice (NMBA 2016). These documents outline the expected standards of practice and requirements for practice, and are based on the universal human rights of people and the responsibility for nurses to maintain the dignity and worth of all those for whom they care.
- As members of a profession, nurses are expected to demonstrate a level of professionalism commensurate with the NMBA professional codes, standards and guidelines, to which they are accountable and responsible. Registered nurses are autonomous in their practice, with knowledge, skills and attitudes that promote client advocacy and client-centred care. The registered nurse needs to portray a professional

image at all times. Some ways in which this image is portrayed are through showing respect for all persons, having excellent communication skills and possessing the requisite skills, knowledge and competence to undertake nursing practice within the frameworks, codes and guidelines described in this chapter.

Suggested responses

REVIEW QUESTIONS

1 How do the Australian National Safety and Quality Health Service Standards (ACSQHC 2017) aid in maintaining client safety?
2 Why is maintaining legal and ethical practice important to nursing as a profession?
3 Explain the difference between observable and non-observable aspects of professional practice.
4 Why are professional boundaries important to maintain ethical nursing practice?
5 Outline the four steps involved in the quality improvement process.

RESEARCH TOPIC

How do the NMBA Registered Nurse Standards for Practice demonstrate professionalism, decrease clinical risk and encourage legal and ethical practice?

FURTHER READING

Clavelle, J., Goodwin, M. & Tivis, L. (2013). Nursing professional attire: Probing patient preferences to inform implementation. *Journal of Nursing Administration*, 43(3), 172–7.
Davis, A., Fowler, M. & Aroskar, M. (2010). *Ethical dilemmas and nursing practice*, 5th edn. Englewood Cliffs, NJ: Prentice-Hall.
Lachman, V. (2016). Moral resilience: Managing and preventing moral distress and moral residue. *MedSurg Nursing*, 26(2), 121–4.
Spigelman, A.D. & Rendalls, S. (2015). Clinical governance in Australia. *Clinical Governance*, 20(2), 56–73.
Sutherland, L., Dampier, S., Sevean, P., Seeley, J. & Ellacott, R. (2013). Professional comportment: Nurses, patients and family survey. *Nursing Leadership*, 26(2), 44–58.

REFERENCES

Aroskar, M.A. (1982). Are nurses' mind sets compatible with ethical practice? *Topics in Clinical Nursing*, 4(1), 22–32.
Atkins, K., De Lacey, S., Ripperger, B., & Ripperger, R. (2020). *Ethics and law for Australian nurses*, 4th edn. Melbourne: Cambridge University Press.
Australian Commission on Safety and Quality in Health Care (ACSQHC) (2017). *National safety and quality health service standards*, 2nd edn. Sydney: ACSQHC. Retrieved from https://www.safetyandquality.gov.au/sites/default/files/migrated/National-Safety-and-Quality-Health-Service-Standards-second-edition.pdf.

———— (2019). *Australian charter of healthcare rights: My healthcare rights*. Retrieved from https://www.safetyandquality.gov.au/sites/default/files/2019-06/Charter%20 of%20Healthcare%20Rights%20A4%20poster%20ACCESSIBLE%20pdf.pdf.

Australian Institute of Health and Welfare (2018). *Australian's health 2018*. Retrieved from https://www.aihw.gov.au/reports-data/australias-health.

Berglund, C. (2019). *Integrating law, ethics and regulation: A guide for nursing and healthcare students*. Melbourne: Oxford University Press.

Clavelle, J., Goodwin, M. & Tivis, L. (2013). Nursing professional attire: Probing patient preferences to inform implementation. *Journal of Nursing Administration*, 43(3), 172–7.

Cusack, L., Drioli-Phillips, P., Brown, J. & Hunter, S. (2019). Re-engaging concepts of professionalism to inform regulatory practices in nursing. *Journal of Nursing Regulation*, 10(3), 21–7.

Daigle, A. (2018). Professional image and the nursing uniform. *The Journal of Continuing Education in Nursing*, 49(12), 555–7.

Davis, E. & Beale, N. (2015) It's time: The poor culture regarding safety and quality in Australian hospitals must be addressed! *Asia-Pacific Journal of Health Management*, 10(3), 36–41.

Ganz, F.D., Wagner, N. & Toren, O. (2014). Nurse middle manager ethical dilemmas and moral distress. *Nursing Ethics*, 22(1), 43–51.

Haddad, L.M. & Geiger, R.A. (2020). Nursing ethical considerations In: StatPearls [Internet]. Treasure Island (FL): StatPearls Publishing. Retrieved from https://www .ncbi.nlm.nih.gov/books/NBK526054/.

International Council of Nurses (ICN) (2012). *Code of ethics for nurses*. Geneva: ICN. Retrieved from https://www.icn.ch/sites/default/files/inline-files/2012_ICN_ Codeofethicsfornurses_%20eng.pdf.

Lachman, V. (2016). Moral resilience: Managing and preventing moral distress and moral residue. *MedSurg Nursing*, 26(2), 121–4.

Mendes, A. (2017). Nursing care and maintaining professional boundaries. *British Journal of Community Nursing*, 22(3), 407–8.

Nursing and Midwifery Board (NMBA) (2016). *Registered nurse standards for practice*. Retrieved from http://www.nursingmidwiferyboard.gov.au/Codes-Guidelines-Statements/Professional-standards/registered-nurse-standards-for-practice.aspx.

———— (2018). *Code of conduct for nurses*. Retrieved from http://www.nursingmid wiferyboard.gov.au/Codes-Guidelines-Statements/Professional-standards.aspx.

Nursing and Midwifery Council (NMC) (2017). NMC and CNOs launch professionalism guide. *Journal of Perioperative Practice*, 27(6), 125.

Petosa, S.D. (2018). Maintaining professional nursing boundaries. *Home Healthcare Now*, 36(3), 154–8.

Roy Morgan (2021). *Roy Morgan image of professions survey 2021*. Retrieved from https://www.roymorgan.com/~/media/files/findings%20pdf/2020s/2021/ april/8691-image-of-professions-2021-april-2021.pdf.

Royal College of Nursing (RCN) (2000). *Clinical governance: How nurses can get involved*. London: Royal College of Nursing.

Sutherland, L., Dampier, S., Sevean, P., Seeley, J. & Ellacott, R. (2013). Professional comportment: Nurses, patients and family survey. *Nursing Leadership*, 26(2), 44–58.

Western Australia Department of Health (2018). *Clinical risk management guidelines: A best practice guideline*. Retrieved from https://ww2.health.wa.gov.au/-/media/Files/Corporate/general-documents/Quality/PDF/WA-Health-Clinical-Risk-Management-Guidelines.pdf.

Wilson, J. & Tingle, J. (eds) (1999). *Clinical risk modification: A route to clinical governance*. Oxford: Butterworth-Heinemann.

Wilson, R.M., Harrison, B.T., Gibberd, R.W. & Hamilton, J.D. (1995). The quality in Australian health care study. *Medical Journal of Australia*, 163, 458–71.

Zanetti, A., Gabriel, C., Dias, B., Bernardes, A., Moura, A., Gabriel, A. & Lima Júnior, A. (2020). Assessment of the incidence and preventability of adverse events in hospitals: an integrative review. *Revista Gaúcha De Enfermagem*, 41. https://doi.org/10.1590/1983-1447.2020.20190364.

Professional experience placements

Nick Arnott, Melanie Eslick and Maryanne Podham

14

LEARNING OBJECTIVES

At the completion of this chapter, you should be able to:

1 Describe the purpose and importance of practice-based learning in undergraduate nursing education.
2 Outline various strategies that can help you prepare for, and achieve optimal success in, your professional experience placements.
3 Apply relevant principles and actions to guide 'scope of practice' decisions as a student on placement.
4 Deploy various organisational and time-management strategies and skills to support the quality and efficiency of your placement experience.
5 Explain the role and safeguards associated with social media use in nursing education and practice.

Introduction

In accordance with the standards for nursing and midwifery education, training and assessment, the Australian Nursing and Midwifery Accreditation Council (ANMAC) requires students to engage in a variety of professional placement experiences as part of an accredited program of undergraduate study, with mandatory hours of activity linked to successful learning outcomes and registration to practise as a nurse in Australia (ANMAC 2017; Ford et al. 2016; Schwartz 2019). Clinical placements are therefore a central component of nursing education, complementing the theoretical foundations and simulation-based learning provided at university and fostering the cognitive, technical and interpersonal skills and confidence required for professional practice (Birks et al. 2017; Cummings & Connelly 2016).

Preparing you for professional practice is the overarching goal of nursing education. While professional exposure and practice-based learning are essential for this, your success in professional experience placements depends on your ability to effectively draw upon and translate all aspects of your learning to the clinical practice context and environment. This chapter provides some specific information and strategies to help you understand and succeed in the clinical-practice component of your course but this should be considered in conjunction with all other learning experiences (including reading the other chapters in this book), rather than as a stand-alone topic or resource. The chapter also introduces the rapidly expanding role of social media in nursing education and practice. Although relevant to a range of content areas covered in this book, the focus on clinical placements is considered an ideal time to highlight the obligations and safeguards for responsible social media use as a nurse.

What are professional experience placements and why are they an essential part of your learning?

As a practice-based profession, learning in the clinical environment forms an integral part of nursing education programs. The clinical environment provides an opportunity for nursing students to learn experientially and to translate theoretical knowledge to a variety of mental, psychological and psychomotor skills that are significant for safe and effective person-centred care (Gaberson, Oermann & Shellenbarger 2014; Elbilgahy et al. 2020). This integration of theory and practice *(knowing, doing* and *being),* accompanied by critical reflection and self-appraisal of your performance, supports your progress or transition from 'becoming' a nurse to 'being' a highly capable and professionally accountable registered nurse (Conway & McMillan 2020).

Clinical placements provide opportunities to develop, apply, reflect upon, appraise and improve your cognitive, technical, problem-solving, time-management, documentation and communication skills (Conway & McMillan 2020; Ford et al. 2016). Levett-Jones, Reid-Searl and Bourgeois (2018) suggest that this knowledge pursuit and clinical application represent a continuous cycle of learning (Figure 14.1), in which the knowledge gained through academic pursuits is applied to clinical realities, and areas requiring further knowledge or practice are revealed through critical analysis and reflection on these clinical learning experiences.

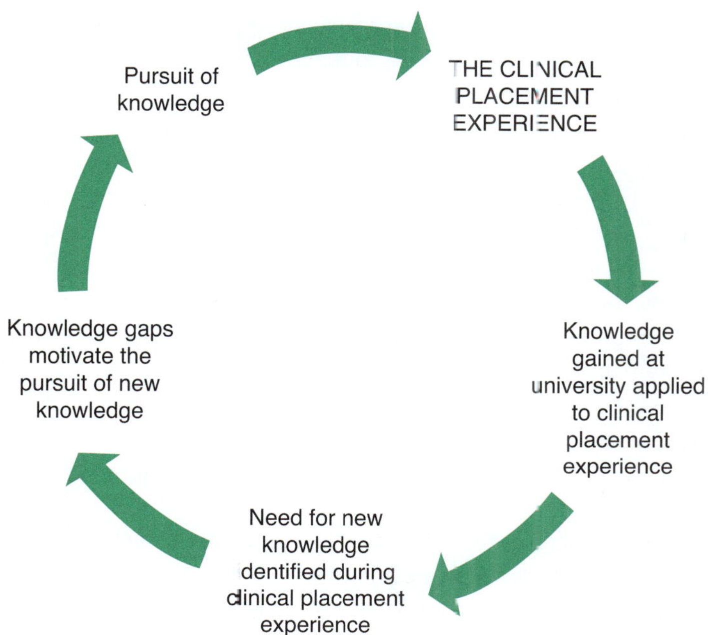

Figure 14.1   The cyclical nature of the pursuit of knowledge and its clinical application

Source: Levett-Jones et al. (2018, p. 5).

The clinical experience component of pre-registration nursing courses is therefore critical to producing reflective, evidence-based practitioners who strive for quality outcomes in the professional practice environment (Birks et al. 2017, p. 21; Schwartz 2019). These placements enable a link between theoretical knowledge and practical application, which is vital for the development of your professional identity and capability as a nurse (Ford et al. 2016; Schwartz 2019; Walker et al. 2014). Clinical placements enable you to immerse yourself in the culture and ethos of nursing, and provide opportunities for professional socialisation, offering realistic and authentic experiences of how nurses think, feel and behave in contemporary practice, as well as the complexities and challenges they encounter (Birks et al. 2017; Levett-Jones et al. 2018). Perhaps most importantly, clinical placements provide opportunities to care for actual clients – to engage with their unique world-views and experiences, and to establish meaningful, person-centred, therapeutic relationships 'underpinned by principles such as trust, empathy, dignity, autonomy, respect, choice, transparency and the desire to help individuals to lead the life they want' (Levett-Jones et al. 2018, p. 7; Stein-Parbury 2018).

Video: Placements

NURSING PERSPECTIVE

My first placement was on a palliative oncology ward. I was looking forward to talking with clients but I didn't know what else to expect. On my first shift, I was assisting my preceptor with an elderly client who was clearly feeling a bit flat – she didn't make eye contact and spoke minimally when we administered her medication. My preceptor had warned me that she'd had trouble forming a therapeutic relationship with this client because she was always 'so miserable'.

Before I left the room, the client asked whether I could wash her hair that day. I'd never bathed anyone before but I gathered my supplies and off we went to the shower, where I hoped I would learn fast. I asked a lot of questions, and by the end we were both drenched and laughing together, and the client's mood completely turned around. I remember thinking that it was amazing how good a hair wash can make someone feel, but also how powerful some chatter and a laugh can be! By the afternoon, the previously bedridden client was up and dressed, wandering down the hall to the common room, much to everyone's surprise.

The next day, I was working with other clients but when I dropped by to say hello the client told me that, many years ago, she had been a nurse too. She then paid me the highest compliment: 'You're very good, you know.' I could have cried – I felt so happy!

That first experience made it clear to me that as a registered nurse my priority would be relationship-building and continuity of care. More importantly, I knew I would be well suited to it. There is no better feeling than working in partnership and sharing a laugh with a client. I now do it daily as an oncology nurse.

REFLECTION 14.1

- What are the strengths you bring to the practice-based learning component of your degree program?
- What are the aspects you are most and least looking forward to?
- What areas (knowledge, skills and/or attitudes) would you like to develop and consolidate further through your exposure to the clinical practice environment?

professional experience placement planned opportunity to put theory into practice, with real people and in real-world settings; clinical placements are designed to build students' knowledge, confidence and professional identity, and to develop and consolidate the capabilities required for registration

block placement a full-time placement for a period of weeks or months, during the study period or over the semester break

distributed placement a part-time placement that operates concurrently with academic classes; the distribution may vary but is commonly one or two days per week over a designated period of time

How and where are professional experience placements provided?

Professional experience placements (sometimes called 'clinical placements', 'practicums', 'fieldwork' or 'work-integrated learning') are usually undertaken across all years of study and are facilitated through **block** or **distributed placement** modes, or a combination (Birks et al. 2017). Research has revealed advantages and disadvantages associated with both block and distributed placement modes; however, Birks and colleagues (2017) found that students' placement experiences and learning success were strongly influenced and determined by individual factors, such as balancing placement expectations with academic workload and other personal, work and family responsibilities, regardless of the placement mode. Achieving a sense of connection and belonging, and feeling accepted, included and valued as a member of the healthcare team, have also been consistently reported by students as being critical to ensuring positive placement experiences and successful learning outcomes (Ford et al. 2016; Paliadelis & Wood 2016).

Multiple-choice question

> ## REFLECTION 14.2
>
> - What do you think are the pros and cons of each of the different placement models – for you, personally?
> - What strategies could you use to help build your sense of connection and belonging in the practice environment?
> - What might you need to consider, plan and do to support your success in the clinical placement program delivered by your institution?

Although some placement decisions are based on pedagogical considerations about how your learning is best served, the climate in which these placements are negotiated is increasingly complex and competitive, influenced by numerous factors that are often beyond the control of the educational institution (Birks et al. 2017; Ford et al. 2016). According to Ford and colleagues (2016), these factors include:

- increased competition for clinical placements across multiple institutions and disciplines;
- constraints on the health setting's capacity to absorb increased student numbers
- limited infrastructure and supervisory resources;
- the availability and preparedness of clinical staff to provide supervision and support
- increased patient acuity;
- diluted skill mix, with fewer registered nurses working alongside enrolled nurses, assistants in nursing and personal care workers;
- escalating staff workloads and
- staff feeling under pressure, unappreciated and unsupported (Ford et al. 2016, p. 98).

The COVID-19 pandemic resulted in these factors being amplified and many placement programs being suspended, deferred or 'reimagined' (e.g. through immersive simulation) in response to logistical and safety considerations (Morin 2020). Many of these factors are obviously outside your direct control; however, having a clear understanding of the context and environment you are entering; being proactive in your learning; and adapting or moderating your attitude, approach and expectations accordingly are important enablers of a positive and successful placement experience.

While ANMAC (2012, 2017) specifies a minimum number of clinical placement hours for accredited undergraduate programs (currently 800 hours), along with guidelines for **supervision** and **assessment** of students in practice, it no longer specifies the types of settings in which placements are to occur. Each educational institution may initiate its own preferences, arrangements and partnerships for the facilitation of professional experience placements; however, most endeavour to provide a broad

supervision all students on placement need to be supervised by a registered nurse; there may be oversight by a clinical educator or facilitator, with day-to-day supervision provided by preceptors, mentors or 'buddy-nurses' from the placement setting

assessment evaluation of your clinical performance designed to enable you to gain a sense of achievement, to gauge your progress and to acknowledge your developing capability for practice; assessment in practice may involve formative and continuous feedback and/or measurement of your knowledge or skills against set criteria, while self-appraisal, peer and supervisor-led assessments may also be used

range of placement experiences throughout the degree program, to reflect the diversity of nursing roles and settings in contemporary healthcare practice. Typically, you can expect to undertake placements in some of the following practice settings or areas:

- general medical or surgical units in public or private hospitals (e.g. cardiac, respiratory, orthopaedics, endocrine);
- specialist or high-acuity units (e.g. emergency departments, intensive care units, coronary care units, operating theatres, renal dialysis, oncology, neurology, and high-dependency units);
- outpatient departments and day-procedure units;
- community and primary healthcare services;
- maternal and child health services, including paediatric, midwifery and neonatal units;
- general practice clinics;
- rehabilitation units or services;
- older persons' services;
- mental health services;
- forensic or prison settings;
- disability services;
- Aboriginal health services;
- refugee health services; or
- rural and remote health services or settings.

NURSING PERSPECTIVE

You are almost certain to have at least one placement in a residential aged-care setting or other service for older persons. Many students initially feel despondent about such placements, especially when comparing themselves with peers who seem to be doing and learning so much more in acute-care environments. However, with the right attitude and a proactive approach, these placements can provide highly valuable learning experiences, for many reasons:

- You get to work with and learn from nurses and personal care assistants who are often experts in many aspects of care that are fundamental to quality nursing practice (e.g. personal hygiene, feeding, pressure-area care, wound management, manual handling, time management and prioritisation).
- You build relationships and empathy with older people, who in fact make up the majority of clients in most healthcare settings.
- You often work directly with people with dementia or experiencing other cognitive decline, which helps to refine your therapeutic and assertive communication skills, and fosters patience, respect and compassion.
- You are taught how to safely mobilise clients without risk of injury to them or yourself.
- You regularly dress wounds such as pressure sores and skin tears.
- You learn about and administer a wide variety of medications for a wide range of conditions.

Achieving positive and successful placement experiences

Most institutions operate dedicated websites or online portals to help streamline the information, compliance, allocation and reporting processes associated with clinical placements. Early access and engagement with such resources are paramount in ensuring your preparation for, and success in, the clinical practice component of your degree program.

Starting out: Safety and compliance

Professional experience placements enable you to put theory into practice, with real people and in real-world settings. Your university and its clinical partners have a duty of care to ensure the safety of students, staff and the people for whom you care. There are several legislative and regulatory requirements that you need to meet before undertaking any placements. These are essential steps towards your future career as a health professional. Compliance is not just necessary for students but is something that every nurse must do to maintain their registration and employment in accordance with the standards, codes and guidelines of the national health practitioner regulation authority (AHPRA) and the Nursing and Midwifery Board of Australia (NMBA), and other relevant national, state or territory regulatory and legislative requirements.

When undertaking clinical placement as a student, the compliance process is designed to protect you and the people for whom you care. It ensures that you are safe *to* practise and helps you to remain safe *in* practice. While many compliance requirements are mandated by national authorities and therefore apply to all nursing students, there may be others specified by your institution that are necessary to meet state, territory or local requirements. As a general rule, you can expect the following requirements to be part of the compliance process for professional experience placements at your institution:

- a national police records check;
- working with children or vulnerable people registration
- current first-aid and CPR certification (a mental health first-aid certificate may also be required);
- current immunisation record or status for specified infectious diseases (this may include COVID-19); and
- medication safety, manual handling, and infection prevention and control training or certification.

Should you have any health conditions or circumstances (or symptoms linked to COVID-19, for example) mandated for disclosure, you may also be required to undertake further health assessment or screening and to have your 'safety to practise' endorsed by a registered health practitioner.

Many of these processes can take some time – for example, some immunisations may involve a course administered over several weeks or months – so it is important that you familiarise yourself with these, and commence the respective processes as early as possible to ensure that all requirements are met within the timelines specified

Multiple-choice question

by your institution. Your entire degree or academic pathway can be compromised if you are not deemed to be compliant to enter practice. It is your responsibility as a student to ensure these requirements remain current throughout your course. Any changes or updates to your information (such as yearly influenza immunisations) should be supplied to your placement team as soon as available.

Along with evidence of compliance, your institution may also require you to read, sign and submit agreements or disclaimers before commencing any placements. This may include a declaration of your medical, physical and psychological capacity to practise safely – linked to a set of 'mandatory functional requirements' aligned with relevant professional standards and regulations. These generally include:

- the *capacity to read* and understand client records, charts, plans, medication orders and labels, and to accurately *write* client notes, charts and reports;
- the *capacity for critical thinking and reflection* to support clinical reasoning and to self-evaluate your feelings, beliefs and practices, and the implications of these for individuals and groups;
- the *capacity to communicate* effectively with patients or clients and colleagues; to accept instruction, feedback and criticism; to question directions or decisions that are unclear; and to resolve any conflict that may arise;
- the *psychological capacity* to demonstrate the professional attributes of honesty, integrity, insight and empathy, to interact with clients, carers and others in a caring and respectful manner, and to exercise self-control in emotionally charged professional situations; and
- the *physical capacity and dexterity* to handle, maintain and operate technical equipment, perform clinical tasks and procedures, and safely assist patients or clients experiencing compromised physical capacity of their own.

Placement allocations and initial preparation

The complexities and constraints involved in the allocation of placements for undergraduate nursing students mean you are unlikely to have much choice about the placement mode/s employed by your institution, and only limited influence over the locations or settings in which these placements occur. It is important, however, that you check your institution's policies and processes for lodging preferences and disclosing any issues up front, so that these can be considered and addressed when placements are being organised. In doing so, you need to think about your specific learning and professional development needs. Some students have (or think they have) a clear idea about the area/s of practice they wish to pursue, and therefore seek placement opportunities in such areas. Our advice is to prepare yourself for a diversity of practice by embracing experiences in a range of different practice areas and settings – especially for your early placements (e.g. first and second year). Try to engage with the diversity of roles, functions and capabilities that are applicable to registered nurses in each environment (e.g. caregiver, collaborator, researcher, teacher, manager, facilitator), so as to extend your preparation and learning beyond direct-care provision and technical skills. Your personal needs and circumstances should also be considered, particularly if these are needs that may affect your ability to safely and successfully complete the placement, rather than general preferences regarding the placement location or setting.

NURSING PERSPECTIVE

I completed my initial nursing training in the hospital system and was convinced (at the time) that this was where I would remain for my entire career. As a new graduate, I was drawn to the fast pace and technical challenges of emergency nursing. I soon found myself working in the emergency department of a children's hospital, which later evolved to a focus on adolescent health, which became the impetus for a subsequent move to the community health sector in a role working with homeless young people. I discovered a strong affinity and passion for community and primary health care, especially the opportunity to support and empower marginalised and vulnerable population groups. This took me overseas, where I spent several years working on aid and development projects across South Asia and the Pacific. Back in Australia, I returned to community health, this time supporting people with a disability as part of the rollout of the National Disability Insurance Scheme (NDIS). By this time, nursing had given me so much, and I decided I wanted to give something back, which led to my next transition – to a nursing education role at an Australian university.

This is just a snapshot of my nursing journey thus far. What stands out to me is that almost everything I have done has been completely different from what I thought I would do, or even realised was possible, when I was a student. My message here is that nursing opens many doors, and it would be a huge shame to close or block those doors too early in your own journey.

Once your placement/s have been allocated, there are some initial considerations, planning and preparation that will help set you up for a positive and successful experience:

- *Where is the placement located?* Is it near home; city, rural or regional; interstate? If away from home, is accommodation provided or subsidised?
- *Do you need and can you get childcare?* Do you have a back-up or contingency plan?
- *What 'type' of nursing is likely on this placement?* Is it hospital or community based? A general or specialty area? Team nursing or mainly solo work? Direct caregiver or care planner/coordinator/facilitator? Fast or slower-paced environment?
- *What types of clients are you likely to encounter?* Older people, children or a mix? Inpatients or day-patients? Acute or chronic conditions? Mental health?
- *What is the workload?* Can you keep doing your paid job? Can you save in advance? Have you negotiated time off if needed?
- *Are there specific learning needs?* Engage in self-reflection on your strengths and limitations; consider feedback or reports from any previous placements; and review materials from any related units of study. Are there particular knowledge or skills you need or would like to develop, practise or consolidate further on this next placement?

REFLECTION 14.3

Regarding the final dot point above, consider developing and documenting some realistic learning objectives for your placement. Sometimes your institution will provide overarching objectives for each placement but try to come up with two or three personal goals for each week, linked to the particular placement context and/or the subject to which the placement is related. Document these goals and regularly discuss and review these with your preceptor or mentor, to evaluate your progress and inform new objectives for the following period.

Try to find out as much as you can about your placement environment in advance, as this will assist you to be as prepared as possible from your first day. Check with your placement team whether it is okay to contact the placement agency and, if permitted, make contact a week or two before you commence to introduce yourself and ask about the arrangements and expectations for the placement. If contact is not possible, review any websites, brochures or other information you can source about the particular organisation or setting. You could also check on social media to find other students who have had that placement or staff who work on the unit, and ask them for advice (being mindful of confidentiality, of course). Some of the things you might want to know include:

- *Hours, shift times and rostering flexibility.* For example, if away from home, can you do an early shift on Fridays so you can travel home for the weekend?
- *Parking/public transport.* What is the best way to get to and from the placement? Is it safe to walk home or use public transport after a late shift?
- *Clients.* Who is a 'typical' client in this unit and what are their common presentations or conditions?
- *Equipment and resources.* Are any specific equipment or resources required for the placement?
- *Revision and practice.* Is there anything you should revise or practise before starting the placement?

Tips for a successful placement

We asked current and former students, preceptors and educators for their top tips for a successful placement. These were their responses:

- Be aware of the facility's (and university's) expectations, guidelines, policies, procedures and key contact people for the placement. Remember, these exist to help you have the best possible (and most successful) experience, and to guide you through any issues that may arise. Your university contacts will be flexible and supportive, but they can only help if you let them know that you need it.
- If relocating for placement, allow sufficient time to settle into your new environment and accommodation before the placement starts.
- Try to get plenty of sleep. You'll be on a steep learning curve so you may be more tired (and/or stressed) than usual. Ensure you have a good diet, especially a hearty breakfast.

- Be involved, enthusiastic and proactive in seeking out learning opportunities. Students can sometimes 'disappear', or say that they are busy doing something else when specific learning or practice opportunities arise. This may be interpreted as a lack of initiative, interest or motivation. It is completely normal to feel nervous or even fearful at times but try to talk this through with your preceptors and educators so that they can provide the support and guidance you require. You need to take responsibility for your learning and be active and engaged in all aspects of the placement experience.
- Maintain a professional approach and work ethic. Be punctual and reliable, and ensure you present to practise in the manner expected (uniform, equipment etc.). Aim to arrive at least 15 minutes early to allow for parking and/or the distance you may need to walk to get to your ward or unit.
- Make time to read client notes from the past few days or a previous visit, to help familiarise yourself with the client's circumstances, plans and status.
- Use a 'planner' to organise your shift. If your facility does not provide such a tool, create your own and stick to it as much as possible. A simple list or table on the back of a handover sheet can work well.
- Think about what you already know and what else you may need to know. Actively seek out and engage with relevant evidence and knowledge to inform your learning and decision-making while in practice. Ask lots of questions. Your preceptors will expect this, and no question is ever considered stupid!
- Keep a notebook. Write down and learn any terms, abbreviations or acronyms used on placement. Keep a list of any medications you see or administer during each shift, and look them up at the end of the day. You are not training to be a pharmacist but having a good knowledge of commonly used medications will help your safety and efficiency in the future. Be sure to record such information in a confidential manner. Only use synonyms or abbreviations that cannot be linked to a specific person. Names, initials, dates, addresses or bed numbers should be avoided.
- Use self-awareness and emotional intelligence to support the provision of ethical, person-centred and culturally competent care (see also Chapter 10).
- Establish and maintain therapeutic relationships with your clients or patients, but remain mindful of privacy, confidentiality and other professional boundaries. Remember that your involvement contributes to client outcomes. Talk to your clients. Ask them about their background and the reasons for being there. Enquire about their experience of being a client and the expectations they have of you and the system.
- Try to write client notes throughout the shift, and watch and practise 'handing over' important information. If it helps your confidence, write a draft of your notes or handover report and have it checked before going ahead.
- Be mindful of the workload of other staff on the unit. Even though the placement is *your* top priority, the registered nurses and other professionals with whom you are working will most likely have other clients and priorities of their own. Try to be respectful of this, especially if you experience some frustration on days when you might feel that your preceptor has not spent enough time with you or you have not had access to the opportunities you hoped for.

- Engage in reflection (both individually and with your peers) – it really is helpful. Make time to think, discuss and write about what you have learnt, done and experienced each day, but be mindful of your obligations regarding confidentiality. List highlights and lowlights, noting how you feel about certain incidents or aspects of your nursing practice and knowledge. Reflect upon your decisions and actions in practice and why these were made or taken. What did you do well? What could have been done differently? What do you need to practise or improve (and how) to address any barriers to success? Where possible, discuss your reflections with your preceptors and seek their feedback to help inform new learning goals and improvement strategies.

NURSING PERSPECTIVE

When I started my first placement on an acute ward, I was worried that my skills (e.g. IV medications, venepuncture, catheterisation) were weak. I decided to be proactive and informed the clinical educator that I would like the opportunity to practise these skills as much as I could during the placement, with any preceptor and any client. On the very first day, I got to insert my first catheter! I was so nervous and shaky, but with guidance and support from my preceptor, the procedure was ultimately a success. About 100 primed IV lines, medication doses and a few successful (and a few missed) bloods later, I realised that I had been hard on myself and that I was in fact very capable – I just needed to step up when opportunities arose to practise and refine these skills. Positive and constructive feedback on my practices and safety from my preceptors definitely helped, too. I received unexpected positive feedback from the clients as well, many of whom said they did not realise I was a student until I told them. A clear sign of my growing confidence and professionalism!

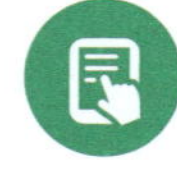

Video: Placement tips

NURSING PERSPECTIVE

One of my clinical placements was on an aged-care ward. A client was admitted, a lovely man, quite energetic when he came in, so I was surprised by his fast decline. His family was with him around the clock. On the third day of his stay, I overheard his daughter tell another nurse that she was worried he did not want to shower, so I took in some hot towels to help him freshen up, and a mouth care tray to show his daughter what to do. When I suggested both, and asked the client's consent, he was pleased and his daughter seemed relieved. I handed the client the towels and he had a quick but dignified freshen up, and then I taught his daughter the steps of mouth care. These tasks took me no more than 10 minutes, but the client's daughter took time to thank me in front of all the nurses that day. The next day her father died, but as she gave me a big hug, she reiterated how much of a difference my help had made to her and her family. Never forget or disregard the needs of family members and loved ones, or the role they play in achieving meaningful client outcomes. Sometimes they just need a job to do in a situation where they have little other control.

Scope of practice

Many aspects of nursing involve enormous responsibility. The outcomes and consequences of certain actions and decisions in practice can literally be a matter of life or death. With the safety of the public in mind, many of the regulatory authorities and frameworks pay particular attention to the profession's **scope of practice**. For nursing, 'scope of practice' involves the full range of roles, activities, responsibilities, functions and decision-making capacity that individual nurses (or nursing students) are educated, competent and authorised to perform (NMBA 2020; Allied Health Professions' Office of Queensland 2014). The scope of practice of an individual nurse may be more specifically defined than that of the profession, with their scope being influenced by the wider healthcare environment; the specific setting in which the nurse works; relevant legislation, policy, education and standards; and the health needs of the population (Levett-Jones et al. 2018; NMBA 2020). In accordance with the NMBA's (2016) Registered Nurse Standards for Practice, scope of practice is not a fixed concept, and nurses are expected to engage in continuing professional development (CPD; see Chapter 13) to update or extend their knowledge, skills and capability for practice.

For nursing students, scope of practice is often thought of as the things you can and can't do on placement. Knowing, understanding and adhering to your scope of practice can be one of the most confusing and contentious aspects of the placement experience. Students often ask why they cannot simply be given a list of things they can do on each placement, but while most institutions will broadly map out the scope of practice for each year of the degree program, different levels of study, practice settings, client groups and clinical contexts make it almost impossible to provide a specific list of roles and tasks. Although you will work under the **direct** or **indirect supervision** of preceptors or educators, you are still expected to be professionally accountable for your own actions and decisions in practice, including any delegations you 'accept' from other registered nurses. Remember, your scope of practice is likely to vary from placement to placement and facility to facility. When making clinical decisions and judgements, key considerations should include the following questions:

- *Have I been 'educationally prepared' for this task?* This may be based on learning at university or education provided 'on the job' by a preceptor or clinical educator.
- *Do I have the capability and support to do this?* Can you effectively integrate the 'thinking' and 'doing' of nursing to safely perform these duties under supervision?
- *Am I authorised to do this?* Is it consistent with relevant legislation, policies, standards or guidelines? Remember, all curriculum and assessment in your undergraduate degree is underpinned by the Registered Nurse Standards for Practice (NMBA 2016), so this should be a key consideration in any scope of practice decisions.

If you are unsure, always seek clarification before making your decision or taking any action.

scope of practice the aspects of practice for which the nurse is educated, competent and authorised to perform

Multiple-choice question

direct supervision when the designated supervisor is present, observes, works with, directs and possibly assesses the student being supervised

indirect supervision when the designated supervisor works in the same area and is accessible but is not always present to directly observe, instruct, support or assess the student being supervised

Short-answer questions
Connecting with practice:
Decision-making
framework

NURSING PERSPECTIVE

On a placement in a rehabilitation ward, I worked as a third member of a team with one registered nurse and one enrolled nurse; there were eight clients between us. It was interesting to watch how the team worked together to efficiently meet the clients' needs by sharing tasks and priorities within their respective scopes of practice. It was also great to work across eight clients, as it put the onus on me to get to know their presentations, some of their history and their immediate needs and plans. The registered nurse monitored vital signs and administered the medications, the enrolled nurse helped with feeding and hygiene, and I floated between the two. Ultimately, working as part of a team meant I was able to learn about all the clients in the section of the ward where I was working and to practise a range of different skills and tasks, rather than taking responsibility for just one or two people. I also felt more confident to ask and answer questions and to prepare and deliver handover: one night I handed over four of the eight clients myself.

Short-answer questions

NURSING PERSPECTIVE

As a student nurse, you may not have experienced death at first hand, so it may be shocking, surprising, terrifying, quiet or uplifting. It may not feel real. If you have lost someone important to you, it may trigger your past grief.

It is important to know that death can be peaceful, and it may come slowly or quickly. Even if the death is shocking – and we have heard stories of students seeing clients bleed out, or semi-conscious clients suddenly throwing their arms in the air, which can be alarming for the family and for staff – it is part of our role to remain calm and to support the client, family and friends through the process.

If you are present when a client dies, remember that the body belongs to a person, and you must respect that person. Sometimes, because you are a student, other nurses might want to protect you from the experience but it is such a key part of nursing that if you feel you can help out or observe, then do so. There are processes to follow, as in all nursing, and you might help to wash the body, or wrap the body in sheets, or clear the room of clutter. Family members might participate, too. You also need to prepare yourself for other nursing tasks that may depersonalise the experience, like placing an ID sticker on the client so they can easily and correctly be identified in the mortuary. There are certain practicalities around death that must occur, including a lot of paperwork. In a busy ward, this may all happen quickly. All the while, the client's family will appreciate appropriate space to grieve, and will likely cry. You might cry too, and so might other nurses, and that is okay: you're allowed to grieve for the client before and after they die. The family will appreciate your empathy. Keep a box of tissues handy and take some deep breaths.

Do not forget that some families have beliefs or follow practices that may be unfamiliar to you, so listen respectfully when they make requests. Some nurses may also hold their own beliefs around death, and these may be front of mind in the moment. Concentrate on being sensitive to the client and the client's loved ones. You can reflect on your own reactions later.

Most importantly, if you feel overwhelmed, tell your preceptor or a nearby nurse, and quietly excuse yourself from the room. Regardless of your reaction or involvement, be sure to discuss the experience afterwards with your preceptor or educator, or a friendly nurse. Journaling can also help to process the heightened emotions that inevitably arise from being present during this extraordinary experience.

And do not forget: just as it is an honour to care for newborn babies, it is a privilege to be involved in end-of-life care.

Organisation and time-management skills

Every day is different in health care and you are likely to face constant and competing demands on your time and attention. These varied, and often unpredictable, demands can make it difficult to identify your priorities, and they commonly contribute to heightened stress, and even burnout over time. Whether it is a change in client needs or status, too many call bells, unscheduled interruptions or the needs of families or co-workers, these priorities and demands will often change rapidly, and you need to be able to constantly reassess the situations, people or events that are clamouring for your attention, and respond appropriately (Elsevier 2016). Following are some tips and strategies for achieving mastery of these essential organisation, time-management and prioritisation skills (Dragon 2019; Elsevier 2016; Leis & Anderson 2020).

Plan your day in advance

While the unpredictable and hectic nature of the environment means this can be easier said than done, even a very loose plan can help you get far more done with much less stress. List the core tasks and activities you need to complete throughout your day and, if possible, estimate the amount of time you will need for each of these. There will be inevitable changes and disruptions but having a plan will help you to be more proactive than reactive, even in the face of unexpected or unscheduled demands. Being proactive might involve a focus on core tasks earlier in the day or making the most of every spare minute you find in your schedule (completing small tasks whenever you can, rather than these accumulating throughout the day). A plan also enables you to schedule time for important administrative responsibilities (e.g. documentation, handover and reporting), which often become an 'add-on' to your day when not considered in advance.

Prioritise: Focus on the most important things first

As you develop your loose plan or schedule for the day, try to rank tasks in terms of their importance. This is not always clear or easy, but prioritising will help you to accomplish the most essential activities for the shift, even if other less-important tasks do not get completed. Prioritisation may help you get through essential tasks first (earlier in the day), but many healthcare activities are actually time-specific (e.g. medications due at a particular time). As such, you may need to consider priorities in two ways: tasks that must be completed at some stage during the day or shift; and priorities for particular blocks of time.

Prioritisation requires conscious decision-making but it is not always easy to choose one task or activity over another. Client safety (the things that are most necessary for client safety and wellbeing) is a key criterion to consider when determining priorities.

Minimise distractions

There are many potential distractions – such as catching up with colleagues or checking social media, personal email and mobile phones – that can consume the time available for other critical tasks. Many healthcare settings do not allow staff to use mobile devices while on shift, but the growing sophistication of these devices means that they are increasingly being used to complement aspects of our work. Either way, it is important that you keep any non-work-related interactions or screen time to your scheduled breaks so that they do not interfere with your professional responsibilities.

Don't let interruptions derail your day

Interruptions are inevitable, but without planning or prioritising, the very first unexpected or unscheduled demand you encounter may very well derail your entire day. Making sense of any interruptions will help you to minimise the disruption they cause. Constantly reassessing the situations, people or events requiring your attention, and re-prioritising your work accordingly, is the key to keeping your day on track. Many interruptions cannot be helped but taking action to minimise some of the avoidable distractions outlined in this section can make a huge difference to your time-management and stress levels.

Keep yourself and your workspace organised

Take a few minutes at the beginning or end of each shift to organise the equipment and materials you require for your work. Keep things clean and ready to use, and try to carry supplies of the things you regularly use (e.g. tape) to ensure they are on hand when needed. Use similar strategies in the client workspace. Use any spare time to restock items that you or the client are likely to need (e.g. gloves, hand sanitiser, tissues, water) so that you do not need to attend to these things when time demands are more critical. Stay on top of your paperwork and other administrative requirements. Try to document in a timely way (as you go) to avoid this becoming an extra burden at the end of the day or shift.

Organisation can also be beneficial when it comes to planning and prioritising your work. For example, changing a client's wound dressing may be deemed a higher priority than assisting them with personal hygiene; however, it may be far more efficient to attend to the hygiene first so as to avoid any inadvertent soiling or contamination of the 'clean' dressing, which may require the task or dressing to be repeated (which could significantly disrupt your schedule).

Be willing to delegate (and to say no)

Effective time management requires you to understand your strengths and limitations, and sometimes this may mean bringing in additional help or resources. You will not always be able to accomplish everything you need to, so whenever necessary, ask your co-workers for help or support. Whether you are giving or receiving a delegation (as a student, delegations will often come your way), you have a responsibility to make sure the delegation is appropriate, clearly understood and accepted (NMBA 2020). Remember, if you are already over-burdened, *it is always okay to say 'no'* when someone else asks you for help.

REFLECTION 14.4

- What organisational and/or time-management challenges do you expect to encounter on placement or in your future practice?
- What organisational and time-management strategies do you already use in your personal, study or professional life? How successful are these strategies? Are there obstacles to using or achieving these? What could you do differently?

CASE STUDY

A 'bad day'

On a third-year placement, I was looking after three clients in a medical ward. One client was a man aged in his late sixties who had recently undergone surgery and radiation for a tumour. His wife told me at the beginning of my shift that they were both having a 'bad day'. The client's mood was gloomy, and he was unenthused about his current liquid diet, but had been told by the dietitian that he was at risk of malnutrition so he had to consume it. His wife was teary throughout the shift. I had worked with them the day before, and we had established a good rapport. Their daughter worked as a registered nurse in the emergency department of the same hospital.

The man's blood pressure had dropped to 94/62, with all other observations within normal parameters. His wife was becoming increasingly anxious, and she called their daughter, who was just leaving her shift, to report the observations over the phone. I told them I was going to take a manual blood pressure reading, and the client's wife started telling me everything their daughter was saying ('He needs fluids!'), in the form of instructions. I asked her, calmly and quietly, to give me a moment, and reassured her that I was doing what needed to be done and that I would ask for a medical review immediately after I had checked the BP manually, which I did. At this stage, I told my preceptor about the situation, recorded the observations and asked the Resident Medical Officer (RMO) to attend as soon as he could.

I continued to explain the situation to the client's wife, who was still speaking to her daughter on the phone, but I wondered whether I should hand them over to my preceptor to do the talking. I knew everything I was doing was within scope, so I decided to continue managing the situation, keeping my preceptor informed. I didn't doubt my own capacity but I was definitely influenced and a little intimidated by the fact that the client's daughter was an emergency department nurse and was giving instructions down the phone, which were making her mother even more anxious.

I knew clearly what I was required to do in terms of process and was confident about implementing that process. I remained calm and polite, reassuring both the client and his wife. However, the man's wife was in tears on the phone to her daughter, so I told them both that I was doing what had to be done, then asked to speak with the daughter. I took the phone to the hallway to advise what I was doing and reiterate that we were on track and that her father was calm. When I told her I was a student, she hesitated a little but I kept speaking confidently about our process and invited her up to the ward.

The daughter came up to the ward, the RMO reviewed the client, a senior nurse inserted a cannula, we administered normal saline according to the RMO's order and I continued to measure blood pressure as per protocol. The client's blood pressure slowly rose back up to within normal parameters. I remained close by and chatted to the family, being sure to advise the client of everything I was doing and why. I usually do this, but I think it was spurred on by the fact that his daughter was there, too. The client said to me later that I was the only nurse he'd had who gave him a running commentary on what I was doing and why. When I described his 117/80 blood pressure as 'beautiful', he laughed, and although his mood was still flat, we shared a few smiles as the shift went on.

Importantly, the man's daughter said I'd done a good job, his wife became calmer, and before she went to dinner she asked if I was on until 10.00 pm because she needed to go home for a rest and knew I'd look after her husband.

QUESTIONS

1 What are the most important capabilities and scope-of-practice issues involved in this situation?

2 With this in mind, how would you approach the situation and what knowledge and/or skills might be necessary for this?

3 Try to revisit the scenario and questions before each placement. How have your responses changed as your scope and capability progress? Are there particular things you would like to learn, practise or improve on your next placement?

Social media: Handle with care

social media the online and mobile tools that people use to share information, network, discuss and debate with others

The Nursing and Midwifery Board of Australia (NMBA 2019) defines **social media** as the online and mobile tools that people use to 'share opinions, information, experiences, images and video or audio clips', including social networking sites such as Facebook and LinkedIn, personal and professional blogs, micro-blogs such as Twitter, content-sharing websites such as YouTube and Instagram, and discussion forums and message boards.

The use of social media by health professionals and, perhaps more critically, *in health care*, has been somewhat contentious. While individuals and organisations are embracing user-generated e-content, concerns about privacy, integrity, safety and reputation have led some to conclude that social media has no place in the health professions. These voices of dissent are rapidly being overwhelmed by the sheer weight of numbers. More than 75 per cent of adults online use social media (Rozenblum, Greaves & Bates 2017), and there is increasing evidence demonstrating the positive influence of these platforms on client, provider and health-system outcomes (Hay 2020; Ferguson 2013; Smailhodzic et al. 2016).

Our professional roles form a significant part of our 'lived experience', and thus it is inevitable that health professionals will make use of these technologies to share information and knowledge, meet and network with contacts, and engage in discourse and debate about their work (Morley & Chinn 2015). There is now a growing evidence base showing that social media and other e-health platforms can play an important and beneficial role in healthcare education and practice, including blended and simulation-based learning (Green, Wyllie & Jackson 2014; Usher et al. 2014); continuous professional development (Morley & Chinn 2015); clinical supervision (Mather, Marlow & Cummings 2013); research and evidence-based practice (Mannix, Wilkes & Daly 2014); clinical information and advice (Appelton, Fowler & Brown 2014); health promotion and self-management (Appelton, Fowler & Brown 2014; Bottorff et al. 2014); peer and social support (Nambisan et al. 2015); and client-experience and quality-improvement endeavours (Nambisan et al. 2015; Rozenblum, Greaves & Bates 2017).

In leveraging these benefits, health professionals (including students) need to maintain professional standards and be aware of the implications of their actions, as is the case for all professional circumstances (NMBA 2019). In response to this, regulatory and professional organisations such as the NMBA, the International Nurse Regulator Collaborative (INRC) and the Australian College of Nursing (ACN) have released policies and guidelines to help guide the ethical and responsible use of social media by nurses and other health professionals, as outlined here (ACN 2015; NMBA 2019; INRC 2014):

- *Benefits and risks.* Understand the advantages and risks of using social media. Acquire skills to use the technology and develop the necessary abilities and judgement to use it properly. Consider social media's constantly changing culture and technology. Continually reflect on the purpose and possible consequences of your online behaviour before you post or send anything.
- *Professional image.* Maintain the same level of professionalism in your online exchanges as in your face-to-face interactions. Keep your personal and professional lives separate by using different accounts.
- *Confidentiality.* Do not share any client information on social media sites. Remember that simply removing names or other identifying details when you post information about a client does not necessarily protect client confidentiality. If you see a confidentiality breach, report it immediately.
- *Privacy.* Protect your own privacy by setting your privacy settings to limit the information you share. No matter what privacy settings you use, it is possible

for other people to duplicate and share your personal information without your knowledge or permission, so things you circulate on social media may find their way into the public domain, irrespective of your original intentions. In such cases, it may well be you, as the original author, who is accountable for any breaches of privacy.

- *Boundaries.* Uphold professional boundaries online by setting and communicating these boundaries for any client interactions. If you interact with clients on social media (there may be a legitimate rationale for this), create a separate professional account for this.
- *Expectations.* Be careful about revealing your identity as a nurse or health professional online. This could lead to others asking for advice, which could confuse the professional relationship. Remember that changing your name online to one that hides your professional identity does not always safeguard you from encountering clients online.
- *Integrity.* Protect your own and nursing's integrity. Do not use social media as a forum to discuss, report and resolve workplace issues. Treat patients, clients and colleagues with the same respect online as you would in person. Before you publicly share information about your profession, your workplace or your colleagues, reflect on your intentions and the possible ramifications. Know that 'liking' someone's disrespectful comments is no different from making one yourself.
- *Organisational policies.* Make sure you are aware of and follow organisational policies concerning social media apps, photographs, computers and mobile devices, including the use of these platforms and devices at work.
- *Accountability.* Take responsibility for your actions. Consider why, how and when you use social media, and encourage your colleagues to do the same. Use your professional judgement and always remember your obligations to clients, colleagues, employers and the public.

Video: Social media policies
Multiple-choice question

REFLECTION 14.5

- What applications, benefits and potential risks do you think the use of social media has for nursing in general, and for your placement settings in particular?
- How will you regulate your social media use as a nursing student (and future registered nurse), and how would you respond to any professional misconduct you may witness by others?

SUMMARY

- Learning in the clinical or practice environment is an integral part of nursing education programs, with professional experience placements being undertaken throughout the degree. The clinical environment allows nursing students to learn experientially and to convert or apply theoretical knowledge to a variety of cognitive, psychological and psychomotor skills that are of significance for safe and effective client care, including cognitive, technical, problem-solving, time-management, documentation and communication skills (Jamshidi et al. 2016). This integration of theory and practice *(knowing, doing* and *being),* accompanied by critical reflection and self-appraisal of your performance, supports your progress or transition from 'beginning student' to a highly capable and professionally accountable registered nurse.

- Clinical placements also enable you to immerse yourself in the culture and ethos of nursing, and provide opportunities for professional socialisation, offering realistic and authentic experiences of how nurses think, feel and behave in contemporary practice, as well as the complexities and challenges they encounter. Perhaps most importantly, clinical placements provide opportunities to care for actual clients – to engage with their unique world-views and experiences, and to establish meaningful, person-centred, therapeutic relationships.

- This chapter has provided a range of information, tips and strategies to help you to prepare for and succeed in your professional experience placements. Safety and compliance, initial planning and preparation, scope of practice, applied learning and skill development, time-management and organisational skills, and communication and feedback have all been discussed.

- While individuals and organisations are rapidly embracing e-content, concerns about privacy, integrity, safety and reputation have led some to conclude that there is no place for social media in the health professions. These voices of dissent are rapidly being overwhelmed by the sheer weight of numbers, with more than 75 per cent of adults online using social media.

- Our professional roles form a significant part of our 'lived experience', and thus it is inevitable that health professionals will make use of social media and other related technologies to share information and knowledge, to meet and network with contacts, and to engage in discourse and debate about their work. There is now a growing evidence base showing that social media and other e-health platforms can play an important and beneficial role in healthcare education and practice, having a positive influence on client, provider and health-system outcomes.

- In leveraging these benefits, health professionals (including students) need to maintain professional standards and be aware of the implications of their actions. Various regulatory and professional organisations have released policies and guidelines to help guide the ethical and responsible use of social media by nurses and other health professionals, as summarised in this chapter.

REVIEW QUESTIONS

Suggested responses

1 What are some of the core safety and compliance requirements that your institution is likely to expect before you can enter the practice environment?
2 What are the three key considerations when making 'scope of practice' decisions?
3 Being a reflective practitioner is integral to your continuous learning and development. How might you develop and apply your reflective practice skills while on placement?
4 What are some of the strategies you could adopt to better manage your time on placement?
5 How can you ensure responsible use of social media as a student nurse on placement?

RESEARCH TOPIC

This chapter has outlined some of the core information, considerations and strategies associated with professional experience placements; however, each university has its own systems, processes, requirements and expectations. It is critical that you thoroughly research or review these things as early as you can to ensure you are absolutely clear about how this component of your course will operate and what is expected of you before, during and after these placements.

FURTHER READING

Collegian (2014). Special issue on social media and nursing. *Collegian*, 21(2), 79–168.

Levett-Jones,T., Reid-Searl, K. & Bourgeois, S. (2018) *The clinical placement: An essential guide for nursing students*, 4th edn. Sydney: Elsevier.

Nursing and Midwifery Board of Australia (NMBA) (2019). *Social media: how to meet your obligations under national law*. Available from https://www .nursingmidwiferyboard.gov.au/Codes-Guidelines-Statements/Codes-Guidelines/ Social-media-guidance.aspx.

REFERENCES

Allied Health Professions' Office of Queensland (2014). *Ministerial taskforce on health practitioner expanded scope of practice: Final report*. Brisbane: Queensland Government.

Appelton, J., Fowler, C. & Brown, N. (2014). Friend or foe? An exploratory study of Australian parents' use of asynchronous discussion boards in childhood obesity. *Collegian*, 21(2), 151–8.

Australian College of Nursing (ACN) (2015). *Social media guidelines for nurses*. Canberra: ACN.

Australian Nursing and Midwifery Accreditation Council (ANMAC) (2012). *Registered Nurse Accreditation Standards 2012*. Retrieved from https://www.anmac.org.au/ sites/default/files/documents/ANMAC_RN_Accreditation_Standards_2012.pdf.

——— (2017). *National Accreditation Guidelines: Nursing and midwifery education programs*. Retrieved from https://www.anmac.org.au/sites/default/files/ documents/National_Accreditation_Guidelines_1.0.pdf.

Birks, M., Bagley, T., Park, T., Burkot, C. & Mills, J. (2017). The impact of clinical placement model on learning in nursing: A descriptive exploratory study. *Australian Journal of Advanced Nursing*, 34(3), 16–23.

Bottorff, J.I., Struik, L.L., Bissell, L.J., Graham, R., Stevens, J. & Richardson, G.S. (2014). A social media approach to inform youth about breast cancer and smoking: An exploratory descriptive study. *Collegian*, 21(2), 159–68.

Conway, J. & McMillan, M. (2020). Professional career development: Development of the CAPABLE nursing professional. In E. Chang & J. Daly (eds), *Transitions in nursing: Preparing for professional practice*, 5th edn. Sydney: Elsevier.

Cummings, C.L. & Connelly, L.K. (2016). Can nursing students' confidence levels increase with repeated simulation activities? *Nurse Education Today*, 36, 419–21.

Dragon, N. (2019). 10 time management tips for nurses and midwives. *Australian Nursing and Midwifery Journal,* 1 August. Retrieved from https://anmj.org.au/10-time-management-tips.

Elbilgahy, A.A., Abdou Eltaib, F. & Lawend, J. (2020) Challenges facing clinical nurse educators and nursing students in Egyptian and Saudi clinical learning environment: A comparative study, *International Journal of Africa Nursing Studies,* 13, 1–7.

Elsevier (2016). Important time-management tips for nurses (Blog post). *Connect.* Retrieved from http://www.confidenceconnected.com/blog/2016/02/09/important-time-management-tips-for-nurses.

Ferguson, C. (2013). It's time for the nursing profession to leverage social media. *Journal of Advanced Nursing,* 69(4), 745–7.

Ford, K., Courtney-Pratt, H., Marlow, A., Cooper, J., Williams D. & Mason, R. (2016). Quality clinical placements: The perspectives of undergraduate nursing students and their supervising nurses. *Nurse Education Today,* 37, 97–102.

Gaberson, K.B., Oermann, M.H. & Shellenbarger, T. (2014). *Clinical teaching strategies in nursing.* New York: Springer.

Green, J., Wyllie, A. & Jackson, D. (2014). Virtual worlds: A new frontier for nurse education. *Collegian,* 21(2), 135–41.

Hay, B. (2020). How social media could drive better care. *The Hive,* 30(Winter), 10–11.

International Nurse Regulator Collaborative (INRC) (2014). *Position statement – social media use: Common expectations for nurses.* Retrieved from https://www.crnbc.ca/Standards/Lists/StandardResources/INRCSocialMediaUseCommonExpectforNurses.pdf.

Jamshidi, N., Molazem, Z., Sharif, F., Torabizadeh, C. & Najafi Kalyani, M. (2016). The challenges of nursing students in the clinical learning environment: A qualitative study. *The Scientific World Journal,* doi: 10.1155/2016/1846178.

Leis, S. & Anderson, A. (2020). Time management strategies for new nurses. *American Journal of Nursing,* 120(12), 63–6.

Levett-Jones, T., Reid-Searl, K. & Bourgeois, S. (2018). *The clinical placement: An essential guide for nursing students,* 4th edn. Sydney: Elsevier.

Mannix, J., Wilkes, L. & Daly, J. (2014). Pragmatism, persistence and patience: A user perspective on strategies for data collection using popular online social networks. *Collegian,* 21(2), 127–33.

Mather, C., Marlow, A. & Cummings, E. (2013). Digital communication to support clinical supervision: Considering the human factors. *Studies in Health Technology and Informatics: Context Sensitive Health Informatics – Human and Socio-technical Approaches,* 194, 160–5.

Morin, K.H. (2020). Nursing education after COVID-19: Same or different? *Journal of Clinical Nursing,* 29(17–18), 3117–19.

Morley, C. & Chinn, T. (2015). Using social media for continuous professional development. *Journal of Advanced Nursing,* 71(4), 713–17.

Nambisan, P., Gustafson, D.H., Hawkins, R. & Pingree, S. (2015). Social support and responsiveness in online communities: Impact on service quality perceptions. *Health Expectations,* 19, 87–97.

Nursing and Midwifery Board of Australia (NMBA) (2016). *Registered Nurse Standards for Practice.* Retrieved from https://www.nursingmidwiferyboard.gov.au/codes-guidelines-statements/professional-standards/registered-nurse-standards-for-practice.aspx.

—— (2019) *Social Media: How to meet your obligations under national law*. Retrieved from https://www.nursingmidwiferyboard.gov.au/Codes-Guidelines-Statements/Codes-Guidelines/Social-media-guidance.aspx.

—— (2020). *Decision Making Framework for Nursing and Midwifery*. Retrieved from https://www.nursingmidwiferyboard.gov.au/Codes-Guidelines-Statements/Frameworks.aspx.

Paliadelis, P. & Wood, P. (2016). Learning from clinical placement experience: Analysing nursing students' final reflections in a digital story-telling activity. *Nurse Education in Practice*, 20, 39–44.

Rozenblum, R., Greaves, F. & Bates, D. (2017). The role of social media around patient experience and engagement. *BMJ Quality and Safety*, 26(10), 845–8.

Schwartz, S. (2019). *Educating the nurse of the future: Report of the independent review of nursing education*. Canberra: Australian Government Department of Health.

Smailhodzic, E., Hooijsma, W., Boonstra, A. & Langley, D. (2016). Social media use in healthcare: A systematic review of effects on patients and on their relationships with health professionals. *BMC Health Services Research*, 16(1), 1–14.

Stein-Parbury, J. (2018). *Patient and person: Interpersonal skills in nursing*, 6th edn. Sydney: Elsevier.

Usher, K., Woods, C., Casella, E., Glass, N., Wilson, R., Mayner, L., Jackson, D., Brown, J., Duffy, E., Mather, C., Cummings, E. & Irwin, P. (2014). Australian health professions' student use of social media. *Collegian*, 21(2), 95–101.

Walker, S., Dwyer, T., Broadbent, M., Moxham, L. & Sander, T. (2014). Constructing a nursing identity within the clinical environment: The student nurse's experience. *Contemporary Nurse: A Journal of the Australian Nursing Profession*, 49(1), 103–12.

PART 3

Being

15 Being a member of an interprofessional team

David Stanley and Karen Stanley

LEARNING OBJECTIVES

At the completion of this chapter, you should be able to:

1 Discuss the principles of interprofessional communication and outline the five competencies of interprofessional collaborative practice.
2 Apply handover frameworks to enhance the transmission of healthcare information to other professionals.
3 Understand the value of teamwork and describe how a registered nurse can participate effectively within interprofessional teams to ensure integrated services.
4 Recognise and understand your own reactions to conflict, and develop strategies for dealing with conflict between colleagues and interprofessional teams.
5 Appreciate the role, responsibilities and competence of your own professional development and the professional development of others in the health service care and provision arenas, through peer learning and mentoring.

Introduction

Communication is recognised as an important factor in interprofessional collaboration and teamwork. The delivery of optimal, person-centred care 'requires healthcare professionals to effectively communicate, cooperate and collaborate with each other' (Stanley & Stanley 2019, p. 63). Interprofessional communication can ensure that information is shared with a collective purpose and clearly defined goals. Thomson and colleagues (2015) demonstrated that having a shared purpose to pursue quality improvement as well as collaboration provides a framework for interprofessional, person-centred care that is highly dependent on effective communication. This chapter outlines the principles of interprofessional communication as well as five competencies that can contribute to collaborative practice. Handover frameworks are explored, along with the value of teamwork. The chapter also examines how nurses and other health professionals recognise and understand conflict, and discusses strategies for managing difficult situations. Finally, professional development is explored through peer learning, mentoring and supervision, with some examples of how this can be achieved.

Communication

The effectiveness of care for clients with complex and long-term conditions is strongly influenced by the quality of communication and the professional relationships of healthcare professionals. It is therefore necessary for them to work together collegially and to ensure that information is communicated effectively. Using effective communication techniques helps to gain cooperation from other professionals while maintaining professional boundaries, and therefore promotes collaborative practice (Brownie, Scot & Rossiter 2016). Professional relationships refer to an alliance between any healthcare professionals, with relationships that are based on a set of boundaries that are deemed appropriate under governing standards (Weller, Boyd & Cumin 2014). According to the Registered Nurse Standards for Practice (NMBA 2016a), it is important that nurses engage in therapeutic and professional relationships within interprofessional teams. This can be achieved through professional collaboration, which can assist with reducing barriers, thereby improving client health outcomes (NMBA 2016a, Standard 2).

Governing standards

Along with other healthcare professions in Australia, nursing is regulated by national law. This refers to the *Health Practitioner Regulation National Law Act 2009* as enacted by the states and territories (see Queensland Government 2009), and provides the legal requirements for registration of health professionals (Berman et al. 2017). In addition, nurses are further regulated and governed by the NMBA, which has approved standards of practice, accompanied by professional codes and guidelines that form the basis of safe and competent practice (NMBA 2018). By adhering to these standards, the nurse ensures the safe delivery of high-quality care and fosters an environment of interprofessional engagement and collaboration between members of the healthcare team (Reeves 2016). The continual process of decision-making for client care can only be achieved through personal accountability and a commitment to uphold the professional regulatory standards of practice for nursing (NMBA 2016a).

Interprofessional competencies

Garvis and colleagues (2016) support the view that competent **collaboration** is necessary to the provision of person-centred care, and discuss key and core competencies in the context of what it takes to be a good collaborator (Stanley & Stanley 2019). Key and core competencies such as trust, respect, effective **communication**, shared knowledge and understanding are identified as essential, because these qualities are needed to build effective **interprofessional** relationships (Stanley & Stanley 2019).

Competency frameworks and clear educational pathways (Rossler et al. 2017) have also been viewed as a way to identify and promote interprofessional competencies.

A recent study undertaken by Stadick (2020) acknowledges the original interprofessional competency framework designed by Bainbridge and colleagues (2010), by confirming the importance of attitudes and collaborative competencies for healthcare professionals such as nurses, doctors and respiratory specialists. According to the health professionals in this study, successful teamwork leads to better client health outcomes due to them collaborating and maintaining their interprofessional relationships (Stadick 2020).

In relation to collaborative practice, the goals are client safety and quality care, which are achieved by effective communication and by:

- *Team work:* Working effectively with other health professionals to achieve the goals of interprofessional practice and person-centred care.
- *Role clarification:* Being clear about each professional's specific role in the clinical team.
- *Conflict resolution:* Actively addressing various points of contention between colleagues and clients in a constructive manner. Also, conducting an appraisal of their role and responsibilities and competencies of their own profession and others in the provision of care.
- *Reflection:* Reviewing practice in order to identify gaps in knowledge and skills and plan strategies that will improve future practice.

Brewer and Flavell (2018) found that these are the competencies that are relevant to interprofessional collaboration and effective communication. Another element that needs to be mentioned in relation to communication is the specific terminology, or jargon, that professionals use 'to describe health practices or apply healthcare principles' (Stanley 2016). Participants in a study by Stanley (2016) highlighted the importance of using a common language that could be understood by all health professionals to ensure that errors were minimised. This is because if the language is significantly different, there is potential for confusion, and this may create barriers between professionals. Therefore, sharing a common language can assist with building effective interprofessional relationships (Rossler et al. 2017; Stanley & Stanley 2019).

collaboration the effective interaction of two or more professionals in health or social care to achieve an optimal outcome for their client or patient

communication the process of transferring information from one person or place to another, using verbal, written or visual methods (Birks, Chapman & Davis 2015, p. 159)

interprofessional two or more professionals in health or social care acting together to achieve an optimal outcome for their client or patient

Short-answer question

Short-answer question

Interpersonal skills

Effective interpersonal skills such as paraphrasing and repeating information for clarity are just two of the ways in which professionals can demonstrate that they are listening and understanding the messages being conveyed. Using positive body language is also useful in reinforcing that the information that is being shared has been received and understood correctly (Brownie, Scot & Rossiter 2016). Transparency and honesty are also qualities that health professionals value, especially as they support the building of respectful professional relationships to encourage collegiality. While Stanley (2016) supported these qualities, honesty appears to be an essential building block for many of the other qualities, as it is attributed to the promotion of trust. Positive results can also be achieved by being open to the other professionals' ideas and engaging in conversations with an attitude of interest and tolerance, and an absence of judgement.

Communication can have a cascading effect, especially in terms of its influence on individuals and interprofessional teams. The quality of communication needs to be clear because it can influence a professional's ability to engage in collaborative health activities. The aim of effective communication is to build rapport with other professionals, which encourages positive interprofessional relationships while maintaining the quality and safety of person-centred care (ACSQHC 2017; Eggins, Slade & Geddes 2016). Brownie and colleagues (2016) also recognised the importance of effective communication within chronic-care practice settings. This is because nurses are not just interacting with clients who have complex and chronic comorbid conditions, but are also part of a multidisciplinary team that includes doctors, social workers, physiotherapists and psychologists. As Brownie and colleagues (2016) asserted, if communication is not effective, it can undermine both professional relationships and the therapeutic relationship, and the quality of care provided to clients, carers and families.

Short-answer question

NURSING PERSPECTIVE

Kim, a registered nurse, listened to the handover tape and discovered that she would be working with the shift coordinator as they were short staffed. She and the shift coordinator had six children to care for in their client load. One was an 11-year-old named Bethany. The tape covered much of the essential care for all six clients but additional information had been handed over verbally, which Kim had missed. The coordinator, Lisa, failed to pass this on. Primarily, it related to Bethany's mother's religious beliefs and a discreet move by the medical team to make Bethany a ward of the state.

Kim decided to check on the welfare of all six clients. Bethany had newly diagnosed acute lymphocytic leukaemia (ALL), and she had recently developed a serious chest infection. To Kim's surprise, Bethany was not receiving any medications and had no IV line. She also found Bethany in her mother's arms, being rocked gently. Kim noticed that on Bethany's medication chart she was written up for IV antibiotics.

'Has Bethany had these medications yet?' Kim asked Bethany's mother.

'Oh no, our religious beliefs don't agree with the administration of drugs of any kind, and I have not allowed it,' the mother replied politely.

Kim thought Bethany looked flushed.

'Can I take her temperature?' Kim asked.

It was 38.9°C.

'Can I give her some paracetamol for her high temperature?' Kim asked.

'No,' said Bethany's mother. 'As I explained, in our religion the use of medications of any kind is forbidden.'

Kim asked if Bethany's mother would use a cool sponge cloth to help cool down Bethany's temperature. Her mother agreed and took the cloth.

Kim was not sure what else to do about the pyrexia, and spoke to Lisa about her concerns. Lisa explained that the doctors were aware of the situation and had sought a court order to compel Bethany's mother to release her into the care of the hospital and to forbid the mother and close family from having contact with Bethany while they treated the chest infection and underlying ALL with aggressive treatments. The doctors had tried to reason with Bethany's mother and were now discreetly planning to treat the child without the mother's consent. Lisa suggested that when Bethany's mother went to the toilet, she should give Bethany some paracetamol for her high temperature. Kim refused, so Lisa asked whether Kim would give Bethany some ice cream, to which Lisa would add some paracetamol solution. Again, Kim refused; she was now very uncomfortable about the unprofessional and inappropriate treatment suggestions of the more senior registered nurse but was too worried to speak to Lisa about it. She was soon in tears in the face of the dilemma. Tony, another registered nurse on the ward, noticed that Kim was distressed and asked her what had happened. Once he was informed of the situation, he spoke with Lisa about her inappropriate requests and supported Kim in her actions.

REFLECTION 15.1

Short-answer question

There are many medico-legal and ethical issues in this scenario. But how might the scenario have played out if Kim had been unable to discuss her concerns with Tony, or if Tony had been unable to offer advice and support?

Handover frameworks

handover a structured approach to transferring information so that the transfer of professional responsibility and accountability for some or all of the client's care can be passed on to other health professionals

Handover standardisation is supported by current literature (Hada, Jack & Coyer 2019; ACSQHC 2017; Eggins, Slade & Geddes 2016). According to Anderson and colleagues (2015), communication tools such as ISBAR (identify/introduce, situation, background, assessment, recommendations; see Chapter 11) have been used to assist professionals to transfer health information successfully and provide continuity of care for clients. Handover frameworks such as ISBAR and the variation, ISOBAR (identification of patient and self; situation and status; observation; background and history; assessment and actions; responsibility, risk management and read-back), have provided healthcare professionals with communication tools to help structure client reports, which can be transmitted efficiently to other professionals. This type of handover has led to improved quality in client care, as it has prevented potential harm to individuals using healthcare facilities by ensuring that accurate and timely information is communicated to members of the healthcare team (ACSQHC 2017, Action 6.7). Handover requires the transfer of professional responsibility and accountability for the care of a client the nurse has been managing or caring for, to another nurse or health professional. Handovers usually happen at the change of a shift, when the person is transferred from another professional group or transferred from a different department or another facility. Handover therefore ensures client safety and continuity of client care, and also provides an opportunity to update knowledge, provide support and share critical thinking (Tollefson & Hillman 2016).

There is evidence to suggest that effective communication and interprofessional 'handovers' have been identified as key activities in promoting interprofessional teamwork and collaboration (Armstrong 2019; Eggins, Slade & Geddes 2016). A study undertaken by Brewer and Flavell (2018) involved evaluating the experiences of students who had completed clinical placements within specific interprofessional community practice settings in Western Australia. Their exploratory case study discovered that the students' experiences of working with students from other health professions, which included psychology, occupational therapy and physiotherapy, were successful. The student placements demonstrated that interprofessional skills and capabilities were learned and developed, which were then consolidated through the positive interactions they experienced. The sharing of essential client information ensured that the continuity of care for clients was appropriately maintained. Communicating the clients' medical treatments and interventions from one group of professionals to another was vital for the progression of the care required by the clients. Innovative learning experiences such as these appear to be leading the way in developing collaborative practice and interprofessional teamwork.

Videos: Communication

Interprofessional teamwork

What is a team?

A team is a group of people who share a common goal and common objectives determined by common needs. To achieve this, each member of the team contributes, in accordance with their competence and skill, and in coordination with the functions of others. Most interprofessional teams fit within this definition. The attributes of effective teams may include:

- a defined or established set of goals and objectives;
- members who have an ongoing relationship;
- a task to focus upon;
- effective communication (Brewer & Flavell, 2018; Mayo & Williams Woolley 2016);
- a willingness to cooperate;
- a focused and single mission;
- the ability to be self-regulating;
- a diversity of styles and life experiences;

- sharing leadership; and
- the ability to listen to each other.

By facilitating the values of respect and mutual understanding between the different professional roles, nurses are able to promote a team-based model of care that promotes positive professional relationships and also ensures that clients receive high-quality care.

Key factors in interprofessional teamwork

Garvis and colleagues (2016) found that key factors are required to promote and sustain interprofessional teamwork. These factors include a willingness to collaborate, trust, mutual respect and communication. This is the case in all practice settings, and as Garvis and colleagues (2016) found, especially so when professionals, such as nurses and childhood educators, work together in childcare practice settings. The culture of an organisation, as well as strong leadership, also influences collaborative working practices (De Brun et al. 2020). Healthcare organisations, by virtue of their diverse clinical environments and multiple clinical practitioners and others, can provide an environment that embraces the important elements of interprofessional collaboration and teamwork, supporting or facilitating interprofessional collaboration and teamwork to flourish (Rossler et al. 2017).

In an ideal organisation, teams should work collaboratively and cohesively to ensure that people pool their skills and are able to contribute their specific talents to the various roles essential for teams to function at their best. Effective teams allow individuals within them to use their skills and knowledge to design creative solutions and to solve complex problems. Effective teams establish goals and set clear objectives, build effective and continuing relationships, focus on the task at hand, communicate effectively (Brewer & Flavell, 2018; Mayo & Williams Woolley 2016), listen to each other, cooperate, self-regulate and share leadership.

Short-answer question

Teams should be able to work interdependently and should also have the ability to engage in civilised disagreement (Stanley 2017; Schot et al. 2020). In keeping with the above list, Dinh and colleagues (2020), Schot and colleagues (2020) and Stanley (2017) suggested that for healthcare teams to function effectively, they need health professionals to employ complementary skills, common goals and a dynamic process of assessment, planning and evaluation of client care. These authors each added that the goal of collaborative working across interprofessional teams can only be achieved with shared decision-making (including with clients), interdependent working and effective communication. This occurs when teams function with:

- participation across teams and inter-agency groups, to ensure integrated services;
- shared decision-making to achieve agreed goals;
- shared or collaborative leadership (De Brun 2020);
- respect for the contribution of other professionals in the provision of services/care; and
- an appraisal of each other's roles, responsibilities and competence (from the perspective of their own professional development and others in services care or provision).

Teamwork is enhanced when interprofessional teams share information in a respectful manner and actively listen; the information is shared in a way that is understandable across the disciplines; and appropriate terminology is used and communicated with other team members in a manner that promotes understanding and positive interactions. This is all enhanced by the application of emotional intelligence (see Chapter 6) and an ability to resolve conflict effectively and appropriately (Stanley 2017).

Multiple-choice questions
Short-answer question

REFLECTION 15.2

At this point, reflect on your own experiences of working with other health professionals – particularly from other health disciplines.

- Were these events positive and easy, or tense and strained?
- What was it about the working relationship that prompted a positive or negative experience?
- Was there a problem that arose in your relationship with an individual, or was it about the quality of your or their communication on a professional level?

Think of a specific event where you worked closely with another health professional.

- What was it about this experience that was either good or bad? What did you learn from the experience?
- What might you do differently, or how might you approach this situation should it occur again?

Conflict resolution

Deutsch (1973) suggests that conflicts of interest exist when the actions of one person who is attempting to maximise their own needs and benefits prevents, blocks, interferes with, injures or in some way makes less effective the actions of the other person. Unfortunately, it is not uncommon for individuals working within interprofessional groups to try to maximise their professional group or personal objectives over the needs of the client or over the efficiency and effectiveness of the group or team. When this occurs, team members need to be able to recognise the clash of goals or the conflict, and plan appropriate **conflict resolution** (Labraguea & McEnroe-Petitte 2017).

conflict resolution an approach to resolving conflict in a structured and well-considered way

Preventing and resolving conflict

In all work situations, there will be conflicts that should be avoided and conflicts that should be managed. When managing conflict, we recommend the following steps:

1 Recognise and accept differences between individuals and groups in terms of values, perceptions, goals, expectations and needs. If any of these are in conflict with the needs of the team, group or client, they should be addressed.
2 Be honest with yourself and with others.

3 Allocate sufficient time and energy to get to know people and their goals and perceptions.
4 Do not assume that you are right and they are wrong, or that your goals are more noble or righteous. Seek clarification.
5 Enable people to express their feelings in suitable ways.
6 Learn from previous conflicts.
7 Respect each other's knowledge, skills and experience, and regard others as a valuable resource (NMBA 2018).
8 Establish a safe environment in which diverse opinions can be expressed, and recognise that there is potential for conflict.
9 Negotiate a solution, build bridges, maintain your composure, facilitate pauses in the conversation, act as a positive role model for conflict resolution, avoid negative negotiation techniques (win–lose) and aim for a win–win resolution.
10 Listen and try to understand.

The following are approaches to conflict resolution that will *not* be effective:

- avoidance;
- force – win at any cost (lose credibility);
- smooth over at expense of self (soothing);
- procrastination (putting the resolution off and hoping it will go away):
  - 'I will wait and see'
  - 'I could ... but I won't ... or maybe I will' – that is, fence-sitting (ignoring self)
  - 'I will do this if you do that' (giving up part of planned goals);
- arguing (looking for an opportunity to escalate the conflict);
- aggression (never a suitable solution in the workplace or in any other environment); and
- complaining or blaming (finding fault – this is a passive–aggressive approach to dealing with conflict, and it is seldom effective).

Managing conflict

There are three main approaches to dealing with conflict:

- *Recognition.* Recognise that interpersonal conflict has occurred (a disagreement or difference of opinion may escalate to destructive conflict) and there is a need for constructive resolution.
- *Acceptance.* Accept that conflict has occurred and that each person owns responsibility for their role in the conflict, rather than blaming the other person.
- *Resolution.* This is more than resolving the conflict: it is about improving interpersonal communication and working relationships, with the employment of strategies such as the use of emotional intelligence and effective interpersonal skills (McKibben 2017).

When managing conflict, it is helpful to ensure that privacy is maintained. There is nothing more off-putting and disruptive than a conflict or openly negative discussion in the middle of a clinical environment. If this occurs, calmly say, 'I appreciate that you have something to say to me, but can we take this to a private space, such as your office?'

It will also be helpful if you can maintain a positive attitude, even in the face of hostile or difficult behaviour (Stanley 2017). Try to be aware of your own and the other person's body language. Try to maintain a confident, assertive, open and relaxed posture. Ensure you start by defining and discussing the problem or concern. Practise active listening and use emotional intelligence (express empathy when needed) to deal with emotional issues and to acknowledge the other person's distress and frustration. Try to establish where your common values lie, so that you can better appreciate the other's perspective (Stanley 2019). Take responsibility for your part in the conflict and use 'I' statements such as 'I feel like this … because of … ', and explain what the consequences are for you as a result – for example, 'I feel disappointed, because you called out to me in a busy ward environment and it disturbed a calm ward setting'. Or 'I feel upset, because you ignored my input when discussing the client's case in the discharge meeting, as it negated my input and potential contribution'.

Try to collaborate and accommodate each other's contribution to resolving the conflict, and maintain an open and honest dialogue. When seeking a resolution, make requests, not demands, for change – and remember that you may need to compromise (McKibben 2017).

Video: Conflict resolution

The power of an apology

Saying you are sorry can be very powerful. If offered sincerely, it can be vital in moving forward. The power comes from expressing regret: saying sorry and accepting responsibility. It is important to offer a reason for the mistake or situation, then find a remedy or try to resolve the issue or mistake as far as possible. When one of the co-authors was working as a hospital manager, it was clear that so many complex and protracted client complaints could have been resolved at the bedside if the health professional dealing with the client at the time had simply been able to say 'sorry'. Often, this was all the client or their relatives wanted to hear – that someone was sorry and would resolve to avoid treating other clients in this way in future. Staff are no different. Many a protracted and difficult staff situation could have been dealt with more simply and quickly if one or other party had been able to accept their part in the conflict and say 'sorry'.

Recommendations for dealing with conflict

Other advice regarding conflict may involve:

- Knowing your own style and ways of dealing with conflict
- Generating a variety of options (ask questions, take time, establish options, listen to objections)
- Knowing your organisation's clinical protocol for the management of aggression
- Attending workshops to develop insights into conflict management and resilience

- Identifying early signs of aggression and dealing with them. Never accept inappropriate behaviour. Speak up, hold people to account and act courageously when appropriate.
- Using evidence-based management techniques and practising using emotional intelligence and empathy.

De-escalation techniques

When dealing directly with conflict, it may be useful to employ specific steps to de-escalate the conflict, including strategies to:

- Use calm, respectful language (avoid swearing or rude and obscene language).
- Use open-ended questions.
- Express your feelings clearly and plainly.
- Let the colleague or client know your concerns.
- Explain to the colleague or client the effect they have on those around them.
- Model calm behaviour.
- Establish rapport and dialogue with the colleague and/or client (Hodge & Marshall 2007).

Peer learning and mentoring

Accessing continuing professional development (CPD) is one way in which healthcare professionals improve, maintain and broaden their expertise, competence and knowledge in practice. Specifically, it enables the registered nurse to update their professional competency, which is required for safe and effective practice. Under national legislation, a registered nurse must complete a minimum of 20 hours of CPD each year (NMBA 2016b; Summers 2015). While there is usually access to continuing education, time and cost can sometimes be barriers. Therefore, taking opportunities through **peer learning**, **mentoring** and supervision can be some ways to remain up to date with current research and best-practice methods (Nokuthula, Ngxongo & Beepat 2018). Learning can also be supported by the establishment of a mentoring relationship. A mentor need not be someone from the same professional discipline, and often mentors are selected by the mentee, rather than appointed.

peer learning an educational practice whereby learners (peers) interact with and learn from each other to achieve their educational or learning goals

mentoring a way of nurturing and supporting health professional colleagues, usually by a more experienced and skilled or knowledgeable professional

The registered nurse needs to:

- reflect on their own contribution to learning;
- address their personal learning needs so that they can improve knowledge, skills and attitudes that enhance collaborative practice;
- seek feedback to strengthen collaboration and team effectiveness;
- evaluate policies and procedures for client care and health outcomes;
- seek out a mentor who can be objective and who can assist in setting realistic goals; and
- learn from peers who use recent evidence for best practice.

CASE STUDY

De-escalating a situation

A woman who has primary responsibility for her grandchild has accompanied the child to a major metropolitan hospital for an operation. The grandmother and child are from a remote community and have never travelled before. The enormous responsibility of supporting her grandchild and consenting to the operation has caused the woman a great deal of anxiety. A registered nurse and a recent graduate have come to give the child their pre-operative medication. As the nurse explains this to the child's grandmother, a social worker arrives to discuss concerns about transportation and accommodation. At this point, the woman becomes distressed and angry saying, 'This is all too much … I don't understand what is going on. The nurse is trying to poison my grandchild and you want me to talk about where I'm staying!'

The social worker shouts at the nurse to stop the medication and calls for the ward manager. The registered nurse tries to explain that she is not harming the child and that the child needs to take the medication before going into surgery.

At this point, the child begins crying and the grandmother becomes more upset. The graduate says calmly, 'Can you take this discussion to the office?' At this point the nurse insists on administering the medication and says that the social worker is holding up the surgery.

QUESTIONS

1   Identify and discuss the problems and concerns in this scenario for the child, grandmother, registered nurse, new graduate and social worker.

2   Discuss possible communication strategies the registered nurse, new graduate and social worker could use to resolve the conflict.

3   What effect does this altercation have on client safety, interprofessional teamwork and the client's grandmother's confidence in the health service?

4   How could this situation have been managed more effectively?

SUMMARY

- Effective communication, teamwork and dealing with conflict can reduce errors, increase client safety and heighten client satisfaction. The role of the registered nurse is to foster professional relationships that affect the delivery of client care, and to ensure safety and quality are maintained. Building and enhancing interprofessional relationships requires the capacity to communicate competently, and to work cooperatively and collaboratively within teams.
- As well as outlining several handover strategies, the general focus of the chapter has been to foster interprofessional teamwork and collaboration, with structured approaches to providing key clinical information being central to the effective transfer of clinical data.

- An important aspect of the chapter has been a focus on the value of understanding what constitutes teamwork, how teams work and why they are vital for safe and effective interprofessional practice.
- Teamwork can produce a climate of conflict. Dealing effectively and productively with conflict can enhance the team's ability to communicate well and to provide safe and effective clinical care. Aspects of this chapter have outlined why it is important to recognise when conflict has occurred and suggested steps to address conflict if it occurs.
- A key aspect of clinical leadership is being a role model for appropriate behaviour and applying the principles of peer mentorship and CPD. Role-modelling these approaches to professional development fosters greater team cohesion and builds respect and resilience in the health service.

Suggested responses

REVIEW QUESTIONS

1   Do you see yourself as a member of an interprofessional team? Reflect on this role and consider whether you communicate differently with members of your own professional discipline. If so, why? How effectively do you communicate? Consider what this chapter has suggested about clear communication.
2   How effective are your interpersonal skills? Do you use active listening, paraphrasing or other communications strategies to ensure your communication is effective?
3   When you are next at handover, focus on how the information is transferred. Was the handover effective or could the communication process have been improved?
4   Do you work as part of a team? How do your team attributes match the attributes of a team described in this chapter?
5   Think about how you prefer to resolve conflict. Do you like to force a win at all costs, do you prefer to avoid conflict or do you look for a compromise resolution?

RESEARCH TOPIC

Interprofessional teamwork is not new but it is also not well developed in many clinical areas. A potential area of research could relate to how professionals from different health disciplines understand each other's roles and work activities. It is assumed that we all know what the other professional disciplines contribute to a client's care. But do we really?

FURTHER READING

Anderson, J., Malone, L., Shanahan, K. & Manning, J. (2015). Nursing bedside clinical handover: An integrated review of issues and tools. *Journal of Clinical Nursing*, 24(5–6), 662–71.

Brewer, M. & Flavell, H. (2018). Facilitating collaborative capabilities for future work: What can be learnt from interprofessional fieldwork in health. *International Journal of Work-Integrated Learning*, 19(2), 169–80.

Brewer, M.L., Flavell, H.L. & Jordan, J. (2017). Interprofessional team-based placements: The importance of space, place and facilitation. *Journal of Interprofessional Care*, 31(4), 429–37.

Nomie, E. & Mullern, T. (2017). Interprofessional barriers: A study of quality improvement work among nurses and physicians. *Quality Management in Health Care*, 26(2), 63–7.

Rossler, K.L., Buelow, J.R., Thompson, A.W. & Knofczynski, G. (2017). Effective Learning of interprofessional teamwork. *Nurse Educator*, 42(2), 67–71.

REFERENCES

Anderson, J., Malone, L., Shanahan, K. & Manning, J. (2015). Nursing bedside clinical handover: An integrated review of issues and tools. *Journal of Clinical Nursing*, 24(5–6), 662–71.

Armstrong, G. (2019). Quality and safety education for nurses teamwork and collaboration competency: Empowering nurses. *The Journal of Continuing Education in Nursing*, 50(6), 252–5.

Australian Commission on Safety and Quality in Health Care (ACSQHC) (2017). *The OSSIE guide to clinical handover improvement*, 2nd edn. Sydney: ACSQHC.

Bainbridge, L., Nasmith, L., Orchard, C. & Wood, V. (2010). Competencies for interprofessional collaboration. *Journal of Physical Therapy Education*, 24(1), 6–11.

Berman, A., Snyder, S., Levett-Jones, T., Dwyer, T., Hales, M., Harvey, N., Moxham, L., Park, T., Parker, B., Reid-Searl, K. & Stanley, D. (2017). *Kozier and Erb's fundamentals of nursing*, 4th edn. Sydney: Pearson.

Birks, M., Chapman, Y.B. & Davis, J. (2015). *Professional and therapeutic communication*. Melbourne: Oxford University Press.

Brewer, M. & Flavell, F. (2018). Facilitating collaborative capabilities for future work: What can be learnt from interprofessional fieldwork in health. *International Journal of Work-Integrated Learning* 19(2), 169–80.

Brownie, S., Scot, R. & Rossiter, R. (2016). Therapeutic communication and relationships in chronic and complex care. *Nursing Standard*, 31(6), 54–63.

De Brun, A., Rogers, L., O'Shea, M. & McAuliffe, E. (2020). Understanding the impact of a collaborative leadership intervention on team working and safety culture in healthcare teams: a realist evaluation protocol. *HRB Open Research*, 2(5), 1–14.

Deutsch, M. (1973). *The resolution of conflict: Constructive and destructive processes*. New Haven: Yale University Press.

Dinh, J.V., Traylor, A.M., Kilcullen, M.P., Perez, J.A., Schweissing, E.J., Venkatesh, A. & Salas, E. (2020). Cross-disciplinary care: A systematic review on teamwork processes in health care. *Small Group Research*, 51(1), 125–66.

Eggins, S., Slade, D. & Geddes, F. (2016). *Effective communication in clinical handover: From research to practice*. Boston: DeGruyter.

Garvis, S., Kirkby, J., McMahon, K. & Meyer, C. (2016) Collaboration is key: The actual experience of disciplines working together in child care. *Nursing & Health Sciences*, 18(1), 44–51.

Hada, A., Jack, L. & Coyer, F. (2019). Using a knowledge transfer framework to identify barriers and supports to effective nursing handover: A focus group study. *Heliyon*, 5(6).

Hodge, A.N. & Marshall, A.P. (2007). Violence and aggression in the emergency department: A critical care perspective. *Australian Critical Care*, 20(2), 61–7.

Labraguea, L. & McEnroe-Petitte, D. (2017). An integrative review on conflict management styles among nursing students: Implications for nurse education. *Nurse Education Today*, 59, 45–52.

Mayo, A.T. & Williams Woolley, A. (2016). Teamwork in health care: Maximizing collective intelligence via inclusive collaboration and open communication. *AMA Journal of Ethics*, 18(9), 933–40.

McKibben, L. (2017). Conflict management: Importance and implications. *British Journal of Nursing*, 26(2), 100–3.

Nokuthula, S., Ngxongo, T. & Beepat, Y. (2018). The influence of peer mentoring on critical care nursing' students learning outcomes. *International Journal of Workplace Health Management*, 11(3), 130–42.

Nursing and Midwifery Board of Australia (NMBA) (2016a). *Registered Nurse Standards for Practice*. Retrieved from https://www.nursingmidwiferyboard.gov.au/Codes-Guidelines-Statements/Professional-standards/registered-nurse-standards-for-practice.aspx.

——— (2016b). *Registration Standard: Continuing Professional Development*. Retrieved from https://www.nursingmidwiferyboard.gov.au/Registration-Standards/Continuing-professional-development.aspx.

——— (2018). *Code of Ethics for Nurses*. Retrieved from https://www.nursingmidwiferyboard.gov.au/codes-guidelines-statements/professional-standards/registered-nurse-standards-for-practice.aspx.

Queensland Government (2009). *Health Practitioner Regulation National Law Act 2009*. Retrieved from https://www.legislation.qld.gov.au/view/html/inforce/current/act-2009-045

Reeves, S. (2016). Why we need interprofessional education to improve the delivery of safe effective care. *Interface: Comunicacao Saude Educacao*, 20(56).

Rossler, K.L., Buelow, J.R., Thompson, A.W. & Knofczynski, G. (2017). Effective learning of interprofessional teamwork. *Nurse Educator*, 42(2), 67–71.

Schot, E., Tummers, L. & Noordegraaf. M. (2020). Working together. A systematic review on how healthcare professionals contribute to interprofessional collaboration. *Journal of Interprofessional Care*, 34(3), 332–42.

Stadick, J.L. (2020). The relationship between interprofessional education and health care professional's attitudes towards teamwork and interprofessional collaborative competencies. *Journal of interprofessional education and practice*, 19.

Stanley, D. (2017). *Clinical leadership in nursing and healthcare: Values into action*, 2nd edn. London: Wiley Blackwell.

——— (2019). *Values-based leadership in healthcare: Congruent leadership explored*. Sage: London.

Stanley, K. (2016). Health professional educators' experiences of interprofessional socialisation within higher education: An interpretative phenomenological study. PhD thesis, Curtin University. Retrieved from https://espace.curtin.edu.au/bitstream/handle/20.500.11937/117/241701_Stanley%202016.pdf?sequence=2.

Stanley, K. & Stanley, D. (2019). The HEIPS framework: Scaffolding interprofessional education starts with health professional educators. *Nursing Education in Practice*, 34, 63–71.

Summers, A. (2015). Continuing professional development in Australia. Barriers and Support. *The Journal of Continuing Education in Nursing*, 46(8), 337–9.

Thomson, K., Outram, S., Gilligan, C. & Levett-Jones, T. (2015). Interprofessional experiences of recent healthcare graduates: A social psychology perspective on the barriers to effective communication, teamwork, and patient-centred care. *Journal of Interprofessional Care*, 29(6), 634–40.

Tollefson, J. & Hillman, E. (2016). *Clinical psychomotor skills: Assessment tools for nurses*, 6th edn. Melbourne: Cengage.

Weller, J., Boyd, M. & Cumin, D. (2014). Teams, tribes and patient safety: Overcoming barriers to effective teamwork in healthcare. *Postgraduate Medical Journal*, 90(1061), 149.

16 Empowering our profession

Nick Arnott and Melanie Eslick

With acknowledgement to Kylie Ward for her contributions to the first edition

LEARNING OBJECTIVES

At the completion of this chapter, you should be able to:

1 Explain the responsibilities we all have for leading and empowering our profession.
2 Discuss various perspectives on leadership and empowerment in nursing.
3 Identify and apply strategies for developing your leadership potential.

Introduction

The challenges associated with delivering quality client care within healthcare systems and environments are characterised by increasing complexity and acuity in client needs, rising consumer (and public) expectations, and increasingly constrained human and financial resources, all of which are everyday realities for many nurses (Courtney et al. 2015). In this context, empowering nurses with the skills, attributes and confidence needed to have control and influence over their own practice is critical. This chapter intends to make more explicit the notions of leadership and empowerment inherent in the other chapters in this book, with a particular emphasis on the responsibility we all have to advance the quality and excellence of nursing practice, to be a voice for our profession and leaders in implementing the changes and improvements necessary to promote optimal health outcomes for local and global communities (Grossman & Valiga 2021; Komives, Wagner & Associates 2016). This chapter presents a range of perspectives on leadership and empowerment in nursing and proposes strategies and ideas for developing your own leadership potential.

We all have a role to play

This chapter is not calling for you to 'do more'; rather, it is looking for a shift in perspective or focus with regard to the role every nurse can play in inspiring a shared vision and creating positive and enabling environments for change (Kouzes & Posner 2018). Put simply, it is not about the *quantity* of time and effort you devote to such things (how *much* you do), but rather the *quality* of that time and effort – being present, proactive and passionate about the changes you want to see (Hougaard & Carter 2017). Khoshmehr and colleagues (2020) contended that the empowerment of novice nurses fosters an emotional commitment to work and increased job satisfaction, thereby influencing responsibility, productivity and the quality of nursing care. In turn, these passionate practitioners help to shape healthy systems, which promote quality and excellence in the pursuit of optimal client outcomes and lead to increased client satisfaction (Khoshmehr et al. 2020).

Empowerment for what?

Nursing is essentially an 'other'-focused endeavour that is concerned primarily with the needs and outcomes of those being 'nursed'. Thus, **empowerment** is first and foremost about acting in the best interests of clients and promoting optimal health outcomes for individuals, families, groups and populations. As a student, 'empowerment' may be viewed mainly in the context of your own learning and performance – the development and application of the knowledge and skills you need to provide the best possible care, support and advocacy for your clients and patients. The pursuit of 'individual excellence' is important; however, the International Council of Nurses (ICN 2017) asserts that a nurse's ability to bring about change is just as important as their knowledge and technical ability to deliver safe and effective care. As a novice nurse, empowering and transformational leadership from your nurse managers and

empowerment the giving of power, authority and opportunities that increase the confidence, autonomy and self-determination of individuals and communities to represent their interests, make decisions, solve problems and drive change

colleagues will benefit your own professional fulfilment as well as your clients' safety and wellbeing outcomes (Boamah et al. 2018).

The achievement of quality client outcomes requires nurses to have the requisite knowledge and skills to deliver and evaluate evidence-based health care and to empower clients and families to make positive changes for themselves, but a nurse's sphere of influence must also extend beyond the 'frontline' (ICN 2017). For example, this influence is also needed in nursing education programs so that the relationship between education, research and practice is fully understood and embedded. It needs to operate at a health systems level, with nurses exercising their voices at the decision-making table and providing stewardship for the complex interactions between policy, regulation and economic factors that underpin these systems. And it needs to be evident in the workplace so that nurses can assume control over their own practices and the unique roles they play, and can operate as full partners and collaborators in the interprofessional or interdisciplinary practice environment (ACN 2015, 2017; ICN 2017).

For nurses to function effectively in dynamic and complex environments and to exert their influence in optimising client outcomes, they need to appreciate the multiple factors that affect their practice, and give due consideration to client, provider and systems issues (Mannix, Wilkes & Daly 2015). Empowerment has been emphasised as having the quadruple aim of promoting optimal health outcomes for individuals and populations, improving the quality and cost-effectiveness of health systems, enhancing client experience and satisfaction, and improving the work life of health professionals themselves (Courtney et al. 2015; Kouzes & Posner 2018; Sikka, Morath & Leape 2015).

What can you do?

Nursing is influenced to some extent by external factors or changes in healthcare systems, policies and settings, but as the single largest group of health professionals, we also have the opportunity – and some would say a responsibility – to be influential in policy, education, practice and research as a means of representing our profession and shaping the system ourselves (Courtney et al. 2015). The dilemma for many nurses is knowing what this means in their own practice. The concepts of leadership and empowerment may resonate even less for students, who often view this as being the exclusive domain of experienced nurses and usually tied to designated roles or positions. However, there have been numerous calls for nurses to be active and influential at all levels (e.g. ACN 2020; Brokaw 2016; Chankova 2020; Doherty & Hunter Revell 2020; Ziel 2016). What might this involve?

In education

In education, leadership and influence is about being an 'active learner'; being deeply engaged in learning resources, content and discussion boards or forums through reading, writing, listening, responding, debating, practising, reflecting and problem-solving. It involves sourcing the best evidence to inform your understanding and application of core concepts and skills. It includes collaborating with peers to facilitate collective learning, progress group tasks or projects, and achieve shared goals. And it requires a commitment to reflecting upon your learning and practice, to seeking out and using feedback to guide necessary changes or improvements, and to contributing to the continuing evaluation of learning and teaching to strengthen these programs for future learners. As your studies proceed, you might volunteer to mentor fellow students, in a simulated practical session, or to conduct peer-based learning. Many universities offer student leadership programs, which introduce leadership concepts, skills and goal-setting before starting in the workforce. These opportunities are discussed later in this chapter.

In clinical practice

It involves working in partnership with clients, families and colleagues in pursuit of shared goals. It includes mobilising skills and expertise to optimise client safety and care, with an emphasis on strategies that empower clients and their support people as 'active participants' in the planning, delivery and evaluation of their care, not just as 'passive recipients' of what we do *to* or *for* them. It requires nurses to source the best evidence to inform these care decisions, and to 'translate' this evidence to the clinical context, including care delivery models and strategies; systems, policies and protocols; and related resources and technology. It covers a mandated responsibility to actively engage in reflection, evaluation and feedback that strengthens your own practice, and drives a culture of innovation and improvement in your workplace.

In the workplace

It is about having a quality improvement mindset and advocating for nurses as active partners in the interdisciplinary healthcare environment. It might involve joining a committee or working group to help design, develop and drive nurse-led solutions or new systems, policies and processes; or being actively involved in evaluation and feedback on the application and effects of these things in your own practice environment. It includes contributing to the recruitment, induction and mentoring of other staff, and recognising and celebrating the achievements and contributions of others as part of a positive, safe and harmonious workplace culture that promotes job satisfaction and retention. This may mean putting yourself forward to act as a preceptor for students, as charge nurse or shift coordinator, or for temporary or permanent management or leadership positions in the workplace.

With other healthcare professionals

More and more, nurses are working as members of *interdisciplinary* teams (also known as *interprofessional* teams), who collaborate to provide the best holistic care for clients by bringing together complementary expertise and skills. This means working in partnership, not just with clients, their support people and nursing colleagues, but also with doctors, specialists and allied health professionals such as dietitians, physical therapists, speech therapists, psychologists, social workers, palliative care specialists and general counsellors. Nurses often forge professional relationships with pathology and radiology professionals, with pharmacists (in both hospital and community settings) and with clients' general practitioners. Interdisciplinary teams provide the best care and health outcomes for clients, regardless of the practice environment (Barnard, Jones & Cruice 2020).

In many clinical settings, nurse practitioners and specialist nurses in fields such as oncology, mental health and rehabilitation may actively participate in *multidisciplinary* teams. Each team member works independently but brings their own expertise and voice to clients' care plans, which are negotiated with clients and discussed at multidisciplinary team meetings, then implemented during diagnosis, treatment and follow-up care (Taberna et al. 2020).

In research

It involves the application or translation of research to different practice contexts and environments, and the identification of clinical problems or questions requiring a research-based response. It may involve a more formal or active role in the research process, including applying to be a research participant, undertaking research training, joining a research team or even leading a project yourself (Holmström 2020). It might also include action research, audits or evaluation processes at the local, organisational or sector level, as part of a clinical, quality or system improvement endeavour. As a student, it involves developing your skills and confidence in sourcing, interpreting and applying research as evidence to support your practice.

In the wider community

It is about paying attention to your professional identity and how you represent yourself and what you do to clients, the public and other health professionals. It might include active involvement in community development or population health endeavours and/or political advocacy through participation in relevant campaigns or causes. It could involve joining a professional society or association to help advance your own career and the profession more broadly through collegiality, leadership, advocacy and mentorship.

Connecting with practice:
NurseStrong
Short-answer question

Leading the way

Although nurses are highly valued by society (Gardner 2017), within the hierarchy of the healthcare system itself they are often rendered submissive and subordinate to the dominant 'medical establishment'. This has largely been the norm since the time of Florence Nightingale, who – despite advancing the unique knowledge and contribution of nursing – argued that the qualities of a 'good nurse' were discipline, obedience and restraint, and carrying out the orders of the doctors 'in a suitably humble and deferential way' (Levett-Jones & Bourgeois 2015). In more recent times, this outdated image of nurses has begun to change, with nurses taking a much more prominent role in the management and organisation of staff (especially other nurses) and the planning and coordination of care delivery in a range of clinical settings and contexts. This was particularly evident in the many diverse roles nurses took up in the public health response to the COVID-19 pandemic (Jackson et al. 2020).

For the past few decades, 'management' skills have been highly regarded within healthcare organisations, but more recently the demand for **leadership** skills has gained prominence (Courtney et al. 2015; Doherty & Hunter Revell 2020). While debates about the relationship between leadership and management continue, it is now widely accepted that leadership requires an extended range of complex skills,

leadership a process, not a position, which shapes and elevates systems and practices by engaging others in the establishment of a shared vision, and motivating others (followers) to willingly act towards achievement of that vision or change

strengths and attributes that are pivotal in shaping practice, and that management is simply one possible role or function of leadership (ACN 2017; Courtney et al. 2015; Daly, Speedy & Jackson 2015).

NURSING PERSPECTIVE

For most people and professions, the concept of a leader is related to their job title. But a leader does not have to be in a formal management position, and within the nursing profession nurse leadership does not equal nurse management.

A nurse manager has an important responsibility for coordinating all the aspects of care delivery; however, a nurse leader does not have to be in a management role to have vision and initiate change. A nurse leader drives organisational change to create a better workplace and better client outcomes.

The ability to lead effectively in a management position is based on several key skills: strategic thinking ability, decision-making, problem-solving, organisation, planning and having a vision of where you want to be.

If you are not in a management position, you still have an important contribution to make and you too can lead client advocacy and provide nurse-led solutions based on the experiences gained during your professional practice. It is about having the confidence to express your ideas and viewpoint, and having the knowledge, passion, expertise, commitment and skill to inspire others to share your vision.

Source: ACN (2015).

Multiple-choice questions
Short-answer question

Nurses may not consider themselves to be leaders, but every nurse has a voice and can use that voice to make a difference. The ICN (2017) describes leadership as a process, not a position, asserting that it is not necessary to have a traditional title or elected position to take the lead and make changes that help other people. According to the ICN, 'leadership is tied to social responsibility and good citizenship', which clearly aligns it to every nurse's 'professional and ethical responsibilities to champion the human right to health' (ICN 2017, p. 52).

Effective nurse leaders require various attributes and skills that enable the nursing profession to flourish and for the ultimate goal of the profession – excellence in safe, person-centred care – to be achieved (Grossman & Valiga 2021; Scully 2015). These skills and attributes include high-level communication skills; awareness of one's values, beliefs, emotions and attitudes; respect and empathy for others; and commitment, passion, flexibility and adaptability to thrive in complex and dynamic healthcare environments (Daly, Speedy & Jackson 2015). Various leadership styles or types have been researched, with **transformational leadership** being identified as central to effective nursing practice (Richards 2020; Scully 2015).

Transformational leaders do not set goals that others are expected to attain but rather motivate followers to shape, alter and elevate their potential for excellence and to 'perform beyond expectations, by creating a sense of ownership in reaching a shared vision', inspiring teamwork and empowering change (Scully 2015, p. 442). This

transformational leadership
a 'selling' leadership style in which the leader recognises the need for change, creates a shared vision and plan, and uses encouragement to enact the change with the support of the followers (members of the group) (Cato et al. 2019)

is in contrast to the more directive, task-oriented and reward-motivated **transactional leadership**, which is perhaps more akin to traditional management models or theories (Richards 2020).

REFLECTION 16.1

What does leadership mean to you?

Leaders need to be able to create safe, effective and encouraging working environments, inspire shared visions, act as role models and stimulate, motivate and mentor others (Daly, Speedy & Jackson 2015; Grossman & Valiga 2021; Scully 2015). In doing this, effective leaders tend to exhibit specific traits, possess certain skills and practise particular habits. Kouzes and Posner (2018) proposed the 'leadership challenge model', which includes the 'five practices of exemplary leadership: model the way; inspire a shared vision; challenge the process; enable others to act; and encourage the heart'. They recently updated and contextualised this model for students, presenting ten commitments or behaviours that enable and exemplify these five practices (Table 16.1) to illustrate how students can develop, practise and exhibit the best in contemporary leadership, both now and as graduates (Kouzes & Posner 2018).

Table 16.1   The five practices and ten commitments of exemplary leadership

Practices of exemplary leadership	Commitments of exemplary leadership
Model the way	Clarify values by finding your voice and affirming shared values. Set the example by aligning actions with shared values.
Inspire a shared vision	Envision the future by imagining exciting and enabling possibilities. Enlist others in a common vision by appealing to shared aspirations.
Challenge the process	Search for opportunities by seizing the initiative and looking outward for innovative ways to improve. Experiment and take risks by constantly generating small wins and learning from experience.
Enable others to act	Foster collaboration by building trust and facilitating relationships. Strengthen others by increasing self-determination and developing competence.
Encourage the heart	Recognise contributions by showing appreciation for individual excellence. Celebrate the values and victories by creating a spirit of community.

Source: Kouzes and Posner (2018, p. 15).

REFLECTION 16.2

How could you implement some of these practices and commitments now?

Video: Nursing leadership

Leadership and empowerment in nursing

While there is often much attention on the stressors and challenges facing the nursing profession, and the health and aged-care systems more broadly, there is also a sense of excitement associated with the influence that nursing as a profession can have on improving the social determinants of health, enhancing client experiences and promoting the health and wellbeing of communities throughout Australia and beyond (Ward 2017).

Against the backdrop of challenges – but also from the position of possibility – the importance of leadership and the development of these capabilities in all nurses is apparent. Put simply, being a nurse means being a leader. While this is true in terms of our professional responsibilities, it is not yet part of the psyche of our profession or who nurses believe they are. There are some nurses who feel that the pressure of being a leader is not for them or that it is someone else's job – perhaps it is part of certain positions but not intrinsic to many roles, particularly direct-care roles. If every nurse embraced a leadership mindset, it could make a tremendous difference to the nursing profession claiming its rightful place as an equal in discussion and debate on future healthcare reforms.

There are more than 410 000 registered and enrolled nurses in Australia (NMBA 2020). Nurses are the backbone of the healthcare system, taking key responsibility for many aspects of care in every healthcare setting. The importance and 'benefits of a well-qualified nursing workforce and high-quality, visible nursing leadership are well documented to lead health and aged care reform in a dynamic and transformational way' (Ward 2017, p. 585; ICN 2016).

Video: Leadership skills

However, nurses remain under-represented, disproportionately represented or simply not represented at all at the highest levels of decision-making (ACN 2015). Representation of the profession is essential at every level of the system (Chankova 2020). The real challenge lies within every nurse. Most nurses choose to become nurses because they are driven to care for people and to make a difference in their lives. These qualities and attributes are key elements or enablers of the remarkable work nurses do and the difference nurses make, yet individual nurses (and the profession more broadly) have often been slow – and even reluctant – to recognise, promote and celebrate this contribution. The community knows the value of nurses: for more than 20 years, nurses have been voted the most ethical and trusted profession (Roy Morgan 2017). However, Ward 2017 asked 'what does this actually mean and why does it not guarantee [nurses] a seat at every decision-making table relating to health [policy], expenditure, resourcing or system redesign?' (p. 585). What will have to happen for nursing to be considered the most important and influential professional group in such reforms by both politicians and policymakers? After all, nurses and midwives make up close to 60 per cent of the healthcare workforce (AIHW 2020), and arguably have the greatest engagement with, and understanding of, the needs and expectations of the people who use (or even depend upon) these services.

Nurses have always been known as the clients' advocates. Advocacy includes directly 'speaking up' for clients, carers and families when they cannot (or lack the confidence to) advocate for themselves, but also the provision of education, encouragement, support and opportunities that empower people to use their own voices. If the nursing profession channelled its ability to advocate for clients into advocating for its own importance, it would likely engage in an entirely different discourse. Sometimes nurses exhibit 'learned helplessness' (Peterson, Maier & Seligman 1993) and speak of being undervalued, underpaid and under-appreciated. Leadership is about understanding nursing's image or identity, impact and worth. Language that keeps nurses 'small', or even invisible, is in direct contrast to the actual difference they make and how the community sees them. Nursing language therefore must be bold, and must more explicitly link nursing literature, knowledge and care to the positive client outcomes and experiences it affords.

Global nursing challenges

The World Health Organization (WHO 2016a) predicted a universal health workforce shortage of 40 million workers by 2030. In 2015, the WHO indicated that there were 20.7 million nurses and midwives worldwide (WHO 2016b). As nurses contend with local pressures such as client flow, demand management, changing healthcare models and settings (e.g. increased focus on community and primary health care), clients with higher-acuity health needs, the increasing burden of chronic conditions and comorbidities, and an ageing population and workforce, it can be easy to forget or ignore the global situation (Cho et al. 2015; Dossey 2016; Thompson 2016). News-media coverage of the COVID-19 pandemic and the plight of nurses around the world has attracted increased attention to the global workforce. Universal health care is an important priority for all nurses, and in the coming years global issues are likely to have a significant effect. In addition to the continuing pressures wrought by the COVID-19 pandemic, responding to the needs of refugees and migrants displaced by issues such as war, climate change, conflict, famine and communicable diseases will challenge every healthcare worker (Dossey 2016; Morabia & Benjamin 2015).

Benefits of effective nursing leadership

In short, leadership is understood to be about motivating others to achieve shared goals (Ward 2017). The literature describes leadership as 'a complex and multifaceted process which involves providing support, motivation, coordination and resources to enable individuals and teams to achieve collective objectives' (Ward 2017, p. 585; Scully 2015). Having effective leaders in nursing makes for a workplace that benefits both staff and clients (Ward 2017). Nursing leadership is essential for 'envisioning' our future and attracting people to the profession. There is a link between effective leadership in nursing and enhanced staff recruitment, retention and, most importantly, client outcomes (ACN 2015; Ward 2017).

How can you foster your own leadership potential?

With these challenges and opportunities in mind, every nurse's leadership potential can be nurtured and fostered through membership of a professional peak body such as the ACN, which has been resolute in its commitment to 'advancing nurse leadership at commonwealth, state and territory levels, as well as developing individual nurses as they acquire the skills and develop the attributes of excellence in leadership' (Ward 2017, p. 586). Creating opportunities for leadership beyond an individual organisation or position remains a priority so that each nurse, irrespective of age, stage, role or experience, can find and exercise their voice (Ward 2017). As a profession grounded in humanistic values and relationships, nurses are perfectly placed to develop leadership capabilities, as leadership is first and foremost about people. Committing to lifelong investment in developing these qualities and abilities, both personally and professionally, should be at the core of every nurse's goals.

NURSING PERSPECTIVE

I became a member of the Australian College of Nursing over 20 years ago and am proud to remain a Fellow. It is comforting to receive and engage with contemporary professional information and resources, and not to be entirely reliant on often delayed or 'sanitised' information from our individual organisations. The opportunity to connect with like-minded people around the country has always been appealing, as is being part of something greater than any one individual. In all my years as a nursing director, employing hundreds of graduates, I have always looked at resumes to see whether someone was a member of a professional body or college (and by this I do not mean our union or federation, as this is an industrial body with a different 'brief' altogether). Such membership shows an understanding of professionalism and of giving back. It also creates opportunities for a nurse to grow and gain a greater breadth and depth of connections and experience. These are the nurses I want caring for my loved ones – those who want to be the best they can be at doing whatever job they are doing right now.

The time to promote nursing leadership by supporting both our emerging and future nurse leaders is now, so that all people can continue to receive accessible, high-quality and affordable care, designed around and responsive to both the local and global needs of individuals, populations and society as a whole (Ward 2017).

Multiple-choice question
Video: ACN membership

We still have to work to break the silence

[Source: This section is reproduced from Aranda, S. (2015). We still have to work to break the silence. *Collegian*, 22(4), 351–2, with permission from Elsevier.]

Recently, as I completed my AHPRA forms online, I ticked for the last time a 'yes' to the question of being employed in a role that required me to be a registered nurse. I had just accepted a new job that required me to give up the paid roles I continued to have in both nursing education and research since moving into my first 'non-nurse' role almost five years ago. Would this mean that next year I might be no longer able to call myself an RN after 37 years? Does this even matter?

In September 2015, Kelley Johnson, the Miss America contestant from the USA state of Colorado, walked onto the stage in scrubs and gave a monologue on her special talent: 'Being a Nurse'.

Video: Kelley Johnson's monologue

For those who didn't see the YouTube clip, she gave a poignant reflection on her experience of making a difference in the life of one dementia patient and how he had taught her about the important contribution nurses make in people's lives, through the lens of being 'Just a Nurse'.

In the days following Kelley Johnson's monologue, she was ridiculed on a national television show called *The View* by women who professed to be leaders among women and examples of how far women have come since the times of our forbears. Johnson was laughed at, her talent of being a nurse compared unfavourably with the talents of singing, dancing and stereotypical desires for world peace. Centre-stage was ridicule of her wearing of a nursing 'costume', her scrubs and of wearing a 'medical' stethoscope, implying that this was an illegitimate tool for someone who was 'just a nurse'. The hosts later gave an apology of sorts, suggesting nurses needed to chill and not be so sensitive, which served only to galvanise nurses and their supporters into social commentary about what being 'just a nurse' really means. The apology suggested that despite increased understanding of and research about the important role nurses have in patient outcomes, social attitudes often reflect nurses as simply there to support the more important medical doctor who does all the real work. The show has continued to lose important sponsors, such as Johnson and Johnson, due to the remarks, the apology and the social media storm that followed.

Video: *The View* on Kelley Johnson

Among the passionate social media commentators who supported the critical role of nurses in the days following was a surgeon by the name of William R. Blythe, who spoke eloquently about nurses' roles across the client-care pathway that rendered his own role into one of minor actor.

Another important friend of nurses, perhaps the person who has most studied what nurses contribute, Suzanne Gordon, took to social media to correct the injustice and to re-activate her previous 'Just a Nurse' campaign from 2001. For several decades Gordon has called on nurses to share with the public what they know and to learn to speak differently about their profession, to help the public better understand their contribution. Her work includes the seminal book she wrote with Bernice Buresh, *From Silence to Voice.* Many nurses see this call to voice as unimportant, their mission being to focus on the wellbeing of patients. I am not of this view as I believe the silence that surrounds the work of nurses has greater impacts than we can imagine. Here are just some of the ways I believe the silence of our nurses' voices has influence:

- Our silence influences who comes into nursing – students are actively discouraged from being nurses, especially when they have the grades to get into seemingly 'more important' professions. I have stood in the line at Open Day and talked to potential medical students about why they are seeking to go into medicine. Almost all of their answers have much more to do with the role of nurses than the role of doctors. As Suzanne Gordon says, shows like *ER* have doctors performing largely nurses' work. Without this there would be very few doctors in the picture.

- Our silence reduces the influence nurses have in changing systems of care. Nurses know how systems work and often do the hard work of changing the way things are done to improve patient outcomes, from waiting times through reduction of complications and prevention of unnecessary death. However, every time a new hospital, government or system advisory committee is announced we search to find the name of the one nurse among the many doctors. Sometimes we do not even see that one nurse, and everyone wonders why the system rarely works or that changes fail to take account of the daily delivery of patient care.
- Our silence influences government policy decisions about things like Medicare billing items, rendering nurses as always subservient to doctors and costing our health system much more than is needed for work nurses are well prepared to, and do, undertake.

REFLECTION 16.3

- What is your reaction to the original monologue and the media scrutiny that followed?
- What could you do to be a 'voice for your profession' in a situation such as this?

The silence and invisibility of nurses for members of the public was brought to the surface for me recently when my niece had a ten-hour operation to remove a very large cancer from her adrenal gland. Post-operatively, the doctors were a minor and intermittent presence at her ICU bed while the nurses did the work of making sure her ravaged body healed without complication. Indeed, the operating consultant had still not visited her at day ten post-op and counting. On her second day post-operatively I observed the acute pain team discussing her pain management. Her Fentanyl epidural was not working well on the right side and they planned to start a ketamine infusion. The team, a man and a woman, talked in depth about the right approach, my initial impression being that they were two registrars or a junior consultant and registrar, such was the tone of the conversation and my own lack of recent experience in the clinical milieu. Towards the end the woman suggested a plan to make some provisional changes possible over the following 24 hours, 'or otherwise I will need to get you back' she said. At this moment I thought, I know now that you are the advanced practice nurse (APN) on the pain team. As she handed him the medical form to write up the medications my suspicions were confirmed. If she were a doctor she would have written the prescription she had devised herself. All of the planning was hers. Her call to not disturb him later by having a backup plan cleverly disguised her attempt to ensure my niece was not left in pain while waiting for a doctor to write a prescription. A couple of days later, when my niece's pain was again unstable, it was this APN who stayed with her through an increase in her ketamine dose to help her manage the auditory and visual hallucinations this caused. My niece could not have got through this with anywhere near the level of skill if not for the presence of this nurse. However, I can bet that most people observing would have thought this skilled APN was a doctor, and nothing about her attire or identification corrected this impression.

This silence and invisibility of nursing leads to misunderstanding by the public of what nurses do. My darling mother, proud of me as she is, once said 'So what is it that you do?' I replied 'These days mostly research', to which she replied 'but it's not real research is it because it doesn't save lives'. At that point in my life I was unable to reply with sufficient thought to this question. Today I would say 'Yes, Mum, it does. Every patient who is better prepared to self-assess their response to treatment and knows about their risk of blood infections after chemotherapy who comes into hospital without hesitation is a potential life saved. Every patient who is supported to stay on chemotherapy or radiotherapy because a nurse has delivered one of the interventions my team has developed has less risk of their cancer coming back and indeed might be saved by this research.'

This leads me back to the beginning. Why is it important to me and to the profession that I remain an RN in both my heart and my title as I move into this next stage of my career, where being a nurse is no longer a requirement of the job? Too many nurses who take up roles outside of nursing are seen to do so because they are 'too good' or 'too smart' to be 'just a nurse'. That is not me. I am as much a nurse in my daily life in my new role as I ever was at the bedside, in the classroom or in my research department. All I have ever done is seek larger canvases on which to try and make a bigger difference to outcomes for patients, especially those who are most vulnerable to the non-system in which health care is often delivered. Too many nurses who leave 'nursing' roles abandon their nurse identity, and it is interesting to me that this does not occur for other disciplines such as medicine, physiotherapy and social work. Indeed, I remember going to a social work alumni dinner at the university some years ago and being surprised by the four sitting members of the Victorian government in the room proudly declaring themselves social workers. I had no idea if there were any government members who were nurses. I am sure there were and are, but the silence of their voice and nursing identity is in contrast to our colleagues in social work.

I do not have room here to explore the question of whether this moving away from nursing identity is because the nurse experiences greater respect and authority for the role taken when the nursing identity is left behind. What I do know is that I have certainly experienced my views being dismissed in the context of the same views being expressed by a doctor and accepted. Short of an 'out a nurse campaign', we must give some thought about how to profile the fabulous nurses who make a big difference as leaders in our world, as one part of giving voice to the contribution of nurses and the skills they gain and have to offer. We need everyone to be part of breaking the silence! For me, being a nurse is and always will be a key part of my identity.

Developing your leadership potential

Grossman and Valiga (2021) contended that leaders are not born; rather, they emerge and continuously evolve through a range of experiences and interactions with a variety of other people. Whether you aspire to a formal leadership position or simply wish to 'do your bit' to advance the profession and strengthen your own practice, it is never too early to develop, nurture and exercise your leadership potential (Broome & Gilbert

2015). This chapter does not profess to be a stand-alone leadership development program but it offers some perspectives, ideas and encouragement to develop your motivation and capability in these areas – particularly as a student, and also beyond.

Self-assessment

Assessment of your leadership potential is one of the first, and regular, steps you should take (Broome & Gilbert 2015). Reflection and self-awareness may be useful in this regard, but you are likely to be best served by the use of structured **self-assessment tools**, which provide validated items, questions and scores or scales to identify your strengths and limitations in certain areas. Compare these with previous assessments and use this information to inform and evaluate personal leadership development plans and strategies (Broome & Gilbert 2015).

self-assessment tools validated tools that guide the identification of your leadership strengths and limitations for the purpose of informing and evaluating your personal leadership development plans and strategies

There is no 'one size fits all' when it comes to such tools. An internet search will reveal a plethora of tools and options, and it is important that you review these carefully (and possibly use some 'trial and error') to identify one that is relevant and meaningful for your particular needs and circumstances. In the 'leadership challenge' model discussed earlier in this chapter, Kouzes and Posner (2018) presented a *leadership practices inventory* for students, which may be a good place to start.

REFLECTION 16.4

- What personal skills, strengths, attributes and characteristics do you possess that will enable you to assume or demonstrate leadership as a nurse?
- What would you like to work on or develop further? How might you go about fostering your leadership potential?

Continuous learning and professional development

Your university may offer a range of leadership development opportunities, including units, modules or programs, both within and external to your actual degree program or school. You may also choose to engage in other learning opportunities, including free online courses offered through global learning platforms such as Future Learn, Coursera or the Khan Academy (an online search will reveal many more); a MOOC (Massive Open Online Course) offered by many universities; or various seminars and short courses offered by professional associations such as the ACN. As the preeminent professional body for policy, governance and leadership in our profession, the ACN hosts the Emerging Nurse Leaders Program, which recognises and develops future generations of leaders in nursing through a range of learning, mentoring and engagement strategies, beginning at the undergraduate level.

There are also several postgraduate courses available at Australian universities for registered nurses (including new graduates) who want to develop their leadership skills.

Leadership development as a student nurse

As a student, you may think that you are entering nursing at the bottom rung of the profession, so it can be hard to work out how you can 'lead' (or be a leader) early in your career. We asked some recent graduates how they developed their leadership skills while at university. This is what they said:

- *Group work.* I hated group work at first. It often required us to work with people we were unfamiliar with, and was frequently linked to assessment tasks, which raised all sorts of challenges associated with different motivations, expectations, standards, and technology literacy. This changed when I was asked to co-lead a group project with another team member. Between us, we were able to use our communication and negotiation skills to establish a shared vision for the project, get input from the whole team about their particular skills and preferences, and then set agreed tasks and deadlines based on what they told us. We did not want to be overly demanding or directive, but we set up an online chat, regularly checked in with team members and offered support and advice to help keep everyone on track. We ended up with a High Distinction for that project, and I always volunteered to be a leader in group work after that.
- *Peer-Assisted Study Sessions (PASS).* When I was a third-year student I worked as a PASS leader, providing online learning, revision and mentoring sessions for second-year students. It was a great opportunity to write learning materials, design activities and coordinate participant engagement and communication via an online platform. I was able to develop and practise a range of valuable skills but I'm certain I learned as much from them as they did from me.
- *Student societies.* The cohort before us had no nursing society so along with a few friends I decided to establish one. The aim of this society was 'to create opportunities for students to get to know each other in social settings; to advance the profile and contribution of the nursing discipline; and to advocate for changes that [helped to] achieve a stronger connection with each other, our campus and the broader university [community]' (Williams & Arnott 2014). Setting up the society was a huge learning curve. We had to communicate with the student union, find funding, draft a constitution and information materials, and recruit members.

It was so worth it, though, and the university now has a vibrant nursing society with growing membership.

- *Faculty committees.* I was elected as a student representative on my faculty's Learning and Teaching Committee, which was responsible for reviewing changes to course content, delivery and assessments. I had always been confident and comfortable interacting with my peers but taking on the responsibility of being a 'voice' for the students really helped to develop my consultation, negotiation and feedback skills. Joining the committee was scary at first but I was able to provide some important insights and network with a range of faculty members, which quickly helped me to gain confidence. Later in my career, I'd like to teach, so it also provided an interesting and informative insight into academic processes.
- *Vice-Chancellor's Leadership Program (VCLP).* The VCLP is a program open to all students at my university, and I started it in my third year. The aim of the program is to identify and develop leadership values, strengths and skills via community activity, such as volunteering and working with other student leaders. The program involved writing a leadership development plan; completing two citations (I did *community and civic,* and volunteered to fulfil that, and *research,* where I did a six-week research internship directly after my final nursing exam); developing my CV and LinkedIn profile; preparing various reflective pieces; and participation in a panel interview. I successfully gained the Vice-Chancellor's Leadership Award and it led to so many other opportunities after university.

Short-answer question

Get involved: Professional nursing associations

Professional associations and societies are not just for registered nurses; they also provide many benefits for students. Professional associations provide an environment of collegiality, leadership and advocacy, which helps in formulating your professional identity as a nurse and in advancing the nursing profession by fostering high standards of nursing practice, promoting safe, ethical and collaborative work environments, enhancing the health, wellness and satisfaction of nurses themselves, and advocating on healthcare issues and policies that affect nurses and the public (Cline, Curtin & Johnston 2019; ICN 2017). These associations may have a general or specialist focus and achieve these outcomes through a range of activities, including the development of policy documents and position statements; publication of professional journals; provision of education and training; organisation and hosting of scientific meetings, conferences and seminars; sponsorship of research, scholarships and award programs; and facilitation of online communities of practice (Cline et al. 2019).

> **professional associations**
> professional groups or organisations that provide an environment of collegiality, leadership, advocacy, continuing education and mentoring to help advance the nursing profession and promote high standards of nursing practice

As a student, you will often receive reduced or subsidised membership fees and full access to resources, events and mentoring while you study, along with opportunities to meet and network with other nurses, students, leaders and supporters. A range of professional nursing associations you might consider joining include:

- your university's nursing society and other university clubs;
- Australian College of Nursing (ACN);
- Australian Student and Novice Nurse Association (ASANNA);
- National Rural Health Student Network (NRHSN);

- Australian College of Critical Care Nurses (ACCCN);
- Australian Primary Health Care Nurses Association (APNA);
- College of Emergency Nursing Australasia (CENA);
- Australia College of Mental Health Nurses (ACMHN);
- Enrolled Nurse Professional Association NSW (ENPA NSW); and
- an Australian branch of the Sigma Theta Tau International Honor Society of Nursing.

Multiple-choice question

Mentoring

mentoring a supportive and developmental relationship between a more experienced or skilled mentor and a less experienced protégé, which exists to enhance professional growth and maximise individual potential

Mentoring programs are becoming increasingly common at many universities, so you may already have had an opportunity to work with an academic or career mentor. Mentoring is also an important feature of the supervisory arrangements and relationships you will encounter in the professional experience placement component of your nursing degree. For those wanting to extend such opportunities, mentoring may also be offered through various industry groups or professional associations.

Engaging with a mentor can accelerate self-development and growth (Broome & Gilbert 2015). The mentor–mentee relationship is defined as a supportive and developmental relationship between a more experienced or skilled mentor and a less experienced mentee or protégé, in which both benefit through the sharing of knowledge, skills, attitudes and experiences to help enhance professional growth and maximise individual potential based on the mentee's goals, career direction and timeframe for professional development (Broome & Gilbert 2015; Burgess, van Diggele & Mellis 2018; Pullen 2016). According to Broome and Gilbert (2015), this relationship generally comprises three core functions: career support (in which the mentor serves as a coach and champion for the protégé); psychosocial support (including acceptance, confirmation and counselling); and role-modelling (providing the protégé with a frame of reference for appropriate professional behaviours and values).

As a student, you may be able to start building your own mentoring skills by participating in peer mentoring through your school or faculty, such as the PASS program mentioned earlier in this chapter.

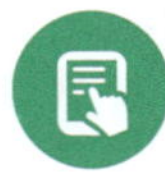

Short-answer question

Volunteering

volunteering unpaid participation in work experience as a means of developing and practising your professional skills and attributes and building your resume

Volunteering is a great way to develop and practise your skills, gain work experience and build your resume while you study. You may already be involved with or know of organisations in your local area but if not, there are national and state-based volunteer registers, like Volunteering Australia, where you can search for volunteering opportunities that suit you. In making your decisions, consider the type of organisation and workplace you would like to join, the tasks you would like to do and who you would like to work with or for, as well as how much time you can offer and how you will fit your volunteering around your studies and other commitments.

Volunteering provides a range of benefits and opportunities, such as working collaboratively with people who share your values to make a difference; learning and developing new skills; gaining workplace experience; establishing professional networks; being part of a community; and increasing your confidence and pride in your achievements (Williamson et al. 2018).

REFLECTION 16.5

- What type of volunteer work would you like to do?
- How might it benefit your future career choices?

NURSING PERSPECTIVE

While I was completing my third (and final) year of undergraduate studies to become a registered nurse, I realised I wanted to work in oncology, so I started looking for volunteering work that could help me reach my career goal. I already volunteered at Cancer Council events, where I met cancer clients and survivors, but I wanted an ongoing role where I could meet some people working directly in this field. I had some experience in social media management, and while I was on a community placement one of the GPs recommended that I contact a small, state-based, not-for-profit organisation to see whether I could help them out.

The organisation raises awareness of melanoma, and supports people at risk of, or affected by, this form of cancer. I contacted the founder and soon started working with her for about eight hours every week. I chose to volunteer there because of the following reasons:

- Its mission aligned with my own interests, values and career ambitions.
- The board comprised oncology clinicians, including doctors and nurses, and melanoma clients, whose experiences and expertise underpin the resources and campaigns offered by the organisation. I was excited by the opportunity to network with and learn from these people.
- It was a small and relatively new organisation, so I could participate and contribute in a variety of ways that I knew would be valuable to it, but would also stretch and challenge me.

I volunteered for a year, and in that time I reviewed and reorganised the website and Facebook page, drafted a social media strategy, created a publishing calendar, helped to draft and design newsletters, and assisted with grant writing. I also helped to organise and host some local events, and to present to and collaborate with the board, staff and other volunteers. These opportunities contributed to me developing a range of personal and professional skills, such as the ability to source and interpret information; develop high-level communication skills with clients, the public and experts in the field; learn new technology skills; self-motivate and work autonomously; manage and prioritise my own time and that of others; and lead tasks and projects through to completion, including planning and coordinating necessary resources.

I really believe that volunteering enhanced my graduate capabilities and leadership potential – and it looks great on my resume. Communicating regularly with leaders in the field broke down my fears about starting out in nursing. It helped me to build confidence and broaden my oncology knowledge, and provided insight into melanoma clients' experiences and needs, preparing me to support and advocate for them in my own nursing practice. Best of all, I detailed my volunteering in my Transition to Practice application, and I attained a place in a graduate-year program in oncology nursing!

Research

Many students think that research is conducted in laboratories by scientists – and some is – but there is a huge body of nursing literature based on research studies designed and administered by nurses who practice nursing in a range of environments. This research creates best practice in nursing, which leads to better client outcomes. Evidence-based nursing care evolves from implementation of the latest research findings, which is another reason nursing is such an interesting job: it is dynamic and requires us to be lifelong learners who continue to develop our knowledge and skills for professional practice.

Research is obviously important in the context of your academic studies and achievement of clinical excellence, but involvement in research as a student can also contribute to the development of your professional capability and leadership skills. So how might you get involved? Here are some suggestions:

- *Participate.* Most academics are also involved in research, and your lecturers may invite you to be a participant in a study – for example, about student nurse perceptions or experiences. Do it! Your participation will most likely be anonymous and you will be asked to sign documentation about your involvement before you do anything. Being a participant in a study will help you understand the research process. After you have gained some insight into how it works, the kinds of research studies you reference in your academic assessments will be less confusing or daunting.
- *Assist.* If you have the chance to assist any of your lecturers in conducting research, ask them what is involved, check that you have enough time and help out. You might search for articles for the literature review part of their study, help to recruit participants or assist with general administration. You will learn about the research process and it will look great on your resume.
- *Conduct.* If you want to pursue research as a career, or even as part of your nursing role, apply for a research internship at your university or at an associated research institute to get a feel for what is required. If you are keen to jump right in, apply for research honours in nursing as an extension to your undergraduate degree.
- *Administer.* If you are organised, interested in client experience, and want to learn about research processes, consider becoming a clinical trials nurse in a hospital or a research institute. Trials nurses recruit clients or participants, liaise with them, educate them about trial participation and interventions, administer medications or other interventions, conduct tests (bloods, ECGs), and monitor and document outcomes, among other things. It is a challenging and varied role that involves liaison with researchers, study participants, and other nurses and health professionals (Holmström 2020).

Short-answer question

CASE STUDY

Research internships

Towards the end of my degree program, I applied for a research internship at an institute for medical research that is affiliated with my university.

I applied so I could experience what biomedical research involves from day to day, and to find out whether a research career would suit me – and, more importantly, whether I would suit it. A list of possible projects and mentors was supplied and I had to secure my internship (and a mentor) by writing a detailed application similar to any job application, in which I needed to clearly outline my interest and capability for this role. The researcher who took me on informed me that I would drive a small research project with her guidance and input, and other help as required, with the end-goal of drafting an article about our findings for submission to (and hopefully publication in) a peer-reviewed journal.

My project involved assessing how 'heart-healthy' Australians are, analysing data from the Australian Bureau of Statistics' National Health Survey on the health of Australian adults against the American Heart Association's benchmark Life's Simple 7 health metric. I began my internship by reading an epidemiology textbook and then started the research process, in which I compared Australian health guidelines against Life's Simple 7's recommendations, read studies from around the world on Life's Simple 7, conducted a literature review, defined the statistical search parameters and analysed and reviewed our findings. I created graphs, tables and charts to make our findings easily comprehensible, then drafted the article for dissemination of these findings. Along the way, I met weekly with my mentor, who guided my inquiries and helped with the data extraction but encouraged me to lead the project. I loved that first glimpse of what research involves and was inspired to become a researcher. But there were other benefits of the internship, too.

My research mentor acted as a career mentor. She knew it could be difficult for nurses to move into research and she welcomed my enthusiasm. On the final day of my internship, she invited me to undertake a research honours program at the institute, working on data relating to a large longitudinal study. Of course, I said yes. So now, as a novice nurse, I have an article being assessed by a prominent Australian medical journal, opportunities to present my research at public health conferences, and an honours research project all of my own to complete part time, over two years. I had been nervous to apply for the internship, assuming it was only for medical students, but I am so glad I did. I learned that I am suited to research, and the internship has developed and refined my skills and shaped my future career.

QUESTIONS

1 What were some of the important leadership and empowerment skills and attributes that were enacted or demonstrated by the intern and mentor in this scenario?

2 How could you use research (not necessarily a formal internship) as a way of developing and practising your own leadership capacity?

Speak up and be heard

This chapter has emphasised the importance of using your voice to make a difference. This might involve having the confidence (and courage) to exercise your professional and ethical responsibility to speak up when something has gone wrong, someone has done the wrong thing or things need to be changed, but it may also involve using your voice in other ways. You can advocate for the nursing profession via social media, sharing evidence-based information and public health campaigns among colleagues and contacts. You can participate in nursing events, such as International Nurses Day, which help to raise the nursing profession's professional profile (ICN 2017). You can speak up to take on leadership roles, whether in study groups or in your workplace. What is important is that all nurses feel empowered to express themselves as professionals, which in turn changes public perceptions of nurses so that we are recognised as healthcare representatives and leaders. You may feel as a student nurse that nursing leadership is years away, but you can begin now by mentoring, volunteering, taking out student memberships of professional nursing organisations and seeking out student leadership programs and opportunities. That way, you will develop confidence as a novice nurse to represent the nursing profession and to seek out leadership opportunities that help to foster change, promote clinical excellence and 'secure nurses' place at the table'.

SUMMARY

- This chapter has detailed the responsibility we all have to advance the quality and excellence of our own practice, and also to be a voice for our profession and a leader in the changes and improvements that are necessary to promote optimal health outcomes for local and global communities. The ICN (2017) describes leadership as a process, not a position, asserting that it is not necessary to have a traditional title or elected position to take a lead and bring about change that benefits others. This chapter has discussed how nurses can be active and influential at all levels, including in education, clinical practice, the workplace, interdisciplinary teams, the research setting and the wider community.
- This chapter has emphasised empowerment and leadership as having four aims: promoting optimal health outcomes for individuals and populations, improving the quality and cost-effectiveness of health systems, enhancing client experience and satisfaction, and improving the working life of nurses themselves. We have examined the idea that 'being a nurse means being a leader', and the importance of this leadership mindset in nursing claiming its rightful place as equals in healthcare governance and reform.

  Leadership is about understanding our identity, influence and worth, and this chapter has called for all nurses to exercise their influence and voice in ways that more explicitly link our contribution to the positive client and system outcomes it affords. The silence that surrounds the work and contribution of nurses influences how we attract and retain future nurses, and diminishes the influence that nurses have on systems of care and the policies, resources and technologies that drive quality and excellence in these systems.

As part of a profession grounded in humanistic values and relationships, nurses are perfectly placed to develop leadership capabilities, as leadership is first and foremost about people. This chapter has discussed how your leadership potential can be nurtured and fostered through membership of a professional association such as the ACN. Such membership helps to foster your own professional growth and development, shows an understanding of professionalism and of giving back, and gives a collective voice to nurses and the knowledge and skills we have to offer.

- This chapter has outlined perspectives, strategies and encouragement for developing your motivation and capability as a leader, both as a student and beyond. Self-assessment, learning and professional development, professional associations and societies, mentoring, volunteering, research and social media have all been discussed as possible strategies or opportunities for developing your leadership potential.

ACKNOWLEDGEMENT

The authors of this chapter would like to acknowledge Sanchia Aranda and Elsevier for the contribution of the section 'We still have to work to break the silence'.

REVIEW QUESTIONS

Suggested responses

1 What is the 'quadruple aim' of empowerment and leadership?
2 What differentiates transformational and transactional leadership?
3 Are the qualities and attributes of a good nurse manager different from those needed to be a good leader, and can leadership be demonstrated outside a formal management position?
4 How do professional associations contribute to empowerment of the nursing profession?
5 What are some of the benefits and opportunities that may come from volunteering while you study?

RESEARCH TOPIC

Search for and review some of the leadership self-assessment tools that are available. You will discover many of these through a simple internet search, but a summary of some common tools is provided in Broome and Gilbert (2015), which is a good starting point. Following this review, select and apply a tool that resonates for you and use this information to develop an initial leadership development plan to guide your proactive development and progress as a student and new graduate.

FURTHER READING

Australian College of Nursing (ACN) (2016). *Nurses are essential in health and aged care reform*. Canberra: ACN. Available from https://www.acn.edu.au/wp-content/uploads/white-paper-nurses-essential-health-aged-care-reform.pdf.

——— (2018). *NurseStrong care packages*. Available from https://www.acn.edu.au/nursestrong.

Daly, J., Speedy, S. & Jackson, D. (2015). *Leadership and nursing: Contemporary perspectives*, 2nd edn. Sydney: Elsevier.

International Council of Nurses (ICN) (2017). *Nurses: A voice to lead – achieving the Sustainable Development Coals*. Available from https://www.icnvoicetolead.com/wp-content/uploads/2017/04/ICN_AVoiceToLead_guidancePack-9.pdf.

Kouzes, J. & Posner, B. (2018). *The student leadership challenge: Five practices for becoming an exemplary leader*, 3rd edn. San Francisco: Jossey-Bass.

Scully, N.J. (2015). Leadership in nursing: The importance of recognising inherent values and attributes to secure a positive future for the profession. *Collegian*, 22(4), 439–44.

REFERENCES

Aranda, S. (2015). We still have to work to break the silence. *Collegian*, 22(4), 351–2.

Australian College of Nursing (ACN) (2015). *Nurse leadership*. Canberra: ACN. Retrieved from https://www.acn.edu.au/wp-content/uploads/2017/10/acn_nurse_leadership_white_paper_reprint_2017_web.pdf.

——— (2017). Nurses: A voice to lead. ACN Fact Sheet. Canberra: ACN.

——— (2020). The importance of value-based health care to patient centred, fiscally responsible health care and the centrality of nursing to its authentic and effective functioning. (White Paper.) Canberra: ACN.

Australian Institute of Health and Welfare (AIHW) (2020). *Health workforce*. Retrieved from https://www.aihw.gov.au/reports/australias-health/health-workforce.

Barnard, R., Jones, J. & Cruice, M. (2020). Communication between therapists and nurses working in inpatient interprofessional teams: systematic review and meta-ethnography. *Disability & Rehabilitation*, 42(10), 1339–49.

Boamah, S.A., Spence Laschinger, H.K., Wong, C. & Clarke, S. (2018). Effect of transformational leadership on job satisfaction and patient safety outcomes. *Nursing Outlook*, 66(2), 180–9.

Brokaw, J.J. (2016). The nursing profession's potential impact on policy and politics. *American Nurse*, 22 September. Retrieved from https://www.myamericannurse.com/nursing-professions-potential-impact-policy-politics.

Broome, M. & Gilbert J. (2015). Developing and sustaining self. In J. Daly, S. Speedy & D. Jackson (eds), *Leadership and nursing: Contemporary perspectives*, 2nd edn. Sydney: Elsevier.

Burgess, A., van Diggele, C. & Mellis, C. (2018). Mentorship in the health professions: A review. *The Clinical Teacher*, 15(3), 197–202.

Cato, D., Walker, K., Anders, D., Fuyang, F. & McFadden, M. (2019). The CNO US Healthcare Immersion Program, Part 1: A transformational leadership model. *Nursing Administration Quarterly*, 43(1), 40–9.

Chankova, S. (2020). Florence Nightingale and the changing face of nursing. *The Economist*. Retrieved from https://theworldin.economist.com/edition/2020/article/17519/florence-nightingale-and-changing-face-nursing.

Cho, E., Sloane, D.M., Kim, E.Y., Kim, S., Choi, M., Yoo, I.Y., Lee, H.S. & Aiken, L.H. (2015). Effects of nurse staffing, work environments, and education on patient mortality: An observational study. *International Journal of Nursing Studies*, 52(2), 535–42.

Cline, D., Curtin, K. & Johnston, P. A. (2019). Professional organization membership: The benefits of increasing nursing participation. *Clinical Journal of Oncology Nursing*, 23(5), 543–6.

Courtney, M., Nash, R., Thornton, R. & Potgieter, I. (2015). Leading and managing in nursing practice: Concepts, processes and challenges In J. Daly, S. Speedy & D. Jackson (eds), *Leadership and nursing: Contemporary perspectives*, 2nd edn. Sydney: Elsevier.

Daly, J., Speedy, S. & Jackson, D. (2015). *Leadership and nursing: Contemporary perspectives*, 2nd edn. Sydney: Elsevier.

Doherty, D.P. & Hunter Revell, S.M. (2020). Developing nurse leaders: Toward a theory of authentic leadership empowerment. *Nursing Forum*, 3, 416.

Dossey, B. (2016). Global health, decent care, and the Nightingale Declaration. In B. Dossey (ed) *Holistic nursing: A handbook for practice*, 7th edn. Burlington, MA: Jones & Bartlett Learning.

Gardner, G.E. (2017). New nursing for a new generation health service: The National Health Forum Oration (extract). *The Hive*, 19, 10.

Grossman, S. & Valiga, T. (2021). *The new leadership challenge: Creating the future of nursing*, 6th edn. Philadelphia, PA: F.A. Davis.

Holmström, R. (2020). Clinical trials: what does a research nurse do? Roles that can change patients' lives, from study coordinator to supporting participants. *Cancer Nursing Practice*, 19(6), 20–22.

Hougaard, R. & Carter, J. (2017). f you aspire to be a great leader, be present. *Harvard Business Review*, 13 December. Retrieved from https://hbr.org/2017/12/if-you-aspire-to-be-a-great-leader-be-present.

International Council of Nurses (ICN) (2016). *ICN Biennial Report 2014–2015*. Retrieved from http://www.icn.ch/images/stories/documents/publications/biennial_reports/ICN_Biennial_Report_2014–2015.pdf.

——— (2017). *Nurses: A voice to lead – achieving the Sustainable Development Goals*. Retrieved from https://www.icnvoicetolead.com/wp-content/uploads/2017/04/ICN_AVoiceToLead_guidancePack-9.pdf.

Jackson, D., Bradbury-Jones, C., Baptiste, D., Gelling, L., Morin, K., Neville, S. & Smith, G.D. (2020). Life in the pandemic: Some reflections on nursing in the context of COVID-19. *Journal of Clinical Nursing*, 29(13–14), 2041–3.

Khoshmehr, Z., Barkhordari-Sharifabad, M., Nasiriani, K. & Fallahzadeh, H. (2020). Moral courage and psychological empowerment among nurses. *BMC Nursing*, 19(1), 1–7.

Komives, S.R., Wagner, W. & Associates (2016). *Leadership for a better world: Understanding the social change model of leadership development*, 2nd edn. San Francisco: Jossey-Bass.

Kouzes, J. & Posner, B. (2018). *The student leadership challenge: Five practices for becoming an exemplary leader*, 3rd edn. San Francisco: Jossey-Bass.

Levett-Jones, T. & Bourgeois, S. (2015). *The clinical placement: An essential guide for nursing students*, 3rd edn. Sydney: Elsevier.

Mannix, J., Wilkes, L. & Daly, J. (2015). Watching an artist at work: Aesthetic leadership in clinical nursing workplaces. *Journal of Clinical Nursing*, 24(23–24), 3511–18.

Morabia, A. & Benjamin, G.C. (2015). The refugee crisis in the Middle East and public health. *American Journal of Public Health*, 105(12), 2405–6.

Nursing and Midwifery Board of Australia (NMBA) (2020). Registrant data. Reporting period: 1 July 2020–30 September 2020. Retrieved from http://www.nursingmidwiferyboard.gov.au/About/Statistics.aspx.

Peterson, C., Maier, S. & Seligman, M.E.P. (1993). *Learned helplessness: A theory for the age of personal control.* New York: Oxford University Press.

Pullen, R.L. (2016). Leadership in nursing practice. *Nursing Made Incredibly Easy*, 14(3), 26–31.

Richards, A. (2020). Exploring the benefits and limitations of transactional leadership in healthcare. *Nursing Standard*, 16(1), 46–50.

Roy Morgan (2017). Roy Morgan Image of Professions Survey 2016: Nurses still easily most highly regarded – followed by doctors, pharmacists & engineers. Retrieved from http://www.roymorgan.com/findings/6797-image-of-professions-2016–201605110031.

Scully, N.J. (2015). Leadership in nursing: The importance of recognising inherent values and attributes to secure a positive future for the profession. *Collegian*, 22(4), 439–44.

Sikka, R., Morath, J.M. & Leape, L. (2015). The quadruple aim: Care, health, cost and meaning in work. *BMJ Quality & Safety*, 24(10), 608–10.

Taberna, M., Gil Moncayo, F., Jané-Salas, E., Antonio, M., Arribas, L., Vilajosana, E., Peralvez Torres, E. & Mesía, R. (2020). The multidisciplinary team (MDT) approach and quality of care. *Frontiers in Oncology*, 10(March).

Thompson, P.E. (2016). New generation leaders: The future for nursing and midwifery. *Journal of Nursing Management*, 24(3), 273–4.

Ward, K. (2017). Guest editorial: Nursing leadership and Australian College of Nursing's (ACN) work in capacity building for the Journal of Nursing Management, *Journal of Nursing Management*, 25, 585–6.

Williams, D. & Arnott, N. (2014). Achieving a sense of 'place': Reflections from a satellite campus, *Places & Spaces – Proceedings of the Teaching Matters 2014 conference*, 56–64.

Williamson, I., Wildbur, D., Bell, K., Tanner, J. & Matthews, H. (2018). Benefits to university students through volunteering in a health context: A new model. *British Journal of Educational Studies*, 66(3), 383–402.

World Health Organization (WHO) (2016a). *Global strategy on human resources for health: Workforce 2030.* Retrieved from https://apps.who.int/iris/bitstream/handle/10665/250368/9789241511131-eng.pdf;jsessionid=EC24FBAF2F30EA76B8776FEC6DBC67D6?sequence=1.

——— (2016b). *Global strategic directions for strengthening nursing and midwifery 2016–2020.* Retrieved from https://www.who.int/hrh/nursing_midwifery/global-strategy-midwifery-2016-2020/en.

Ziel, S.E. (2016). Nurses as leaders in healthcare design: A resource for nurses and interprofessional partners. *Interdisciplinary Journal of Partnership Studies*, 3(2), Article 8.

Preparing for the transition to registered nursing practice

Jackie Lea

The author acknowledges that an earlier version of material contained in this chapter appeared in Lea (2013).

LEARNING OBJECTIVES

At the completion of this chapter, you should be able to:

1 Demonstrate an understanding of the process of transition to registered nursing practice.
2 Identify ways to manage the transition to professional nursing practice effectively, including caring for yourself.
3 Reflect on the professional roles, responsibilities and autonomy required of beginning registered nurses.
4 Develop and refine a professional portfolio that reflects your beginning registered nursing status, including preparing an application for a new graduate nurse position.

Introduction

What do you expect the first year of professional nursing practice to be like? What will this time be like for you, personally and professionally? This chapter aims to start you thinking and reflecting on how you will manage the change, the skills you need to refine and the self-support strategies you need to develop in your final year so that you are well placed for a successful transition to professional registered nursing practice.

There are many things you can do to enable yourself to be as ready as possible. This chapter focuses on preparing you to enter the nursing workforce. For the beginning registered nurse, this process is known as the transition to professional practice. In examining this transition, concepts related to the theory of professional socialisation and the reality shock that can occur for new graduate nurses as they enter the workforce are examined to help you understand what you may experience during this transition. In addition, the expectations of new graduates about their identity, autonomy and professionalism as they enter the nursing workforce are investigated. Finally, this chapter explores how to prepare for the graduate year, through professional portfolios and resumes, refinement and drafting applications for graduate nurse positions.

The process of transition to registered nursing practice

transition a passage from one life phase, condition or status to another; transition refers to both the process and the outcome of complex person–environment interactions, may involve more than one person and is embedded in the context and the situation (Chick & Meleis 1986, pp. 239–40)

Whether you have previous experience in nursing, perhaps as an assistant in nursing, an endorsed enrolled nurse or an international nurse, the journey of **transition** to a new role can be like a rollercoaster of emotions – especially in the first three months, which can be a particularly stressful time. A transition is movement and adaption to change (Kralik, Visentin & van Loon 2006, p. 326), and the transition to professional nursing practice has been described as 'a process of making a significant adjustment to changing personal and professional roles at the start of one's nursing career and generally thought to encompass the first 12 months as a graduate' (Duchscher 2008, p. 442).

Professional socialisation

The process of transition from student to graduate nurse is an intense period of socialisation into the workplace culture. In nursing, professional socialisation is 'a process where a student or nurse acquires the knowledge and skills needed for practice' (Oermann 1997, p. 10). This process enables an individual to develop a self-concept associated with a role and then to acquire the role behaviours and expectations needed to carry out the role in practice. For each new role that is acquired, a re-socialisation process or role transition will occur. In nursing, re-socialisation, or role transition, often occurs with a change in focus of a role. Moving to a nursing management role or from community nursing to an acute setting, or vice versa, are two examples.

The role transition or re-socialisation occurs for new graduate nurses entering professional practice when there is a need to adapt to the workplace nursing role learned in the educational setting. As a new graduate nurse, you may also experience frequent re-socialisation, because graduate nursing programs in Australia may require graduates to rotate through different clinical areas, where you must learn to adapt to different clinical roles, management styles, client-care practices and staff personalities.

Transition models

A large body of evidence describes the transition to professional practice and what that experience is like, and it is recommended that you should do your own investigation around this concept. See, for example, evidence from Kralik, Visentin and van Loon (2006), who suggested that the transition process of becoming a registered nurse has four identifiable phases. The first phase involves the predictable, structured and familiar life of a student, which provides security and a recognised identity, plus a range of friendships and relationships in which you as a student are accepted. An ending to being a student, which is characterised by disruption, ambiguity, loss of identity, insecurity and marginalisation, indicates the second phase. A limbo phase follows, wherein becoming a registered nurse may be disorientating and disempowering, and may involve feelings of confusion, powerlessness, isolation and insecurity. The final phase is characterised by graduate nurses becoming acclimatised to a new role and identity, with experiences related to renewal, transformation, familiarity and reconnection with colleagues.

It is not possible to set boundaries on the time taken to move through these phases, as transitions do not always follow the same trajectory. However, people can move back and forward through transition phases, depending on what is occurring in their lives (Fedoruk & Hofmeyer 2012, p. 5). For you as a student nurse, **professional socialisation** and subsequent role acquisition will occur initially in the educational setting. This is followed up in the practice setting, where an awareness of the nursing role – which can only be shaped by experience – is developed.

One of the best-known models of re-socialisation and the transition into nursing, which describes the *reality shock* experienced through the transition from the educational setting to the workplace for new graduate nurses, comes from Kramer (1974). The model describes the fears and difficulties experienced by new graduate nurses in adapting to the work setting, which remain applicable to the transitions that occur for new graduates today. Winter-Collins and McDaniel (2000, p. 106) discuss four phases of reality shock that are experienced sequentially by newly graduated nurses and that are identified by Kramer's 1974 model; these are represented in Figure 17.1. The first stage is *the honeymoon phase*, which is characterised by excitement and euphoria when obtaining your first nursing job. *The shock phase* constitutes the second stage: as a graduate, you may discover that your goals may not be able to be met because of your inexperience or because of the organisational nature or culture of the environment. This shock phase is often characterised by feelings of depression, outrage and fatigue. It is followed by a *recovery phase*, wherein you gain some perspective of the job. The fourth and final phase is the *resolution phase*, where you acquire a nursing self-identity.

professional socialisation
a process whereby an individual learns the roles and values of a profession, with the aim of developing a professional identity; in nursing, professional socialisation is 'a process where a student or nurse acquires the knowledge and skills needed for practice' and also where they 'internalise the norms and values of the nursing profession into their behaviour' (Oermann 1997, p. 10)

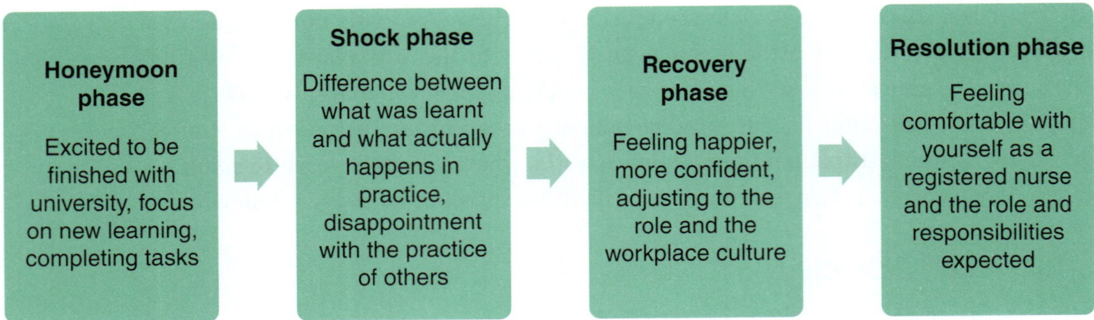

Figure 17.1   Reality shock model

Source: Adapted from Winter-Collins and McDaniel (2000, p. 106).

The stages of transition

The concept of 'reality shock' continues to serve today as a construct for understandings of the initial transition to professional practice, in a theory of the stages of transition that is specific to new graduate nurses. The theory includes transition shock (see Figure 17.2), which occurs when new graduates move from the protected academic environment to the unfamiliar and 'expectant' context of professional practice (Duchscher 2009, p. 1111).

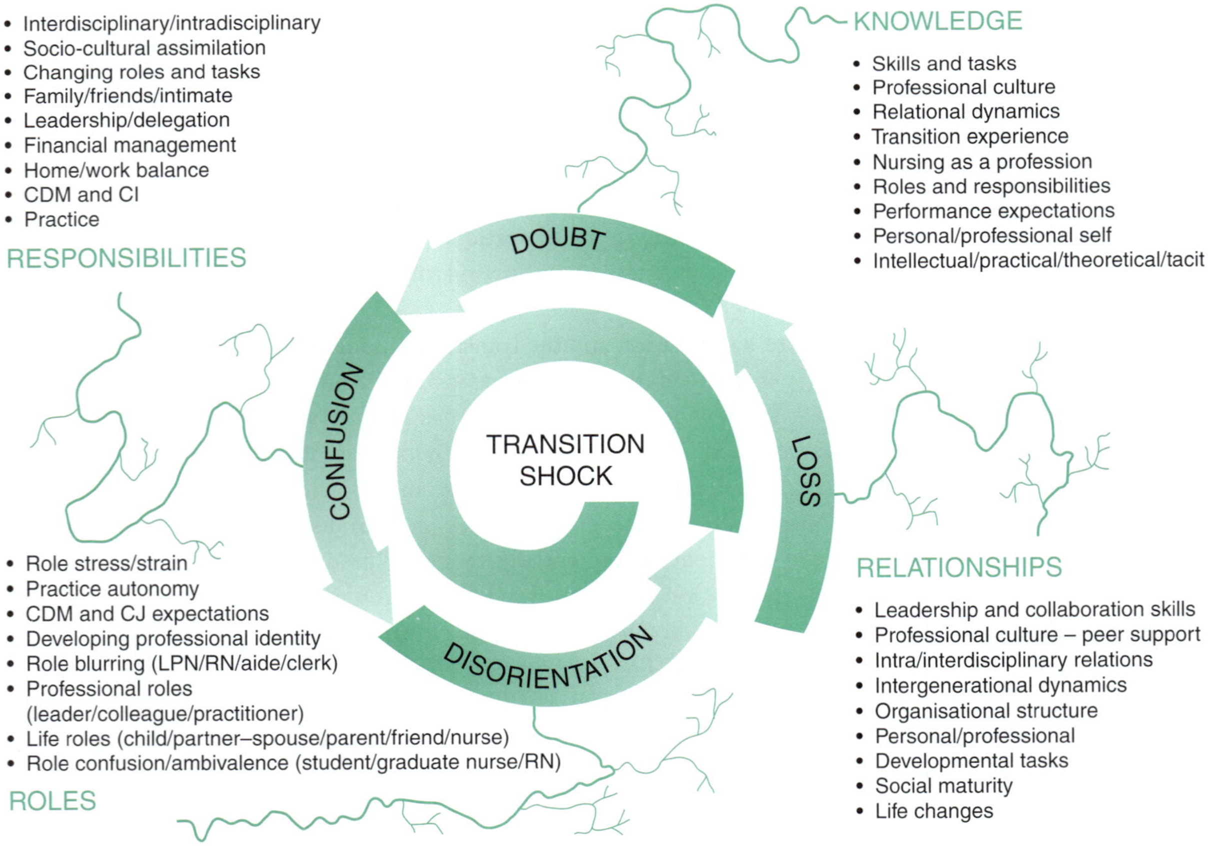

Figure 17.2   Transition shock model

Source: Duchscher (2009).

Duchscher's (2008) model for new graduate nurse transition illustrates three stages of doing, being and knowing through which new graduate nurses progress within the first 12 months of practice. Duchscher identified that the time taken for new graduates to move through these stages is different for each new graduate, and that it is influenced by the clinical context, practice situations and/or events (2009, p. 1111) (see Figure 17.3)

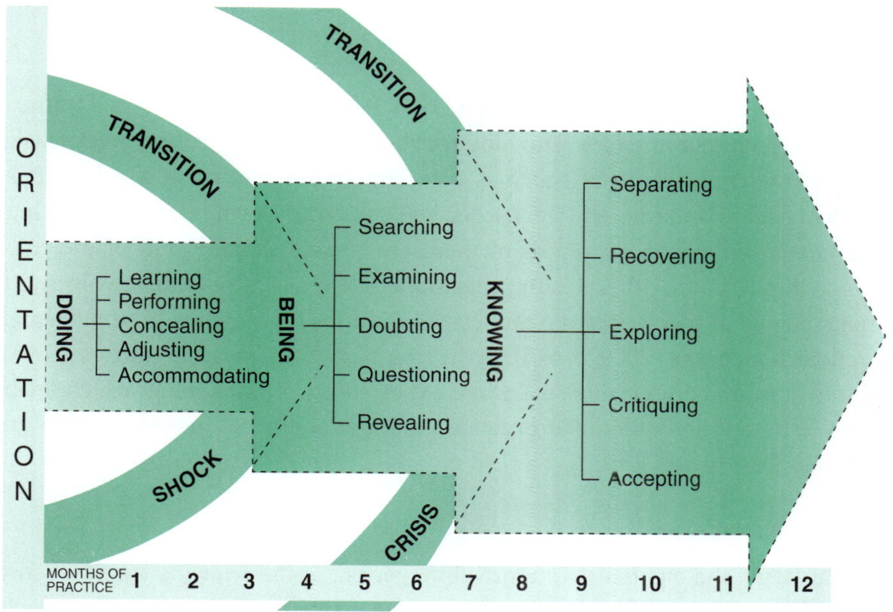

Figure 17.3   Stages of transition theory

Source: Duchscher (2008, p. 443).

Stage 1: Doing

The first three to four months of transition are represented by the *doing* stage, which is the period of 'in-between-ness', when you are moving from the known role of the student to the less familiar role of professional practitioner (Duchscher 2009, p. 1111). The first stage of changing roles, responsibilities relationships and levels of knowledge is characterised by feelings of disorientation, loss, doubt and confusion. The adjustments in the first one to four months are the result of emotional, physical, intellectual and sociocultural changes, and are associated with feelings of overwhelming stress and anxiety that often correlate with a lack of practice experience and confidence, plus insecurities about communicating and relating to colleagues. Fears are related to being exposed or thought of as clinically incompetent, failing to provide safe care to clients and not being able to cope with designated roles and responsibilities. Physical adjustments are influenced by the energy consumed in trying to perform in a new role, at the level expected and without revealing any difficulties. The expectation of making advanced clinical judgements and clinical decisions, the physical demands of adjusting to shiftwork, coupled with changes to living arrangements and personal relationships, contribute to new graduates'

Short-answer question

physical exhaustion (Duchscher 2009, p. 1106). This adjustment is about new graduates learning to trust their professional selves, distinguishing themselves from others, being accepted into the nursing culture, balancing personal and professional work life, and seeing and doing in the real world, as opposed to what was learned in the education setting (Duchscher 2009, p. 1108). In this first one to four months, considerable stress can be experienced in supervising, delegating and providing direction to other personnel and in relating to other professionals – for example, communicating with physicians and senior staff.

Stage 2: Being

The *being* stage is the four to eight-month period. Recovering from the initial transition shock, this stage commences with doubts about your abilities, and peaks with a crisis of confidence due to insecurities regarding **competence** and a fear of failing clients, colleagues and oneself (Duchscher 2009, p. 446). During this time, graduates experience an increased awareness of themselves professionally, and of the role of the nurse in relation to other health professionals. A sense of self-trust evolves as the graduate begins to seek validation and clarification for their own clinical judgements and actions (Duchscher 2009, p. 446). In the later part of this stage, graduates generally relax into 'a more comfortable space' and experience a 'reawakening', which enables them to be in new and unfamiliar practice situations and plan long-term career goals (Duchscher 2009, p. 447).

competence the combination of skills, knowledge, attitudes, values and abilities that underpin effective and/or superior performance in a profession or occupation area (ANMAC 2020)

Multiple-choice questions

Stage 3: Knowing

This final stage, the eight to 12-month time period, is the *knowing* stage, when the graduate is moving out of the learner role into one that has more expectations attached to it.

Signs of progress include being able to answer questions, assist others with their workload and the advancement of organisational and prioritisation skills.

REFLECTION 17.1

Drawing on your experience from clinical placements, reflect on the following questions and record your responses in your reflective journal or professional portfolio.

- How much support and what type of support do you expect you will need in your first year of professional practice? List some key words associated with support that illustrate what support and a supportive clinical environment might look like for you.
- What are your expectations of health service staff regarding provision of support in your graduate year, in terms of structured support, the content, number and frequency of education days, expectations of feedback from your registered nurse peers and how you would expect any feedback to be given?

CASE STUDY

Easing the transition

In an Australian study, Lea and Cruickshank (2015) used a case study research methodology to investigate the support needs of new graduate nurses making the role transition into rural practice settings. New graduate nurses were interviewed about their support needs at various times throughout the graduate year. Although their study was conducted in rural areas, and Duchscher's (2008) work was the result of studies conducted in metropolitan areas of Canada, the Lea and Cruickshank findings support and confirm the stages of transition theory posed by Duchscher (2008, 2009) as an accurate representation of the continuum of transition experienced by new graduate nurses in rural practice. Both studies advocate that new graduate nurse support mechanisms need to consider the distinct stages of transition through which graduates progress to professional nursing practice. In addition, the evidence presented by these authors recommends that transition-to-practice programs offer an incrementally staged workload and responsibilities that recognise the graduate's beginning nurse status.

QUESTION

In the *being* stage of the stages of transition theory posed by Duchscher (2008, 2009), she referred to graduates experiencing *a tenuous sense of self-trust*. What do you think Duchscher meant by this term, and what behaviours might it describe in relation to new graduate nurses?

Video: Transitioning

Strategies to successfully manage the transition to the first year of professional practice

The evidence pertaining to the new graduate entering professional practice (Bennett et al. 2012; Chang & Hancock 2003; Cubit & Ryan 2011; Duchscher 2001, 2008; Kelly 1998; Oermann & Garvin 2002; Ostini & Bonner 2012; Walker et al. 2017) is that the amount and quality of support in the first three months is crucial to a successful transition to professional nursing practice because this first three months is when the new graduate nurse is likely to experience a rapid personal and professional transformation. Organisational support strategies to ease the transition comprise structured support systems such as graduate nurse programs or transition-to-practice programs. Also advocated to ease the transition are self-support and personal support measures that are related to the personal qualities or resilience of the new graduate nurse. These include strategies such as reflective practice through debriefing and journaling, seeking support via a mentor, seeking feedback and gathering strategies for looking after yourself.

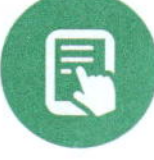

Short-answer question

Graduate nurse programs

Graduate Nurse Programs (GNPs) or Transition to Practice Programs (TTPPs) are structured support systems designed to provide a nurturing environment, professional role-modelling and consolidation of skills. It is widely recognised that the new graduate needs to be 'guided, advised and mentored' (Schwartz 2019, p. 45) through the first year of practice, and TTPPs are a way to achieve this. TTPPs aim to assist with professional socialisation in response to the reality shock of entering the nursing workforce by providing a 'mediated' entry. They share three primary goals: to develop a competent and confident registered nurse, facilitate professional adjustment and develop a commitment to a career in nursing (Levett-Jones & Fitzgerald 2005, p. 41). It is also believed that structured support assists with the application of knowledge, and the further development of clinical reasoning and decision-making (Clayton, Broome & Ellis 1989; De Bellis et al. 2001; Nayak 1990; Seright 2011), and has been shown to enhance client safety, reduce attrition and work stress for new graduates (Meyer Bratt 2013).

Structured transition programs vary in nature and duration within health services across Australia; not all programs are the same, and nor do they offer the same level of support (Schwartz 2019). Preceptoring and mentoring are the clinical support models generally used to support new graduates within these programs. The desirable qualities required of a preceptor or mentor include being a role model, having clinical expertise, being able to assist with the application of theory to practice and having a willingness to provide supervision and teaching (Hardyman & Hickey 2001, p. 59).

Health services – both public and private – usually have a 12-month transition program for new graduates, which may include rotation to different clinical areas, sometimes of three months' duration, although evidence (Walker et al. 2017, Chang & Hancock 2003; Newton & McKenna 2007) suggests that new graduates are better served by a program that has fewer rotations, to ease the re-socialisation that occurs with changes in clinical areas. TTPPs are mainly offered in hospitals (Schwartz 2019) and may be offered in specialty areas of practice, but these are dependent on the size of the health services and the resources available to provide support programs. In recent years there has been an increase in TTPPs offered in primary care, aged-care and day-procedure settings; however, while the support can sometimes be more personalised in these settings, they often lack the resources needed to provide structured and consistent mentoring and support for new graduates. Many health services do not provide a guarantee of permanent employment once the TTPP is completed, and at the completion of the program continued employment may be dependent on available permanent positions at the health agency. You may need to reapply for a position, or you may be transitioned by the agency into a permanent position. Second-year graduate programs are becoming popular across Australia, so there may be an opportunity to apply for a second-year graduate position. Should you wish to remain employed in the agency, you will need to investigate the employment status of graduates at the completion of the program before you start it, so that you can plan your future and seek out employment and career opportunities.

It is advisable to seek employment though a formal structured graduate nurse program; many health facilities do not employ new graduate nurses unless they are on a TTPP. However, some agencies and clinical workplaces employ new graduate nurses without a structured program in place and ensure that the graduates are afforded the support of a formal program; these include practice nursing, some aged care providers and non-government organisations. In choosing where to undertake your graduate program or where to seek employment, factors that influence the undergraduate nurse's decision are locality, the reputation of the healthcare facility, rotations offered to specialty areas and familiarity with the healthcare facility, as well as decisions related to and influenced by the origins of the new graduate – for example, a desire to return to a rural environment upon graduation (Lea et al. 2008).

Short-answer question

Wherever you apply for your graduate year, it is important that you investigate the agency of choice. Most agencies and health services have information available online about their graduate programs but it is also a good idea to investigate programs during clinical placement by talking to new graduates who are already employed at your agency of choice, or make an appointment to speak to the new graduate coordinator about the program on offer or the employment opportunities available. Do not be frightened to ask about the programs, and how they are structured, and ask current new graduates whether the programs delivered what they said they would. You need to make an informed decision about your future, so it is important to gather as much information as you can to help you decide what will suit you.

Some health services provide a highly structured TTPP that involves graduates completing academic modules of study and assessments relevant to the clinical context or specific to the health service. These types of structured theoretical TTPPs may be located in rural and or remote practice environments, within the private healthcare sector or in specialty clinical contexts where specific and specialised learning needs to occur. Often, these types of TTPPs have reciprocal arrangements for recognition of prior learning (RPL) into postgraduate programs (e.g. postgraduate certificate) or honours programs offered by partner higher-education institutions.

Questions to ask before making any decision to accept or apply for a new graduate position could include:

- How many positions are available in the health service and where are they located? That is, in which geographical area, because some health services may have smaller rural sites and/or multipurpose services as part of their graduate programs.
- Are there support opportunities for new graduates not employed within a TTPP?
- What is the structure of the TTPP? For example, does the program require completion of academic assignments, case study presentations or other structured assessments by participants?
- Are there any reciprocal arrangements for RPL for completion of the program into postgraduate programs?
- What type of support is offered at the ward or unit level?
- How many days of orientation at the ward or unit level are provided?
- What are the structure, content and frequency of education days?
- What career support and development are provided?
- What employment opportunities are available at the completion of the program?

REFLECTION 17.2

- Write a list of all the agencies and clinical areas you think you may want to work in after your graduation.
- Write a list of the positive aspects of these agencies for graduate employment; include aspects that will affect your personal life as well as your career.

Strategies for you

It is extremely important as you prepare to enter the workforce as a beginning registered nurse that you take time to develop personal self-support strategies that will assist you to fit into the organisational culture and that will give you the best chance of a successful transition.

Mellor, Gregoric and Gillham (2017) identified that, in order to fit into the organisational culture, new graduates need to be able to understand the nature of transition; recognise and regulate emotions; manage distress and foster courage; self-assess progress and performance; and focus self-care needs on developing their resilience. They add that it is important for nursing students to learn to manage stress by reflecting on clinical scenarios; being able to recognise when help is required; and taking control of seeking help. Johnstone and colleagues (2007) found in their study of new graduate nurse support that the greatest sources of support for new graduates was 'self-support'. Graduate nurses themselves are often best placed to decide what support they need; however, their ability to seek support depends on their confidence and their support-seeking behaviours. Lea and Cruickshank (2017) reported that experienced nurses were concerned when new graduate nurses did not seek support or ask questions.

It is therefore important that you reflect on your personal support strategies and identify those you need to develop prior to completing your program. Strategies such as journaling and debriefing are good ways for students and new graduates to enhance critical reflection and process critical incidents. Journaling can be initiated at any time, and it is good practice to try to do this every day. If not available to you, formal debriefing can be sought through your university lecturers if you are a student, and through the new graduate coordinator, or the nurse unit manager or other work colleagues with whom you feel comfortable. Set professional goals for your own practice and learning needs, and implement self-support strategies using a framework for learning objectives, such as the SMART framework – Specific, Measurable, Achievable, Realistic and Timely.

Your personal support strategies should also include maintaining, cultivating and making time for personal friendships and family relationships. These support systems have been important to you as you have studied for your degree, and they will be just as important as you make the transition to professional practice. Many new graduates find the transition journey isolating (Lea & Cruickshank 2015), and any TTPP should include social events and social networking opportunities to assist new graduates to form new friendships; make the effort to attend these events if they are offered to you. Making time for yourself through exercise, good sleep and rest habits, a balanced healthy diet, social outings and hobbies will help you to develop your resilience and manage the emotions that arise during your transition, and will also assist you to achieve a work–life balance that is important for good health and a happy life.

Professional roles, autonomy and responsibilities of the registered nurse

As a healthcare professional, you will be part of an interprofessional team, and as a student in the final year of your studies, it is expected that you be aware of where you fit into the team, and that you are working to become part of the team. You will be working collectively and ultimately, as a new graduate, will be accepted as part of the team. To be accepted, new nurses have to demonstrate that they have proficient clinical skills (Walker et al. 2013), are useful and can take a share of the workload, and also be mindful of the professional attributes and work ethic expected, such as punctuality and respect for their peers. In addition, having a degree of social intelligence, being able to ask for help from one's team or supervisor, and having resilience and flexibility have been found to be crucial for new graduate success during the transition (Walker et al. 2013)

It is important to realise that in many contemporary healthcare organisations there may be four generations of nurses working side by side. Each generation will bring varied life and work experiences to the workplace. Different generations of nurses can make a significant contribution to your professional learning and development during your transition to professional practice; however, as a graduating nurse, this can also make your transition complex, as you will need to learn and navigate the different values, attitudes, educational experiences and work habits of your team members.

Interprofessional and multidisciplinary teams

As a student of nursing, you are being prepared to work in the contemporary healthcare environment, and it is imperative that you recognise the significance and responsibilities of being an active participant in multidisciplinary healthcare teams (see Chapter 15). Being a registered nurse requires much more than an ability to perform clinical skills or a set of procedures (Cashin et al. 2017). The registered nurse must also have good communication skills and be able to work in and with teams (Schwartz 2019). During your education program, you will no doubt have experienced working with students from other health disciplines, with the aim of assisting you to function within the interprofessional team and hopefully become aware of everyone's role in the team, each profession's scope of practice and how to communicate effectively with team members. This will also have been reinforced and perhaps consolidated during your clinical placements. As a new graduate, you may experience further consolidation of your teamwork skills through interprofessional education or simulated learning experiences provided by your employer.

Communication

Communication is one of the important components of effective teamwork. As you enter professional practice you may not feel confident in your communication with senior nurses or with members of the multidisciplinary team. One of the key issues faced by new graduate nurses in their first year of practice is the difficulty in communicating with medical staff. Having **clinical conversations** with medical staff about client conditions, reporting assessment findings and approaching medical staff to review a client are examples of the difficulties new graduates experience that can cause significant stress for them (Lea & Cruickshank 2015).

As a health professional, you need to be an assertive communicator and a good listener when working as part of a team – these skills are crucial to the quality and safety of health care. Each state or territory health department, health service or agency will have a framework that it recommends to assist staff to engage in appropriate and timely communication, to ensure quality and safety, and to reduce errors. Many resources are available with frameworks to guide clinical conversations, and your education program should prepare you to use a framework (see ACQSHC 2020). However, many students do not get enough practice in the conversations that they will need to be able to have as a graduate nurse. When reflecting on your competence or capability and readiness to enter professional practice, this should be a key area of focus. In your final clinical placement, two of the important areas in which to refine and develop your practice and confidence should be clinical handover and clinical conversations with other health professionals, clients and their families.

clinical conversations the conversations we have as health professionals with other health professionals, whether face to face, by telephone or information and communications technologies (ICT), to hand over care, discuss care regimens and report assessment findings; these conversations should follow a structured framework, such as ISBAR (see Chapter 11)

Video: ISBAR
Connecting with practice:
Communicating for safety

CASE STUDY

Research highlights: Clinical conversations

Lea and Cruickshank (2014, 2015) found that one key area of difficulty for graduates as they make the transition to professional practice is communicating with medical staff. Having clinical conversations with medical staff about client conditions, reporting assessment findings and approaching medical staff to review a client were all cited in their research as causing new graduates significant stress in all stages of the transition to registered nursing practice.

QUESTION

Why might new graduates find clinical conversations challenging? Do you find this aspect of practice challenging? What could you do to improve your practice and confidence in this area of nursing responsibility and accountability?

Managing expected roles and responsibilities

This section looks at leadership, management and delegation. Research with new graduate nurses (Lea & Cruickshank 2007, 2014; Parker et al. 2014) identified that the first year is hard to navigate. Being familiar with the models of care and managing time and the new responsibilities and accountability associated with registered nursing status, together with pressure on the new graduate to be work ready, have been found to affect new graduates' experience of transition (Kelly & Ahern 2009; Parker et al. 2014).

Delegation

As a new graduate, you may be required to delegate or assign tasks to personal care assistants, assistants in nursing, enrolled nurses and/or students of nursing. There will also come a time when you may find yourself in the team leader role or in charge of the ward or unit. This is not ideal in your first few months as a registered nurse, but it does happen – particularly in the fast-paced, ever-changing workplace, with its demanding workloads. New graduates can find it extremely difficult to delegate during their graduate year (Lea & Cruikshank 2015) and it is ideal for graduates to be assisted to adopt these responsibilities incrementally through workplace learning models such as mentoring and during workshops during TTPP education days. As a key responsibility of registered nurses, delegation skills cannot be taught in theory alone; rather, learning and practising this responsibility needs to be a focus of your final-year clinical learning experience. When delegating, it is important to consider the needs of the people in your care and the stability or acuity of their health condition, as well as the complexity of the task being delegated and the expected outcome of the delegated task. As a registered nurse, you will be accountable for the decision to delegate, and you should only delegate to staff whom you know have had appropriate education and training, and who are competent to perform the task. This involves making sure that you know that the person to whom you are delegating – the delegatee – understands the nature of the task and what is expected of them in performing the task, and also that the delegate knows their limitations or scope of practice and is aware of how to seek advice. During your clinical experiences, observe and consider which tasks and activities your registered nurse role model delegates.

Providing workplace learning support

One of the difficulties of the registered nurse role about which new graduates express surprise is the expectation that they will provide clinical learning support to new learners in the workplace. For many graduates, this can result in feelings of being overwhelmed and out of their depth, and many feel unprepared for this role. However, the role and responsibilities of being a registered nurse include mentoring nurses and others, such as enrolled nurses, assistants in nursing and students of nursing, and all beginning registered nurses will eventually have to assume this role. This is one aspect of being a registered nurse that you should be investigating now – perhaps look for appropriate role models while you are on clinical placement so that when the time comes, you can model your own professional practice in this area. Additionally, once you are established in the registered nursing workforce there will be many professional development opportunities for you to develop skills in providing workplace learning support through attendance at workshops, or through completion of online study modules or formal postgraduate study.

REFLECTION 17.3

- As a student, when you have a difference of opinion with colleagues or fellow students about work-related issues, how do you or would you communicate with them about this?
- As a new graduate nurse, how would you deal with having a difference of opinion with work colleagues?
- What factors would influence your communication as a new graduate nurse?
- As a new graduate nurse, from whom could you seek support from when dealing with the difference of opinion?
- In your final clinical placement, what strategies might you employ to help you build or develop skills in professional communication with colleagues?

Short-answer question
Multiple-choice questions

Developing and refining a professional portfolio reflecting beginning registered nursing status

A professional portfolio is a reflective and personal statement about you, your competence and your development as a nurse. It provides evidence of your competence and details the strategies you have devised for your continuing development as a health professional. As a student of nursing, you may find that the development of a portfolio is an assessable task in preparation for the portfolio you should keep as a registered nurse. At different stages of your nursing career, you need to choose what to include in your portfolio that best represents you and your achievements or plans. While there are very good guidelines on what to include and how to present your portfolio, there is no right or wrong content. You may choose to develop and present your portfolio as an e-portfolio – an electronic collection of evidence that shows your learning journey as a nurse over time (see Chapter 9). Your evidence may include writing samples, photos, videos, research projects, observations by mentors and peers and/or reflective thinking. The key aspect of an e-portfolio is *your* reflection on the evidence, including why it was chosen, how it demonstrates your beginning competence and developing capabilities and what you learned from the process of developing your e-portfolio.

What you choose to present should be clear and concise, and the justification, evidence or plan should be convincing. The following section outlines the key elements of a professional portfolio for a beginning registered nurse, which you will need to update every year to demonstrate your continuing competence and your learning and currency of practice.

Your status

- Provide a curriculum vitae or resume at the beginning, using a framework. There are many modified templates available online that are free to use. Many universities also provide these career-planning resources and tools.

- It is a good idea to complete a self-assessment of your capability as a registered nurse against each of the Registered Nurse Standards for Practice (NMBA 2016). However, in your portfolio you must go on to provide justification for and supporting evidence of your achievements to support your claims. As a new graduate, this may include assignment feedback and marks or unit grades from units over the course of your study, as well as your clinical practice reports. Make sure that your evidence is only about you, how you perform as a nurse and what steps you take to ensure that you are capable or competent in each of the standards. Do not include any client information such as client notes or client data.
- Include goals for your professional development using a framework (e.g. SMART). Goals for your professional portfolio should not be focused purely on the attainment of clinical skills or tasks, but rather on development of professional capability across all domains, career development and continuing education. For example, you may wish to have as a goal to develop skills and confidence in providing workplace learning support, so your strategy could be documented as 'to attend in-service education on models of clinical education, complete online learning modules on being a mentor and volunteer to be a mentor for new staff'. In subsequent years, your goal may change to become a clinical nurse educator, so your strategy may be to enrol in postgraduate study that will prepare you for this role.
- Throughout the graduate year, on completion of your graduate year and then every year thereafter, continually update your portfolio with any new evidence to support your proof of competence in each of the Registered Nurse Standards for Practice. For example, add any feedback from performance appraisals, recognition awards, self-assessments, record of in-service education, mandatory education, and conference and seminar attendance. In addition, if you undertake further formal study, you can use assignment feedback and unit grades to prove your continuing professional development.

Connecting with practice:
Portfolio development

Basically, the professional portfolio showcases who you are as a professional nurse and provides evidence to answer the question 'Why should the Nursing and Midwifery Board of Australia (NMBA) approve me as a registered nurse?' The NMBA can ask to see your professional portfolio at any time – that is, it can conduct an audit of your portfolio, so that you must present the evidence to prove your capability, competence and currency of practice as a registered nurse. Failure to provide the required evidence when being audited will mean you will not be registered, and may not be able to work as a nurse. It is therefore extremely important to keep your portfolio up to date. Your portfolio will also serve you well when applying for nursing positions.

NURSING PERSPECTIVE

Talk to any nursing student, and you will find that many have the goal of travelling and working overseas as a nurse. Although nursing has always been thought of as a career choice that enables you to travel, it is not as easy as packing your bags and heading off once you have completed your course. There s a significant process to work through in order to be able to work in another country as a registered nurse. Depending on where you want to travel, you may need to pass a standardised examination designed to assess knowledge skills and abilities to provide safe and effective care (e.g. the NECLEX in the United States) and you may need to prove your language proficiency, as well as provide extensive evidence of what your pre-registration education consisted of, in terms of hours of theory and hours of practice in specific clinical contexts, before you will be eligible to be registered or licensed to practise as a nurse in another country.

It must also be acknowledged that your educational preparation here in Australia prepares you for practice in Australia, ensuring that you meet the Australian Registered Nurse Standards for Practice and the professional accrediting bodies' minimum educational requirements. Although Australian-prepared nurses are well regarded overseas, there is no guarantee that you will be able to work as a nurse in another country, as you will still need to provide documentary evidence to prove your competence against your country of choice's competency standards and meet its minimal educational requirements.

Following are some hints and tips to assist you if you are contemplating travelling overseas to work as a nurse:

- Investigate the country's requirements a long way in advance of the completion of your educational program. For example, some countries require specific theoretical and clinical experience in some clinical areas – paediatrics is a common requirement – and without this you may not be eligible to register. If you know this in advance, you can discuss with your academic institution how you can meet specific theoretical or clinical hours in the specified area.
- Investigate whether there is an exam you need to pass as part of the registration process so you can prepare for it well in advance.
- Some countries prefer a minimum of one year's postgraduate experience before you can apply.
- Register in Australia as a registered nurse first before you apply for overseas registration.
- Keep all your university or education provider records (copies of unit grades, clinical placement records etc.) in your portfolio so you can produce evidence of your education if needed.
- Most registering authorities require official documents – signed with a university seal – from your educational institution to prove hours of theory and clinical experience. This takes time for universities to complete, and the wait will be even longer if the request goes to the wrong department or person. Make sure you send your request to the person responsible for the nursing pre-registration program in the institution where you studied. Send an email first asking about the process, and keep all emails so that you can follow up if needed.
- It can take at least three to six months for overseas registration to be approved, so make sure you have left enough time for this before travelling.
- Keep your professional portfolio updated while you are overseas so that you will have no trouble proving your competence or currency of practice when you return to Australia. Also, make sure that you maintain your Australian registration at all times – *do not let it lapse*.

SUMMARY

- The transition to professional practice is a process of change and adjustment from the familiar life of a student to the role of a professional registered nurse. Transition involves the new graduate nurse progressing through several stages during the first 12 months of practice.
- Graduate nurse support programs are designed to support the transition and to provide the new graduate nurse with structured support to ease them into the expectations of the registered nurse role. Development of self-support strategies is important for new graduate nurses, for resilience and to adapt to the organisational and workplace culture of health care.
- Delegation, communication, teamwork and providing workplace learning support are some of the professional roles and responsibilities expected of beginning registered nurses. These higher-order skills need to be developed prior to graduation and will be refined further throughout the first year of professional practice.
- As a registered nurse, it is a requirement of the NMBA that you provide evidence of your capability or competence, continuing education and currency of practice, and that you keep a professional portfolio that is regularly updated and able to be produced upon request to prove that you meet the registration standards for the nursing profession.

REVIEW QUESTIONS

Suggested responses

1 Outline the stages of transition to professional nursing practice and provide an example of feelings that a new graduate might experience at each stage.
2 The delegation of care is an important responsibility for the registered nurse. Name some key functions or activities that the registered nurse could delegate.
3 Why is it important to have a professional portfolio?
4 To enter the workforce as a registered nurse, do you have to be on a graduate program?
5 Research indicates that communicating with medical staff is a key area of difficulty for graduates. What are the three specific areas that new graduate nurses struggle with and need learning support with?

RESEARCH TOPICS

- Investigate the evidence surrounding the experience of new graduates as they enter professional practice.
- What does the term 'interprofessional team' refer to? Reflect on your clinical experiences and write about the other health professionals in the team and their roles.

FURTHER READING

Andre, K., Heartfield, M. & Cusack, L. (2017). *Portfolios for health professionals*, 3rd edn. Sydney: Elsevier.

Ankers, M.D., Parry, Y.K & Barton, C.A. (2018). A phenomenological exploration of graduate nurse transition to professional practice within a transition to practice program. *Collegian*, 25, 319–25.

Australian Commission on Quality and Safety in Health Care (2020). *Communicating for Safety*. Available from https://c4sportal.safetyandquality.gov.au.

Nursing and Midwifery Board of Australia (NMBA) (2020). (Website.) Available from https://www.nursingmidwiferyboard.gov.au.

REFERENCES

Australian Commission on Safety and Quality in Health Care (ACSQHC) (2019). *Action 6.7: Clinical handover*. Retrieved from https://www.safetyandquality.gov .au/standards/nsqhs-standards/communicating-safety-standard/communication-clinical-handover/action-67.

Australian Nursing and Midwifery Accreditation Council (ANMAC) (2020). About ANMAC. Retrieved from https://www.anmac.org.au/about-anmac.

Bennett, P., Barlow, V., Brown, J. & Jones, D. (2012). What do graduate registered nurses want from jobs in rural/remote Australian communities? *Journal of Nursing Management*, 20, 485–90.

Cashin, A., Heartfield, M., Bryce, J., Kelly, J., Thoms, D. & Fisher, M. (2017). Standards of practice for registered nurses in Australia. *Collegian*, 24, 255–66.

Chang, E. & Hancock, K. (2003). Role stress and role ambiguity in new nursing graduates in Australia. *Nursing and Health Sciences*, 5(2), 155–63.

Chick, N. & Meleis, A.I. (1986). *Transitions: A nursing concern*. New York: Elsevier.

Clayton, G., Broome, M. & Ellis, L. (1989). Relationship between a preceptorship experience and role socialisation of graduate nurses. *Journal of Nursing Education*, 2, 72–5.

Cubit, K. & Ryan, B. (2011). Tailoring a graduate nurse program to meet the needs of our next generation nurses. *Nurse Education Today*, 31, 65–71.

De Bellis, A., Longson, D., Glover, P. & Hutton, A. (2001). The enculturation of our nursing graduates. *Contemporary Nurse*, 11(1), 84–94.

Duchscher, J.E.B. (2001). Out in the real world: Newly graduated nurses in acute care speak out. *Journal of Nursing Administration*, 31(9), 426–39.

—— (2008). A process of becoming: The stages of new nursing graduate professional role transition. *The Journal of Continuing Education in Nursing*, 39(10), 441–50.

—— (2009). Transition shock: The initial stage of role adaptation for newly graduated registered *nurses. Journal of Advanced Nursing*, 65(5), 1103–13.

Fedoruk, M. & Hofmeyer, A. (2012). *Becoming a nurse: Transition to practice*. Melbourne: Oxford University Press.

Hardyman, R. & Hickey, G. (2001). What do newly qualified nurses expect from preceptorship? Exploring the perspectives of the preceptor. *Nurse Education Today*, 21, 58–64.

Johnstone, M., Kanitsaki, O., Currie, T., Smith, E. & McGennisken, C. (2007). Designing and delivering clinical risk management education for graduate nurses: An Australian study. *Nurse Education in Practice*, 7, 247–57.

Kralik, D., Visentin, K. & van Loon, A. (2006). Transition: A literature review. *Journal of Advanced Nursing*, 55(3), 320–9.

Kramer, M. (1974). *Reality shock: Why nurses leave nursing*. St Louis, MO: Mosby.

Kelly, B. (1998). Preserving moral integrity: A follow-up study with new graduate nurses. *Journal of Advanced Nursing*, 28(5), 1134–45.

Kelly, J. & Ahern, K. (2009). Preparing nurses for practice: A phenomenological study of the new graduate in Australia. *Journal of Clinical Nursing*, 18(6), 910–18.

Lea, J. (2013). An Investigation into the Provision of Support within Transition to Practice Programs for New Graduate Nurses in Rural Health Settings. Doctoral thesis, University of Canberra. Retrieved from https://researchprofiles.canberra.edu.au/en/studentTheses/an-investigation-into-the-provision-of-support-within-transition-

Lea, J. & Cruickshank, M.T. (2007). The experience of new graduate nurses in rural practice in New South Wales. *Rural and Remote Health*, 7, 814.

—— (2014). The support needs of new graduate nurses making the transition to rural nursing practice. *Journal of Clinical Nursing*, 24(7/8), 948–60.

—— (2015). Supporting new graduate nurses making the transition to rural nursing practice: Views from experienced rural nurses. *Journal of Clinical Nursing*, 24, 2826–34.

—— (2017). The role of rural nurse managers in supporting new graduate nurses in rural practice. *Journal of Nursing Management*, 25(3), 176–83.

Lea, J., Cruickshank, M., Paliadelis, P., Parmenter, G., Sanderson, H. & Thornberry, P. (2008). The lure of the bush: Do rural placements influence student nurses to seek employment in rural settings? *Collegian*, 5, 77–82.

Levett-Jones, T. & Fitzgerald, M. (2005). A review of graduate nurse transition programs in Australia. *Australian Journal of Advanced Nursing*, 23(2), 40–5.

Mellor, P., Gregoric, C. & Gillham, D. (2017). Strategies new graduate registered nurses require to care and advocate for themselves: A literature review. *Contemporary Nurse*, 53(3), 390–405.

Meyer Bratt, M. (2013). Nurse residency program: Best practices for optimizing organizational success. *Journal for Nurses in Professional Development*, 29(3), 102–10.

Nayak, S. (1990). Strategies to support the new nurse in practice. *Journal of Nursing Staff Development*, 7(3), 64–6.

Newton, J. & McKenna, L. (2007). The transitional journey through the graduate year: A focus group study. *International Journal of Nursing Studies*, 44, 1231–7.

Nursing and Midwifery Board (NMBA) (2016). *Registered nurse standards for practice*. Retrieved from http://www.nursingmidwiferyboard.gov.au/documents/default.aspx?record=WD16%2f19524&dbid=AP&chksum=R5Pkrn8yVpb9bJvtpTRe8w%3d%3d.

Oermann, M. (1997). *Professional nursing practice*. New York: Appleton & Lange.

Oermann, M. & Garvin, M. (2002). Stresses and challenges for new graduates in hospitals. *Nurse Education Today*, 22, 225–30.

Ostini, F. & Bonner, A. (2012). Australian new graduate experiences during their transition program in a rural/regional acute care setting. *Contemporary Nurse*, 41(2), 242–52.

Parker, V., Giles, M., Lantry, G. & McMillan, M. (2014). New graduate nurses' experiences in their first year of practice. *Nurse Education Today*, 34(1), 150–6.

Schwartz, S. (2019). *Educating the nurse of the future – report of the independent review into nursing education*. Canberra: Department of Health.

Seright, T.J. (2011). Clinical decision-making of rural novice nurses. *Rural and Remote Health*, 11, 1726.

Walker, A., Costa, B.M., Foster, A.M. & de Bruin, R.L. (2017). Transition and integration experiences of Australian graduate nurses: A qualitative systematic review. *Collegian*, 24(5), 505–12.

Walker, A., Yong, M., Pang, L., Fullarton, C., Costa, B. & Trisha Dunning, A.M. (2013). Work readiness of graduate health professionals. *Nursing Today*, 33(2), 116–22.

Winter-Collins, A. & McDaniel, A. (2000). Sense of belonging and new graduate job satisfaction. *Journal for Nurses in Staff Development*, 6(3), 103–11.

Conclusion: What now? Where to from here?

Penny Paliadelis

18

LEARNING OBJECTIVES

At the completion of this chapter, you should be able to:

1 Identify how you are developing your identity as a nurse.
2 Understand the range of career pathways and options available to nurses.
3 Appreciate the value to your nursing career of lifelong learning.
4 Contribute to and support the next generation of nurses.

Introduction

The focus of this book has been on exploring the concepts, knowledge and skills that are relevant to contemporary nursing practice, with a strong emphasis on 'meaning-making' – what things really mean; how this meaning is established; why particular knowledge is necessary or important; and how all of this informs your road to nursing, your continuing learning, practice and professional identity-formation, and your conception of what it really means to be and act as a nurse.

This final chapter weaves together some of the key focus areas that have made up this 'journey', using stories from practice that may provide you with some further insights to guide you on your path to becoming a skilled and experienced nurse.

The second part of this chapter focuses your attention on the fact that, once you enter the profession as a beginning-level nurse, this is not the end of your journey; in fact, it is only the first stage of your career. There are many options and learning opportunities that can further your career and assist you to develop into an expert nurse across a range of settings.

The last section of this chapter focuses on how you can contribute to the further development of the nursing profession by role-modelling and promoting nursing, mentoring and supporting others, and developing and sharing your skills and knowledge with new generations of nurses.

Nursing is a diverse and varied profession that is at times rewarding, challenging, happy and sad. Nurses are the most vital cog in the development, delivery and leadership of health services to meet the current and future health needs of society. You have chosen a rewarding and exciting career!

Stories from practice

Humans are 'hard-wired' to learn from stories. Throughout history, stories have been shared through fables, fairy tales and anecdotes to convey meaning and promote learning (Paliadelis et al. 2015). In healthcare contexts, storytelling is the foundation in which nurses learn from and about their clients and each other. Nursing 'handover' is a form of structured storytelling that conveys meanings relevant to the care of clients, to provide continuity of care from one nursing shift to another (Paliadelis & Wood 2016). Several stories from practice are provided in this chapter to illustrate and expand upon some of the important messages in this book:

Video: Storytelling

- developing as a professional nurse;
- being ethical and responsible;
- understanding the contexts of practice; and
- working effectively in a healthcare team.

Nursing professionalism

The first two stories presented here encourage you to think about your identity as a professional nurse. What does it mean to be professional and why is it important?

The first story is from a nursing student:

> I was on my second week of placement in a day procedure unit of a regional hospital when on the television it was reported that there had been a shooting in the town, and that one person was dead and the alleged shooter was injured. The staff and clients were aghast, and conversations ensued about who was dead and who the shooter might be. This speculation is understandable in a regional town, but what followed was a shock to me.
>
> Throughout the morning, the television announced 'breaking news', and soon the identities of the victim and the shooter became known. The staff were openly discussing the matter in front of, and sometimes with, the clients in the unit. I became increasingly uncomfortable with the level of detail and the opinions that were being expressed about the victim and the shooter, both of whom were local. Soon, one of the nurses commented that she had received a text message from a relative who worked at the local paper, asking whether the shooter was badly injured and whether there were any more details. This prompted even more speculation, and one nurse volunteered to go and talk to a friend who worked in the emergency department to find out more.
>
> This situation left a bad taste in my mouth, as I believe that nurses should behave professionally and ethically, regardless of their personal feelings – meaning that they should not do or say anything that might be construed as discrimination or disrespect. According to ethical principles and codes of conduct for nurses in Australia, nurses are required to provide care to those who need it, in a fair and equitable way. The comments of the nurses on that day, and their open conversations in front of me (the student) and clients, were not professional or aligned with the code of conduct, in my view. Both the victim and alleged shooter had families and friends, and I felt that this breach of professional conduct may undermine respect for nurses.
>
> This event taught me an important lesson about how I will conduct myself when I become a qualified nurse. Even when my private views might make it difficult, I will always strive to treat people fairly and with respect, and be mindful of principles of ethics and confidentiality.

Before you reflect on this story, please read another (more positive) story from a newly graduated registered nurse that also touches on professionalism as well as the value of teamwork:

> I was caring for a single woman aged in her forties who was diagnosed with a mental health disorder and who provided information on her admission that she was in substantial debt because she was 'not good with money' and 'liked to shop'.
>
> Her parents came to the hospital and were obviously distraught about their daughter's situation.
>
> When they left, they took their daughter's purse containing her credit cards and some cash. This caused the client to become very upset, as she claimed that while she had asked her parents to help her to manage her finances better, she did not want them to take over and restrict her access to her money.
>
> I was not sure what I should do and how to do it in a professional manner, so I reported this situation to the nurse in charge and the admitting doctor, as I needed advice about how to address the client's concerns. The nurse manager and the admitting doctor were very helpful. They explained that they would refer the matter to the Mental Health Review Tribunal and involve the hospital's social worker to talk to the client and her parents.

The social worked arranged for the client to see a financial adviser to educate and empower her to manage her money once her condition stabilised. She was much happier after the meeting and her parents were calmer.

I learned a lot from this situation: first, that I was right to advocate for my client, but that as a nurse I cannot 'fix' it all by myself. I need to call on other health professionals with specific expertise. I have developed my understanding of what it means to be a nurse and deal with situations like this, in which I have to weigh up ethical, professional and personal perspectives to give the best care I can. I have learned that having professional colleagues to call on for support and advice makes my role more effective.

Both these stories revealed lessons learned about what it means to act in a professional manner as part of the wider healthcare team. The first story was about learning from a negative or confronting experience that suggested a lack of professionalism, while the second story was about developing a sense of being a professional within a team.

REFLECTION 18.1

- During your clinical placements, have you experienced both positive and negative situations, in relation to professional behaviours, from which you have learned? What have you learned?
- Once you take up your role as a new registered nurse, how will you identify a positive role model to help you transition into the workforce? What attributes will you look for?

According to Karnick (2014), nursing continues to struggle to be viewed as a true profession that is separate from medicine and with its own body of knowledge. This author suggests that one of the reasons why nursing is such an elusive profession is that historically it has been defined by other, older professions, such as medicine, which has led to a tendency to link nursing with traditionally feminine roles. However, as nursing has evolved and developed its own theories, education, research and practice principles, the profession of nursing has emerged, as well as standards of practice that define and clarify what it means to be a professional nurse. Hoeve, Jansen and Roodbol (2014) and Milton (2018) agreed, suggesting that professionalism is enhanced when nurses increase their visibility and are able to articulate the skills and knowledge they contribute to the health system. Similarly, Buresh and Gordon (2006) suggested that nurses are their own 'worst enemy' when it comes to promoting themselves and the value of what they do. These authors made the case that nurses are reticent to come forward, to speak out professionally, and to celebrate and share their unique knowledge. The challenge for new generations of nurses is therefore how to break with tradition and to act as champions, by promoting nursing as a skillful, knowledge-based profession.

However, in today's world, events such as the COVID-19 pandemic have led to a greater appreciation of the professional role of nurses, globally. This was communicated by the Chief Nurse of Australia, Alison McMillan, in a press conference held on 14 June 2020, which was picked up by a number of news broadcasts. Such opportunities to speak about the vital role that nurses play in caring for our society during difficult times demonstrate the skill and value of nursing as a profession.

Ethical practice and responsibility

As discussed in this book, ethical practice, responsibility and accountability are all core requirements of professions.

In the nursing profession in Australia, we have codes of ethics and conduct, professional boundary guidelines and standards of practice developed by the Nursing and Midwifery Board of Australia (NMBA). These codes, guidelines and standards help to guide nurses and are underpinned by ethical practice principles that are embedded in all pre-registration nursing curriculums.

Ethical dilemmas do not just refer to the 'big ticket items' such as elective abortions, assisted dying, reproductive technologies and genetic testing; more often, ethical dilemmas for nurses occur in everyday practice situations. Understanding the requirements of ethics in the workplace means being able to identify and talk about ethics in the workplace, and also put them into practice. This means having professional integrity and showing a consistent, personal commitment to applying professional ethical codes and standards in all work situations. It also means ensuring that all dealings with colleagues and clients are carried out in accordance with professional and ethical standards and associated legal requirements. Integrity is commonly described as 'doing the right thing even when no one is watching'.

Connecting with practice: Integrity

Similarly, concerns over professional boundaries or conduct are often linked to nurses' desire to care for and assist their clients, which can lead to overstepping boundaries on occasion, so it is important to remember that we need to remain compassionate and professional at all times, while not becoming too involved in the lives and concerns of our clients.

The following stories will provide food for thought:

A registered nurse, Jason, with more than ten years' experience and a postgraduate certificate in aged care, is working on the aged-care assessment team and on this particular day he is scheduled to assess a 91-year-old woman who is living with her daughter. As soon as he arrives to meet the client and her daughter, the client says: 'I do not want to go to an old people's home. My daughter is happy to care for me for the rest of my days.'

Jason has forgotten to bring the standard assessment form with him, so he asks the kinds of questions that are contained on the form and jots down the answers on a sheet of paper.

After assessing that the client has difficulty with mobility, is unable to dress herself and has some degree of cognitive impairment, Jason assesses the daughter's carer strain index, then says to the client: 'You know, you really need to start thinking about entering a residential aged care facility, as you are a lot of work for your daughter, and not as able as you think you are.'

The client and her daughter both become visibly distressed, and Jason replies that he knows that these are hard decisions but he is telling them this because he is thinking of both their best interests.

On returning to the assessment office, Jason fills out the standard aged care assessment form with the information he has gathered, in some places constructing responses to questions that he did not ask directly. He completes the form by recommending that the client requires long-term residential care.

Jason believes that his expert knowledge underpins this decision, as he has seen many examples of carer strain and truly believes that the best way forward is for this client to go into a care facility.

Now consider this dilemma:

> Emma is a second-year registered nurse who has worked in several clinical settings, from the emergency department to community mental health. For the past six months, she has been working in the orthopaedic ward and is loving it. After returning to work following days off, Emma finds that she is caring for a young male client, Mark, who has two broken arms and multiple rib fractures following a motorbike accident. Mark needs assistance with all activities of daily living but despite his injuries he is chatty and upbeat.
>
> Emma finds that whenever she has a spare minute she gravitates towards Mark and they laugh and chat. His accident occurred a long way from his home and he has no family or friends nearby to visit him regularly. Emma feels she is positively contributing to his care by keeping him company whenever she has a chance, as most of the other clients on the ward are elderly.
>
> After six days of work, Emma has two days off, and Mark tells her how much he will miss their chats. He asks her to pop in to see him as a visitor if she has time and to bring him a couple of beers. Emma thinks about whether this is appropriate, but decides to do it anyway, believing that she is being compassionate and caring holistically for her client.
>
> On returning to work, she is approached by the nurse unit manager to explain her actions, which have been reported by a concerned colleague as a breach of professional boundaries.

From these two examples, it is clear that nurses confront 'everyday' ethical and professional dilemmas on a regular basis, and the right decisions are not always easy and clear-cut. In the first example, did Jason really 'know best'? Was the construction of answers to questions that were not directly asked of the client and family unethical? In the second example, was Emma overstepping professional boundaries, and why is maintaining a professional relationship so important?

Other examples of everyday ethical issues include those relating to consent, autonomy and equity of access to health care. The global COVID-19 pandemic has certainly highlighted the ethical dilemmas that can arise when healthcare systems are overwhelmed, such as how equitable access to care and treatment is decided and how decisions are made about distribution of scarce personal protective equipment to frontline healthcare workers. Considering the ethical dimensions of healthcare can often lead nurses to question aspects of the system in which they work, as well as their own practices. With an ageing population, these dilemmas include issues of client cognitive ability and their right to self-determination (Seaman & Erlen 2013). It is therefore vital that, as you commence your nursing career, you are familiar with your ethical and professional obligations and that you have reflected on how you intend to work within these parameters in practice.

Contexts of practice

Nursing is a diverse profession, in which members can be found in many contexts. Broadly, nurses can pursue a career in clinical practice across acute and sub-acute areas. They can be in leadership, management or governance roles, in health promotion, community care, or research and educational roles. Throughout their career, nurses can move across and between these contexts to experience a range of careers within one discipline. There are opportunities and challenges that come with every role, and the examples contained in the following story will assist you to think about your career choices for the future:

> As a registered nurse with more than 20 years' experience, I sometimes reflect on my career and the range of settings in which I have worked. One memory is particularly strong, and I often share it with students and newly graduated nurses.
>
> I started my nursing career in a very large and specialised metropolitan hospital, working my way around a few medical and surgical wards before I was accepted to work in the intensive care unit (ICU). I came to love the specialised nature of the ICU, the interaction between the intensivists, registrars and nurses, and the support of the technical team who set up, maintained and provided advice and access to specialised medical equipment such as ventilators, balloon pumps and extracorporeal membrane oxygenator (ECMO) machines.
>
> After several years, my family and I decided to make a 'tree-change' and move to a rural setting. I was lucky to be offered a position in a small rural hospital (with 24 beds), and the nurse manager seemed happy to have me, as by this stage I had further qualifications in coronary care and intensive care nursing.
>
> After a week of orientation and another week of work on the ward, I was asked to be 'nurse in charge' of the hospital and manage the emergency department. My questions of the nurse manager caused eyebrows to be raised and some laughter when I enquired about who the medical officer-in-charge and the registrar were. I was informed that there was no medical officer or registrar, and that I was 'it'.
>
> The nurse manager went on to say that the on-call doctor, made up of a roster of the town's five general practitioners (GPs) hated to be called out for non-emergencies. As it happened, that night three people involved in a multi-car road trauma were brought in. Two were serious but stable, while one was critical and required ventilation. The on-call GP was grateful for my expertise in setting up the emergency ventilator and between us we organised the client to be airlifted to a larger hospital with the facilities to care for him.
>
> Once the emergency was managed, I was asked to clean and reassemble the ventilator so it would be ready for whenever it might be needed again. It was then that I realised that I had no knowledge of how to do this – in my experience, this was managed by a team of technicians.
>
> From this experience, I quickly developed a much greater appreciation of the roles of rural registered nurses, many of whom work in small and remote facilities with few experienced colleagues to call on for support. They manage great diversity in their practice, from such things as serious road trauma to chronic conditions or sprained ankles. They are generally the only health service open 24/7, and they require advanced clinical judgement skills, calmness and competence to practise effectively in such contexts. So if, as a nursing student, you have the opportunity to undertake a placement or work in a rural setting, jump at the chance! It will give you a new appreciation of the scope of nursing practice, skills, knowledge and commitment of experienced rural nurses that will hold you in good stead for many other contexts of practice.

It is clear from this story that rural nursing practice differs considerably from nursing practice in large tertiary hospitals. A greater understanding of the roles, responsibilities and education needs of rural nurses is provided in an interesting article by Byrne and colleagues (2020), which reported on the evaluation of an exchange program between rural and metropolitan-based nurses in Queensland.

Healthcare teams

Nurses are equal members of the healthcare team, made up of various health professionals and support staff across a range of clinical settings. Understanding how effective healthcare teams work is essential to a successful nursing career. This story from a nursing student highlights the elements of effective teamwork:

> It was towards the end of a busy eight-hour shift in the emergency department when an older female client was brought in by ambulance after being found unconscious at home. The team of nurses and doctors had been given only fifteen minutes' warning; however, the entire team was ready and waiting for the arrival of the client. What impressed me about this incident was the incredible teamwork between the doctors and nurses involved. Roles are closely linked, and collaboration and communication are vital in an area such as emergency, in order to provide effective, safe care to clients in critical conditions, as well as decreasing waiting times and managing stressful clinical incidents (Kilner & Sheppard 2010, p. 127).
>
> I noted that the environment was well laid out with equipment within easy reach of all the staff, and although the area was quite small, the team members were used to working in and around each other and did so cohesively with a minimum of fuss. When the client was brought in, she had regained consciousness, but was unable to verbally respond to questions.
>
> The ambulance officers were able to provide a little background history and we were advised that she had been found on the floor of her home by a neighbour. She had been on the floor for some time – possibly overnight – although it was not clear whether she had had a fall or possibly a stroke. The team of nurses and doctors immediately started to work on the client together, while at the same time working autonomously in their own roles. On arrival, the client was cold to touch, centrally cyanosed and bradycardic, but able to maintain her own airway. Within fifteen minutes of the client's arrival, her heart rate began to drop dangerously low, to between 20 and 30 beats per minute. Doctors gave the order for adrenaline and atropine, and CPR was commenced. The entire team worked on the client, alternately administering drugs to correct her bradycardia and doing CPR.
>
> What stays with me about this incident is the calm environment in which the team worked. As a student, I was encouraged to observe and, where needed, to participate in the resuscitation. As the resuscitation progressed, the doctors made the decision to intubate. The more senior doctor said that intubation was not necessary, as the client was elderly and they felt intubation was unnecessarily invasive. The junior doctor felt intubation was the next step in the resuscitation as the client had begun to lose her airway patency. A compromise was reached, and a nasopharyngeal airway was inserted instead.
>
> During this time, several of the client's family members arrived. The senior doctors spoke to the family and explained the situation to them. The family was obviously distressed by the event but when the doctors discussed intubation and further monitoring in intensive care, the family made it clear that the client would not appreciate such invasive measures. While the family was extremely distressed, they chose to abide by the client's wishes, and the doctors withdrew all life-sustaining treatment. It was ultimately a really good example of great teamwork and also the ethical responsibility of both the doctors and nurses involved to continue life-saving treatment until such time as the family could make an informed decision, based on the client's wishes.

It is clear from this example that the roles of all the team members are closely linked, and that effective collaboration, and communication are based on mutual respect and trust, particularly in an area such as the emergency department, where time is of the essence, in order to provide effective, safe care to critically ill people (Schmutz et al. 2018). Hunziker and colleagues (2011, p. 2381) observed that social aspects, interactive patterns and the personal qualities of various resuscitation team members, including their clinical skill, previous experience, communication styles and leadership skills, have an influence over how resuscitation progresses – particularly the outcome. Therefore, it is important to understand the key factors that enable effective teamwork and to strive towards achieving them in health workplaces

REFLECTION 18.2

- How might you develop your ability to work effectively in cross-disciplinary teams?
- What do you do to build your understanding of the scope and roles of other healthcare professions?

Nursing careers

Have you thought about your nursing career? What opportunities do you see ahead? What interests you? Where do you see yourself in five to seven years' time? All of these questions need your consideration as you embark on your nursing career.

As discussed earlier in the book, nurses work across a very wide range of contexts and have rewarding careers in clinical practice, education, research, management, leadership and health promotion roles across the lifespan and in a range of public, private and not-for-profit organisations.

The world of nursing work is changing, and career opportunities available in the future were not even imagined ten years ago. An example of the expanding roles for nurses was discussed in a national forum held in 2017, facilitated by the Australian College of Nursing (ACN), which brought together key stakeholders such a regulators, educators, researchers and professional nurses to debate and explore the best way forward to enable nurses to work in advanced practice roles, prescribe medications and work more autonomously in the future.

Advanced practice roles already exist in New Zealand, the United Kingdom and a number of other countries, and they have expanded the scope and autonomy of nursing practice in many instances. In Australia, the nurse practitioner role is the only recognised advanced practice role at present but forums such as the one facilitated by the ACN are raising awareness of the broader role that nurses could play in the delivery of health care in this country.

Lifelong learning

Education and lifelong learning support your career development and the creation of new and expanded nursing roles. So, as you embark on your career, you need to be aware of the options that exist to continue your education.

When commencing work as a beginning-level registered nurse, it is easy to think that you have completed your education. However, it will not be long before you realise there is so much more to know and learn. The two major reasons for continuing to learn are personal and professional development, and these often overlap. Lifelong learning is the motivation to continue to learn and to seek informal or formal education in a self-directed manner. Lifelong learning opportunities can include training, coaching or mentoring, and there are many advantages to lifelong learning. For example, having additional qualifications can lead to promotion, enhanced work opportunities and increased income.

In Australia, a wide variety of options can help you to develop your knowledge and expertise, and possibly specialise in a particular area. Some of the popular options for further study are postgraduate certificates, postgraduate diplomas or master's-level degrees in a certain specialty, or in research, education or leadership and management fields. Most universities and many private providers offer a range of programs and courses, from short professional development modules to fully accredited programs that expand your expertise beyond nursing into midwifery, the paramedical field or other health professions. Some nurses seek to specialise in areas such as mental health, aged care, intensive care, renal nursing, rural nursing and nursing education. There are a range of master's-level programs that prepare nurses to become nurse practitioners.

Nurses who wish to focus on research often undertake doctoral research and commence an academic role or work as part of a clinical research team. Those who aspire to leadership roles may study a range of nursing leadership programs or complete a master's in business administration (MBA). In today's technological world, lifelong learning has been made easier and more accessible by online learning opportunities. Most education providers in Australia now offer online study options, which enable learners to study in the comfort of their homes and at their own pace. Nurses can now work full-time and still pursue learning opportunities.

The point is that there are now so many options for nurses to enhance their skills through formal education or professional development opportunities, to advance their careers and meet their career goals. As discussed in this book, nurses are not just 'doers' – they do not just complete a series of clinical tasks; they are 'knowledge workers' who bring expertise and clinical judgement to ensure that those with whom they interact – be they clients, students, colleagues or the wider community – have access to effective nursing knowledge and care. It is important to maintain an open mind to lifelong learning and remain flexible, which are key factors in job satisfaction.

REFLECTION 18.3

- What areas or topics in your undergraduate studies would you like to learn more about?
- What personal interests would you like to pursue?
- What new skills would you like to develop?

Giving back

There are many ways in which nurses give back to the nursing profession. Nurses are active members of the community; they serve as role models; and they are looked up to by their clients as well as the wider community.

Nurses have a strong influence through the support they give. They are accustomed to helping all kinds of people from all walks of life, such as clients for whom they care and health professionals with whom they work on a daily basis. Nurses provide clients with a high level of care and support and are there around the clock whenever the client needs them. Many nurses also volunteer their time to give back to the community.

CASE STUDY

The nursing journey is a lifelong learning journey

Jane Summers had dreamed of becoming a nurse when she was at primary school. 'I always wanted to be able to look after people and care for them,' she said. After finishing high school, Jane enrolled in a Bachelor of Nursing degree and became a registered nurse.

Jane found her job very rewarding, but at the same time she found that the long hours and hard work were sometimes exhausting. Over time, Jane came to realise that she needed to continue learning and so she enrolled in an online Master of Nursing degree at a regional university. Jane now works in a nursing management position at her local hospital and says that her education has allowed her to have a positive effect, and it contributes on a daily basis to her being able to do her job.

Jane also gives back to the nursing community and the wider community. She has taken on the role of a casual lecturer at the regional university where she studied, and she is now sharing her knowledge and skills with nursing students. The rewards of Jane's career in nursing have been multifaceted, as she says that not only is she a role model for the nursing students and the staff at the hospital, but she has also set a good example for her own family.

QUESTION

Have you considered other roles in the healthcare industry? What sort of additional training would be required for these positions?

NURSING PERSPECTIVE

Eva Ballai has over 25 years' experience in health care, spanning frontline, senior management and board-level positions. A Lieutenant Specialist Nursing Officer with the Australian Defence Force and former Treasurer of Special Olympics Australia, she has an extensive operational and strategic understanding of healthcare settings, particularly aged care.

Eva Ballai fled war-torn Yugoslavia with just two suitcases – one filled with clothes, the other with nursing books. The registered nurse came to Australia in 1992 as a refugee. At just 25 years of age and already heartbroken at having to leave her parents behind, Eva's qualifications were not recognised in Australia and, with limited English skills, she had no idea how she would build a new life.

However, she set to work, pursued her goals and has spent every minute since trying to make a difference. Today, Eva has a successful nursing career in which she proudly wears three important professional 'hats'. As operations manager for Sydney-based aged care group Synovum Care, Eva is also a Commissioned Nursing Officer in the Australian Defence Force and the volunteer director of the Australian Foundation for Disability Board. The three roles might seem an unusual combination, but they enable Eva to care for society's most disadvantaged and vulnerable citizens.

'I know it sounds cheesy and I'd like to say joining the Australian Army at 40 was a mid-life crisis, but it wasn't,' she said. 'I think I was ready to give back and I just wanted to say thank you to Australia for giving me a second chance in life. Nursing is my life and it's my character – I just like helping people.'

Eva first went to the Gold Coast in 1992 because her uncle and aunt lived there. 'When my father died the following year, I couldn't even go home to bury him because I was afraid something would happen as I was a political refugee. It wasn't easy,' she said.

Eva started studying at TAFE to improve her English skills. She then found herself moving from the role of student to that of teacher, helping a class full of prisoners who were completing their Year 12 certificates. It did not take long for Eva to find a job as a nursing assistant at a local nursing home. Then she enrolled in a Bachelor of Nursing degree at Griffith University, eventually completing her Australian qualification.

Eva spent many years working in acute-care settings, and she returned to Griffith University to study for an MBA advanced. Eva said this course proved vital to her success in running aged-care facilities.

Eva has come such a long way, and has helped so many people, since leaving behind her homeland with those two suitcases 25 years ago. She remains passionate about nursing. Eva's advice to other graduates is straightforward: 'Follow your passion, love what you do, love your work and have a passion for humanity.'

Source: Rogers (2017).

SUMMARY

- This final chapter has brought together the major focus areas that have made up this 'journey'. The first part of the chapter focused on nursing professionalism and the importance of recognising your professional identity, as well as your ethical practice, responsibility and accountability as a registered nurse.
- The world of nursing work is changing, and career opportunities available in the future were not even imagined ten years ago. This section of the chapter looked at the career options open to nurses – for example, 'advanced practice nursing' and 'nurse prescriber'.

- The second part of the chapter focused on lifelong learning, including the advantages of continuous learning and the many options for informal and formal learning that are available and accessible to you for your professional and personal growth.
- The final section emphasised the concept of giving back to the profession – the many and varied ways in which nurses can contribute to society, and the importance of contributing to the further development of the nursing profession.

We wish you well as you embark on your nursing career, and encourage you to share your knowledge, and continue to learn and grow, to become the best professional nurse you can be.

FURTHER READING

My Heath Career (2020). *The best things about nursing.* Available from
https://www.myhealthcareer.com.au/nursing-career.

Rawson, H. (2020). Surprising careers in nursing. (Blog post). Deakin University.
Available from https://this deakin.edu.au/career/surprising-careers-in-nursing.

Rispel, L. (2020). Our climate and health emergency – future role for global public health.
European Journal of Public Health, 30(Supplement_5).

REFERENCES

Buresh, B. & Gordon, S. (2006). *From silence to voice*, 2nd edn. Ithaca, NY: Cornell University Press.

Byrne, A.-L., Harvey, C., Chamberlain, D., Baldwin, A., Heritage, B. & Wood, E. (2020). Evaluation of a nursing and midwifery exchange between rural and metropolitan hospitals: A mixed methods study. *PLoS One*, 15(7), e0234184.

Hoeve, Y.T., Jansen, G. & Roodbol, P. (2014). The nursing profession: Public image, self-concept and professional identity – a discussion paper. *Journal of Advanced Nursing*, 70(2), 295–309.

Hunziker, S., Johansson, A., Tschan, F., Semmer, N., Rock, L. Howell, M. & Marsch, S. (2011). Teamwork and leadership in cardiopulmonary resuscitation. *Journal of the American College of Cardiology*, 57(24), 2381–8.

Karnick, P. (2014). The elusive profession called nursing. *Nursing Science Quarterly*, 27(4), 292–3.

Kilner, E. & Sheppard, L.A. (2010). The role of teamwork and communication in the emergency department: A systematic review. *International Emergency Nursing*, 18(3), 127–37.

Milton, C.L. (2018). Will nursing continue as the most trusted profession? An ethical overview. *Nursing Science Quarterly*, 31(1), 15–16.

Paliadelis, P., Stupans, I., Parker, V., Piper, D., Gillan, P., Lea, J., Jarrott, H.M., Wilson, R., Hudson, J. & Fagan, A. (2015). The development and evaluation of online stories to enhance clinical learning experiences across health professions in rural Australia. *Collegian*, 22(4), 397–403.

Paliadelis, P. & Wood, P. (2016). Learning from clinical placement experience: Analysing nursing students' final reflections in a digital storytelling activity. *Nurse Education in Practice*, 20, 39–44.

Rogers, M. (2017). Political refugee dedicates nursing career to giving back. *Griffith News*, 12 September. Retrieved from https://news.griffith.edu.au/2017/09/12/political-refugee-dedicates-nursing-career-to-giving-back.

Schmutz, J.B., Lei, Z., Eppich, W.J. & Manser, T. (2018). Reflection in the heat of the moment: The role of in-action team reflexivity in health care emergency teams. *Journal of Organizational Behavior*, 39(6), 749–65.

Seaman, J.B. & Erlen, J.A. (2013). 'Everyday ethics' in the care of hospitalized older adults. *Orthopaedic Nursing*, 32(5), 286–9.

Index